P9-CCY-114

Coyote
Medicine

❦

Lessons from
Native American
Healing

Lewis Mehl-Madrona, M.D.

A FIRESIDE BOOK
PUBLISHED BY SIMON & SCHUSTER

FIRESIDE
1230 Avenue of the Americas
New York, NY 10020

Copyright © 1997 by Lewis Mehl-Madrona
All rights reserved, including the right of
reproduction in whole or in part in any form.

First Fireside Edition 1998

F*IRESIDE and colophon are registered trademarks of*
Simon & Schuster Inc.

Designed by Brooke Zimmer
Text set in Adobe Granjon
Manufactured in the United States of America

3 5 7 9 10 8 6 4 2

The Library of Congress has cataloged the Scribner
edition as follows:
Mehl-Madrona, Lewis, 1954–
Coyote medicine : Lessons from Native American
Healing/Lewis Mehl-Medrona.
p. cm.
Includes index.
1. Alternative medicine — United States. 2. Indians
of North America — Medicine. I. Title.
R733.M443 1997
615.8'82'097 — dc20   96-32714
CIP
ISBN 0-684-80271-6
0-684-83997-0 (Pbk)

For Archie Price, my grandfather,
who loved me deeply and unconditionally
and who was always there when I needed him
and
for my wife, Morgaine.
Without her love, support, and personal sacrifice,
I would never have realized my dream to finish my
medical training and to become board-certified.
Neither would this book have ever happened.
For all these reasons, I thank her.
But most of all,
I thank her for my son, Takoda, who is a ray of sunshine,
and who has brought great joy to my life.
Through her love for him, he has become true to the
meaning of his name, "a friend to all."

Acknowledgments

I wish to acknowledge and thank all the medicine people who allowed me to study with them and who taught me so very much about being both a doctor and a healer. I have changed names, places, descriptions, and dates to protect the identities of those doctors, healers, patients, and friends who shared life's journey with me. I have reconstructed dialogues and other details based on my memory of events that took place long ago. I have followed the advice and counsel of Dr. Bruce Gibbard, chairman of the Vermont Psychiatric Association's Committee on Patient Confidentiality, on how to write case material to protect the patients involved, and I thank him for his helpful lectures and discussions on these important concerns.

I would also like to acknowledge the help of a number of conventional physicians who have helped me with that aspect of my journey, including Dr. John Renner, Dr. Carl Whitaker, Dr. Marshall Klaus and his wife, Phylis Klaus, Dr. David Cheek, Dr. Laura Frankenstein, Dr. Mark Mengell, Dr. Karl Knobler, Dr. C. J. Singh Wallia, Dr. Paul Skinner, and the faculties of the Departments of Family Practice and Psychiatry at the University of Vermont College of Medicine.

Finally, I am grateful to Gail Ross and Howard Yeun, who helped me down the path of actually finishing a book.

Contents

Coyote Medicine

FOREWORD

by Andrew Weil, M.D.

IN THE PROLOGUE to *Coyote Medicine,* Lewis Mehl-Madrona writes that he "became convinced years ago that the ancient and modern approaches to illness can and should be integrated in a way that offers patients the benefits of both." He was way ahead of his time. Integration of "conventional" and "alternative" medicine is now much in fashion, but this is a very recent change, forced upon the medical profession by powerful economic forces. Our health care system is in total economic collapse, the logical result of medicine's decision in the early part of this century to wed itself to technology. Now, as the century closes, high-tech treatments are simply too expensive to deliver to people who need them. No one can pay the bills, and hospitals all over the country are facing bankruptcy.

At the same time a vast and powerful consumers' movement has developed away from conventional practice and toward alternative medicine. Recent surveys show that as many as one in three American patients are now going to alternative providers; significantly, most of them do not tell their regular doctors they are doing so. What patients want is doctors who will take the time to listen to their stories and explain their treatment options, who will not just offer drugs, who are conversant with nutritional influences on health, who can make intelligent recommendations about the use of dietary supplements, who will not ridicule herbal medicine, Chinese medicine, homeopathy, and other unorthodox therapies, who are sensitive to mind/body interactions. They want doctors who will look at them as more than just physical bodies. Obviously, our medical schools are not turning out graduates who can meet these demands.

Out of desperation about the economic catastrophe befalling it, the medical profession is at last opening to new ideas and practices. About twenty medical schools in the United States now offer elective courses in alternative medicine, a few have centers for the study of complementary therapies, and my own institution, the University of Arizona, has started a Program in Integrative Medicine that will soon begin training doctors to combine the best ideas and practices of conventional and alternative medicine. These developments would have been unthinkable even five years ago.

Integration has become a rallying cry of those urging on this reformation. For too long, they say, doctors have regarded patients only as physical bodies, ignoring their minds and spirits. As a result of popular books and television programs, the public has become very enthusiastic about mind/body medicine, not realizing how little of it has penetrated the conventional system. I can see endless possibilities for teaching, research, and practice that take account of emotional and psychological influences on health and illness; in these areas, our work is cut out for us.

But what would it mean to try to incorporate a spiritual perspective into medicine? If doctors routinely ignore the mental/emotional components of human beings, they regard spirituality as completely beyond the pale of scientific medicine.

Throughout the 1970s I traveled around the world looking at healing practices in other cultures. During that time, I visited many Native American practitioners in North and South America. Always I was struck by the fact that when Indians talk about medicine men and medicine women, their use of the word "medicine" means more than our use of it. In the Native American conception, Medicine (I will use a capital *M* here) includes not only our medicine (with a small *m*) but also much of what we call religion and magic. In the ancient world, medicine, religion, and magic were not separate; in our world, they have fallen apart, which is our loss.

Good doctoring requires all the wisdom of religion, all the techniques of magic, and all the knowledge of small-*m* medicine to be most effective. One way to bring that perspective back into our health care institutions is to look to Native American Medicine as a resource. Lewis Mehl-Madrona has much to offer here, since he combines the heritage and experience of a Native American healer with very thorough training in conventional allopathic medicine. On top of that, he has great passion about replacing the reigning biomedical model with a new paradigm, and he is a good writer.

Coyote Medicine is not medicine of the past, of cultures that are fading. It is also medicine of the future that must be taught in medical schools, practiced in clinics, and brought to all those who seek true health.

Tucson, Arizona
April 1996

"Epi," I called out. "And give me a number eight ET tube."

An ambulance had rushed in a fifty-two-year-old man. He hadn't been breathing when the Emergency Medical Technicians arrived at his home. By the time they got him to the ER, he was still warm—"organized electrical activity, but no pulse," as one EMT reported. That gave us enough hope to proceed. The patient was large, diabetic, and known to have heart disease. He had had two prior heart attacks.

At his home, the EMTs had given him three doses of epinephrine and two of atropine, both used to try to get his heart working again. They had shocked him twice with a defibrillator before packing him into the ambulance, then shocked him again on the way to our hospital. CPR was still in progress when they arrived. The smaller EMT was standing on the stretcher to push on the patient's chest. He was dwarfed by the patient's huge abdomen. The man's face was blue and his lips had turned an even darker shade of purple.

I was readying equipment to intubate him (a procedure that involves inserting a tube into the trachea to ease breathing). The nurses and EMTs were dragging him from the ambulance stretcher onto the ER bed. "Suction," I yelled, placing the suction catheter tip between his lips to draw out food and mucus. With that gone I opened up the laryngoscope, inserted its blade between the man's teeth, and pulled his jaw open. My task was to pass the endotracheal tube between his vocal cords (not into the esophagus, as sometimes happens) so that our team could deliver pure oxygen to his lungs. His massive tongue was in the way, but a few adjustments of the blade enabled me to slip the tube safely past it to the man's lungs. I pulled out the stylet and inflated the cuff to keep it in place. Soon the patient was being properly ventilated by the respiratory therapist.

We continued to give him epinephrine and CPR. I grabbed a central line kit and tore it open. We needed IV access to his heart to be sure that the epi had a chance to be effective. I could get the quickest access by putting a needle into the internal jugular vein in his neck. Once I had a good blood flow back into the syringe, I threaded a wire through the needle, pulled the wire through, made a nick in the skin with a scalpel, and then threaded the needle through a very large catheter called a percutaneous sheath. Blood followed. Suddenly we had three large ports to connect to fluids and medicines. We continued our massive doses of epinephrine, and finally the man's heart started pumping. We had a pulse! The EMT stopped CPR; the pulse continued. He climbed off the patient's chest. A nurse inflated the blood pressure cuff. Now we had blood pressure, too—albeit a low one.

"Dopamine drip," I called out, and other nurses ran to start it. (Dopamine is a hormone used to raise blood pressure above critical limits.) Another large dose of epinephrine raised the man's blood pressure enough to pump some blood to his brain.

He survived long enough to make the helicopter trip to another hospital, one with a surgeon waiting to perform a coronary artery bypass graft. But there, on the operating table, the patient died. The power of emergency medicine had kept him alive for a time but was no match for his chronic diseases. Clearly what he had really needed was help years before to change his diet and his life.

Since graduating from Stanford University School of Medicine in 1975, I have practiced scientific and emergency medicine for over two decades, in hospitals from California to New York. I have the utmost respect for what we can do with patients in extremis. But I have also come face-to-face with the many limits of modern medicine. As wonderful as our scientific tools are, we remain unable to heal many of the patients who suffer from chronic illnesses.

During these same twenty years I have also observed, assisted with, and finally led Native American healing ceremonies. I came to realize, during medical school, that my Native American heritage was worthy of study and attention, and had a very important lesson to offer contemporary medicine, indeed our whole society's attitudes toward illness and the recovery of health.

For a Native American, a healing is a spiritual journey. As most people intuitively grasp (except maybe doctors, who are trained to disbelieve the idea), what happens to the body reflects what is happening in the mind and the spirit. People *can* get well. But before a person can do so, he or she must often undergo a transformation—of lifestyle, emotions, and spirit—besides making the necessary shift in the physical body.

Healing and doctoring are distinct pursuits. Having tried both, I saw years ago that both were tremendously—and differently—powerful. It is no exaggeration to say that healers and doctors inhabit different worlds. Nonetheless, I became convinced years ago that the ancient and modern approaches to illness can and should be integrated in a way that offers patients the benefits of both. Modern doctors must learn to take their patients on spiritual journeys. Those who do not will miss out on some of the most incredible tools consciousness has developed for our benefit.

Personal transformation is no match for emergency trauma care. There are still a few old men and women who know the ancient bone-setting and wound-cauterizing techniques, but that kind of medicine is dying out along with its practitioners. And if the man with diabetic dehydration, renal failure, and pulmonary embolism had sought out a shaman instead of an ER, he would most likely have died. Ceremonial medicine isn't designed to deal with that level of complication. It can deal with very serious and chronic disease, however. I have seen cancers, neurological disorders, anginas, glandular and other disease cured without (or sometimes in spite of) surgical or pharmaceutical interventions. We all carry within our souls the capacity to heal ourselves.

There are different ways to tap into the soul's riches. I have learned the Native American way; I believe patients and practitioners alike have much to gain by taking a look at our traditions. Within my ancestors' model, there are many more functions for medicine than objectifying the body's parts. For a Native American healer, the first step in treating a person is to listen. We climb into the world of the patient and see things through his or her eyes. This means we listen without judging or categorizing—we never simply take a history of prior complaints, procedures, and allergies.

The next step is to have the patient create a metaphor for the illness. With such a concrete image of the illness, a healer can construct a ceremony to fight it. The ceremony can take many different forms. What kind of ceremony to conduct depends on the images the patient has used to describe the illness. The exact details of the ceremony cannot be specified in advance. *They emerge from listening to the patient.* The patient must be central to the ceremony, not a passive onlooker.

As a modern medical doctor and a Native American trained in the practices of traditional healing, I can provide a unique and accurate perspective on both Western and Native American medicine. I'd like to bridge the gap between the old and the new, so that each culture may profit from the wisdom of the other. The foundation of this bridge is the Native American concept of interconnection between body, mind, and spirit. By realizing that most everything in our lives, including disease, is simultaneously a physical, emotional, social, and spiritual phenomenon, we will be closer to attaining true health and contentment.

Should conventional doctors be more like shamans? Should they care for the souls of their patients? Does every community need a healer as much as it needs a doctor? Should medicine men and women teach in medical schools, alongside priests, ministers, and Buddhist nuns? I hope to give you some perspective from which to consider these questions as I tell the story of my own twin journeys through the worlds of medicine and the spirit.

CHAPTER ONE

Why Are You Here?

I STARTED medical school expecting to become a research scientist. While still in college, I had joined a professor in his efforts to study biological membranes using a then-new technique called magnetic resonance imaging (now referred to by its acronym, MRI). As a member of his research team, I was named as a co-author of a paper he published on the work, and I imagine my acceptance into Stanford in the early 1970s was based partly on my participation in this new line of research. Indeed, I soon found a professor in my new California home with whom I intended to continue these studies. What I never expected was to become a clinician, focused less on research than on seeing patients.

At Stanford I actually started clinical work immediately. I had pushed myself to finish high school before turning sixteen, and as an undergraduate at Indiana University I had persuaded professors to let me take medical and graduate school biochemistry courses. These gave me advanced standing when I entered Stanford at age eighteen. As long as I took a necessary pharmacology course concurrently, I was ready to start seeing patients on clinical rotations. I was on track to finish medical school in June of 1975, with the required nine-quarter minimum. A decade later I learned I was Stanford's youngest ever peacetime graduate, at twenty-one years of age.

The challenging part for me was not in learning about pharmacology and anatomy but in understanding other doctors. There were numbing lists to memorize, of course, of nerves, muscles, bones, blood vessels, symptoms, diseases, drugs, and side effects; but compared with the knottier puzzles of philosophy or higher mathematics, nothing taught was all that difficult. There was plenty to memorize, but all memorization takes is time. The problem for me was that my interpersonal skills had languished in my race through high school and college. Thankfully, I had a new wife to coach me in the car on the way to dinner parties and social events. Professionally, though, I was on my own.

Medical students on clinical rotations were expected to examine patients and entertain a diagnosis. We would discuss our potential diagnoses, and the treatments and medications they implied, with the faculty physician. The challenge was to show that we had considered every possible diagnosis and had either ruled it out or planned the necessary tests to confirm or disconfirm its existence. Although most patients suffer from common diseases, we relished considering all the outlandish possibilities. First prize went to those who, in the end, turned in exactly the diagnosis our faculty physician had already reached—we had to learn his or her style and mimic it. At nineteen, much to my own detriment, I was still young enough to be idealistic. I thought it was more important to think for myself than to try to think like someone else.

I also thought other doctors shared my own ideal of medicine: that its purpose was to restore unwell persons to health. Imagine my surprise on hearing a renowned professor of internal medicine begin a lecture by noting that the physician's job lay in "slowing and making less painful the patient's inexorable and inevitable progression toward death and decay."

Despite this my first rotation—three months in neurosurgery—was challenging and rewarding. I had already done work in college on the neural functions of rats. I was studying a particular brain rhythm, hoping to show that a molecule called serotonin triggered it. To do this, I implanted electrodes into rats' brains, then measured what happened when I introduced serotonin to different sites of their limbic systems. If the rhythm was produced by the serotonin, I would have strong evidence that serotonin was a neurotransmitter—a message sent by a nerve to the cells in the vicinity. Neurotransmitter molecules are the only verbs a nerve has at its command; which molecules are produced, and how many, determine a message's content. At the time, scientists were certain of only two neurotransmitters; we have since identified twenty-six. These few molecules and the simple messages they carry from one to another of our three billion brain cells are the vital chemistry behind human thought.

Although this wasn't the concern at the outset, neurotransmitter research eventually had the practical yield of all sorts of drugs. Now we know, for instance, that serotonin depletion often accompanies depression. Drugs that increase the availability of serotonin, like Prozac, are common treatments for depression. Prozac, which belongs to a class of drugs known as serotonin reuptake inhibitors, works by blocking the enzymes that cause serotonin to be reabsorbed.

I found that rat brains produced the theta rhythm I was interested in when serotonin was introduced to certain sites "upstream" of the hippocampus—which, in plain language, meant that serotonin was indeed a neurotransmitter, at least for rats. This was a publishable result. With my professor's advice and assistance, I finished my first solo paper and published it in a neurosurgery journal. I was very proud to become a part of a centuries-old tradition of expanding the known limits of scientific knowledge.

Since I already loved research, it was no surprise to find the datagathering aspect of the neurosurgery rotation appealing. But I was unprepared to find how much I enjoyed simply working with people, practicing clinical medicine. Even if I was still more comfortable in a lab than on a ward, two months into the rotation I was starting to consider a career that wasn't pure research but combined research with clinical work. Perhaps I would become a pediatric neurosurgeon. Three months later I was on my second rotation, in urology, about to meet the four very sick men who would challenge my career plans even more profoundly.

It was a foggy April morning outside the renal room of the Intensive Care Unit at San Mateo County Medical Center (SMCMC), a major teaching hospital of Stanford University. A nurse introduced me in a perfunctory manner to the first three of the four men inside. There was little hope for them. The fourth man—whom I will call Juan Martinez—had a chance to survive. He was a forty-two-year-old carpenter from Los Gatos, in the foothills of the Santa Cruz Mountains. He had lost one of his kidneys in a San Jose hospital. After the operation, his remaining kidney had stopped working. When Señor Martinez's twenty-three-year-old daughter offered him one of her healthy kidneys, he had been transferred to SMCMC's renal room to be evaluated for a transplant.

My job was to begin a pre-transplant evaluation of Sr. Martinez to decide if there was any reason not to proceed with the surgery. I wondered what had happened to the man before he lost his kidney—what had brought him here. I started by asking when he had last been well. We had to speak up to be heard over the bustling doctors, the efficient nurses, the constant drone of the voice of the paging operator (these were the days before beepers). Only his three drugged roommates were quiet.

The carpenter was lying on his back, holding himself perfectly still, looking more like a quadriplegic than a dialysis patient. His face had the texture of an onion skin. His muscled arms lay uselessly on the sheets.

He took longer to answer than I expected; he seemed to be searching for an answer to a question much bigger than mine. Finally he said, "I was never sick."

"What do you mean?" I asked. He was avoiding looking at me, focusing instead on the grains in the ceiling panels overhead.

"There was nothing wrong with me," Sr. Martinez said flatly. His usually dark Hispanic complexion was blushing ocher, and he began to cry quietly. His jaw continued working after he spoke, as if there were more to say but no words with which to say it. I glanced out the window. The morning's fog had dissolved into a light rain, unusual weather for April in San Mateo. Water ran slowly in crazy currents down the window panes. I found myself shivering.

"What do you mean, there was nothing wrong with you?" I asked when it was clear that the carpenter wasn't going to go on. He was clutching the bedsheet.

"They said I had protein in my urine—but I didn't feel bad or nothing," the man said without emotion. His face was expressionless except for the silent tears in the corners of his eyes.

"And then?"

"They ran some tests. Then more tests. They took a biopsy of my kidney, and I got this infection that almost killed me." The man gazed down the length of his sheet-covered body. "It did kill my kidneys," he said. His jaw stopped working and his lips began to quiver. Our conference was interrupted by an officious nurse who had come to change his IV. Feeling worried and confused about what had happened to her charge, I left her to the task.

LATER THAT MORNING I read his chart in the conference room behind the nurses' station. Just a few months earlier, he had been framing houses in the canyons outside San Jose. On weekends he went hunting and fishing in the northern California wilderness. His doctor had discovered the traces of protein in his urine during a routine insurance physical. Proteinuria can be a normal enough finding in a person who has been exercising strenuously, but it can also be an early sign of serious kidney ailments and autoimmune diseases.

Although Sr. Martinez had no symptoms of any of these problems, his internist ordered a full workup. A series of ordinarily innocuous medical procedures had led, for Martinez, to the worst possible complications. After his doctors biopsied a kidney, Martinez got an infection, then began to hemorrhage. His doctors repaired that damage by removing the injured left kidney; Martinez's right kidney responded by shutting down. He developed sepsis, an infection of the blood that can spread anywhere in the body. Doctors at SMCMC managed to clear up the infection but couldn't get the right kidney working again. Martinez's best hope now was a new kidney. As for the biopsy that had kicked off the whole process, it had been inconclusive. Nobody had any idea why Martinez had once had traces of protein in his urine, and now nobody was trying to find out. That problem—if it had ever been a problem— no longer seemed important.

I sat in the conference room looking out the hospital's narrow windows at the rain and thinking about the man in the room on the other side of the nurses' station. His old charts and records were heaped on the table before me. I thought of the dark forests of northern California, where Sr. Martinez had hunted, of the deep lakes the forests held, of the ancient trails that led up past the timberline into a world of rock and ice and snow—a world Juan Martinez might never see again. Then I reread his chart, hoping for some clue to his predicament.

I was still searching when a resident in urology, Musaf Habra, walked in and set two Styrofoam cups of tea on the table. Dr. Habra was a Saudi general practitioner who wanted to teach at the Saudi Medical Center in Riyadh after he finished training as a urologist at SMCMC He was the sort of gentle man whose constitutional kindness can be mistaken for weakness. He had won my admiration at a recent party, where he played the violin with a sensitivity that was anything but weak.

"Reviewing Señor Martinez's case?" he asked, nodding at the charts on the table.

"Trying to make sense of it," I said.

"Sense?" Dr. Habra gave me a quizzical look. "What 'sense' are you looking for?"

"I'm not sure," I said. "The logic behind the biopsy, I suppose. I'm trying to understand how this could have happened."

He shrugged and pushed one of the cups of tea toward me. "His doctor wanted to know what was causing his proteinuria," Habra said in a matter-of-fact tone that served to mask what he thought about the whole thing.

"But he says he wasn't sick," I countered. "And I can't find anything in his chart that indicates any other symptoms or diseases."

"He didn't have symptoms. He had proteinuria . . . " Habra thought a moment and lowered his already quiet voice. "And he had the 'advantage' of the best preventive health care in the world."

"You wouldn't have biopsied him in Saudi Arabia?"

"*I* wouldn't have biopsied him *here*," Habra replied. He raised his eyebrows. "But you Americans are so much more advanced than we Saudi." He winked. "Wanting to know the answers to everything can be deadly." He parodied his own accent a little, lending it a playful hint of intrigue.

I agreed with Habra's critique but was hurt to be included by him among "you Americans." Of course I was one, but I didn't identify at all with the culture that lay behind the unnecessary renal biopsy that had destroyed the carpenter's health. I wanted Habra to see me as something more than just another American. I was a *Native* American, for one thing, and I hoped that somehow made me different.

It seemed to me my medical student friends and I were more like Habra than he knew. A small group of us were naturally drawn together—Native Americans, Hispanics, and Asians—because we all had different cultural perspectives from those prevalent at Stanford. Though we didn't have strong social ties, we did hang out together in school. It took the edge off our feeling of not belonging. Some of my fellows had come to Stanford straight from their reservations and found themselves in an entirely new, often incomprehensible culture. Spurred by my new friendships, I began to reconsider my own Native American heritage, which my mother had long ago turned her back on.

While I was thinking about what Dr. Habra had said, David Vickory breezed into the conference room. Dr. Vickory was a decisive, energetic man with an encyclopedic knowledge of kidneys. In his late thirties, Vickory was juggling two ambitious careers, running a busy research lab and simultaneously winning a reputation as one of the best nephrologist—kidney specialists—in the country.

"Well, boys," he said, rubbing his hands together as if they were cold, "what do you think of my man, Martinez—is he a good candidate for transplant, or what?"

Dr. Habra thought for a moment. "There is the matter of his infection—" he started.

"We've licked the infection," Dr. Vickory interjected. "His fever has long since lifted. He's ready for the knife. Unless . . . " He turned a chair backward and straddled it. "Unless you've found something I missed." His tone was challenging. He waited barely an instant and turned toward me. "You look troubled, Dr."—he glanced at my name tag— "Mehl. Did *you* find something I missed?"

I told him I hadn't.

"And yet," he continued in his light, teasing tone, "you do look troubled. Our man is stable. We've cleared his infection. We've got a kidney standing by. And still something worries you."

"Actually," I said slowly, "I'm struggling to understand how he got here in the first place."

Vickory's face went blank for a moment, and his cheerful demeanor vanished. "You have a question about how patients get infections?"

On one level, it would be a ridiculous question for a medical student to ask: even premeds know that microbes cause infection. But on another level, the question was worth pondering. Why did this particular patient succumb to microbes when most others do not? The first question would be too basic and the second too philosophical to warrant discussion in the urology conference room. Vickory was trying to figure out which of these transgressions I had made.

I saved him the trouble. "Of course I know what causes infection. I was wondering why we did a renal biopsy on a healthy man."

"He wasn't healthy," Vickory corrected. "He had proteinuria. That's something we work up. It's the standard of care, as you know—or should know." He could probably see the beads of sweat on my forehead starting to form. I hadn't started out to challenge his authority, but I could see Vickory was thinking I had.

"His proteinuria wasn't causing him any problems," I countered. I could see Habra pursing his lips and shaking his head, but I couldn't understand this taboo on discussing the biopsy. Vickory, after all, was not the one who'd ordered it, so even if it had been a mistake, it wasn't his. "It just seems like they could have waited to see if there were any real problems before going for a piece of the guy's kidney."

"Is that the way it seems to you, Dr. Mehl?" Vickory asked. "Well, maybe . . . " He stroked his chin with his thumb and forefinger and pretended to think about it for just an instant. "But those of us who study kidneys for a living have found that guys who have protein in their urine usually do have a real problem. Maybe someday you'll show us how to identify the lucky ones who don't. Until then, we're just going to have to stumble along doing biopsies. We know from experience that we'll find a lot of renal disease that way. We also know that in a few cases—not many, but a few—there'll be infection." His voice was intentionally slow and flat. "It's unfortunate, but it's life. And it's irrelevant to the business at hand—which is whether or not to give Martinez a new kidney. That's the question on the table this morning," he said, rapping hard on its Formica surface with two fingers. "So you let me know if you see any reason we shouldn't transplant this guy. Until then, Dr. Mehl—" Vickory nodded dismissively and walked out of the room.

I felt stunned and embarrassed. My heart had hammered through every long second of his speech; I wasn't used to conflict, and it frightened me. I was young, I worried what people might think of my youth, and I wanted desperately to do well to compensate. I was scared of Vickory. How could I have had the audacity to challenge him?

"Be careful," said Habra. "If you keep acting like that, you'll never graduate." I was surprised to hear no trace of sympathy in his voice. Although I had not expected him to stick his neck out to defend me from Vickory, I thought at least he would be a confederate afterward. He shook his head as he gathered up the charts. "You might consider which you want to do, debate the philosophy of medicine or become a doctor anytime soon."

"I want to do both," I muttered in a voice barely audible over the background noise of the hospital.

"Good luck," he said without inflection. It was hard to tell whether he meant what he said or precisely the opposite.

WHEN HABRA AND I went back to see Señor Martinez later that day, we found him lying deathly still on his back, moving only his eyes—from Habra to me and back again. He looked bewildered while Habra spoke to him.

"We can give you a transplant," Habra told him, "if that is what you truly want. But I insist that your daughter talk to the psychiatrist. She must know what she's risking. She must know what the chances are that you'll reject her kidney. She must know what she's getting into, and I must know that she knows or I would never forgive myself."

Habra had surprised me again. In the few months I'd spent on rotations, I hadn't come across any other doctors who would consider holding this kind of conversation with a patient, acknowledging that it was possible for the physician to be emotionally affected by a treatment's outcome. But if Martinez was surprised or moved by hearing a doctor mention his own feelings of guilt or responsibility, he didn't show it. His eyes continued to float like the bubbles in his leveling tool, looking for a spot on the ceiling to comfort him.

"Tell your daughter to give me a call," Dr. Habra said, placing one of his cards on the bedside table. He searched the corners of the room for clues about how to proceed. "I am sorry for your misfortune," he told the carpenter shortly, standing up from the bedside chair. "We will see you in the morning and talk again then." Martinez managed a nod.

Habra rubbed his eyes as we made our way to the next bed, where lay Dr. Jackson, a forty-eight-year-old professor of English from the University of California at Santa Cruz. His story was nearly identical to his neighbor's, beginning with proteinuria and ending with two useless kidneys. Dr. Jackson's infection, however, was out of control, and dialysis was failing to cleanse his blood adequately. Habra and I had been asked to determine if surgical removal of his kidneys and debridement of the region (cleaning out the infected tissue) might help. It might, we decided, and should be tried, because it was his only chance to beat the infection. But even this radical treatment might fail. Unless our debridement was accompanied by a miracle, Dr. Jackson did not have a very good chance of leaving the hospital alive.

Neither did a fifty-one-year-old store clerk, Mr. Brasher, nor a thirty-seven-year-old postal worker, Mr. Brown—two more men who had begun with protein in their urine and no other symptoms, who had run the gamut from biopsy to infection to the loss of kidney function. We trudged past their beds, murmuring short greetings and shorter good-byes.

When we finished rounds, we ducked into the cafeteria. Habra bought himself a Coke. "What are the odds," he said, "that in any one morning we would do four such similar consults, that four men who had been well before visiting their physicians would all be lying in the same room together?"

"I don't know," I responded carefully. I wanted to know what Habra thought, but after the episode with Vickory, I was reluctant to set anybody else off. "It seems like something must be wrong with three people dying because of their physicians' best efforts."

Habra nodded. The rain had stopped and the sun was starting to shine. We walked outside. "But what exactly went wrong?" Habra asked. "No one amputated the wrong leg or prescribed incorrectly. No one missed a disease or made the wrong diagnosis. Perhaps Vickory is right—perhaps this is the price we pay for good preventive health care."

"You don't believe that," I ventured. The chairs were still too wet for us to sit down.

"No," Habra said, "but you can't quote me. Anyway, my opinion carries no weight."

"But why is Dr. Vickory so defensive?" I asked. "He didn't make any mistakes."

"He has to defend his colleagues," Habra suggested. "After all, they were faithfully following the guidelines of our profession." We were leaning against the rough concrete walls of the building. We could see planes landing and taking off through the mist covering the San Francisco Bay.

"But is this what good care is?" I asked, genuinely agonized. "If you kill the patient, can you call the operation successful?" I finished my tea. Squirrels were climbing up and down the trees, and birds squawked overhead.

"Who can say?" Habra said as he opened the door to the hospital. "Maybe Vickory's right. Maybe finding the treatable cases justifies the losses, maybe those men we saw today are a statistical anomaly. We are simple soldiers on one battlefield. Maybe we cannot understand the war?"

"Like hell," I shot back, smiling.

"At least you're in a better mood," he said. "There's nothing I hate worse than a mopey intern."

MY GREAT-GRANDMOTHER was a traditional healer in a rural area of Kentucky. I carry vivid memories of her but not of her theories and practices, since she died when I was five. I wish now I could ask her all kinds of questions that I wasn't concerned with then. What I do remember seeing was a number of very sick people coming to her to be healed. When I was older, I watched healings led by the local Christian snake handlers. I didn't know what magic these writhing, agile beasts worked. But magic it was, as far as I could tell.

At the time I was never much interested in the cause-and-effect relationships of anyone's "miracle" recovery. Nor was anyone else I knew. Where I came from, faith healings were accepted as natural occurrences—nothing to arouse either doubt or skepticism. Later, my curiosity would come to rest in the concept of human transcendence, in the movement beyond illness that healing occasions. I would learn that healing sometimes calls for people to ascend the greatest heights they are capable of reaching. And then sometimes healing seems as natural and commonplace as weeds in a garden.

Before a person can be healed, one medicine man told me years after medical school, he or she must answer three simple questions: "Who are you?" "Where did you come from?" and "Why are you here?" This California elder believed that anyone who could give clear answers to these three questions would be well.

The third question seemed easiest to answer—Why was I at SMCMC? I knew that the study of medicine would allow me to pursue my interests in biology, physiology, and psychology. So far these expectations were satisfied. I was only surprised to find, in medical school, that few shared the awareness and acceptance of healing I had known in Kentucky. Why could faith healing occur in the hills of my youth but not in a progressive hospital? I took it for granted that there was a spiritual component to illness, and wellness too, and that doctors would respect it. But I had no thought at that point of integrating my interests, of using the healing traditions of people like my great-grandmother alongside the scientific approach of modern medicine.

It wasn't until I experienced the shock of seeing four devastated but previously healthy men together in the same renal room that I began to think the healing traditions of my childhood might have something to offer the professors of Stanford. There must be an alternative, I thought. I was too naïve to recognize that even the idea of healing—without drugs, surgery, or other invasive care—was considered déclassé and counter to the conventions of medical school.

Now, sometimes invasive procedures are entirely appropriate. But they aren't always. Too many of the doctors I was encountering lacked the critical insight of the healers I was later to meet, that a disease may bring balance to an otherwise untenable situation. Medicine people are careful not to act until they are certain of the consequences of their actions. Disturbing the body's balance without forethought can have disastrous consequences, as Martinez was learning, whether or not his doctor ever did. The true healer recognizes that every action produces a result, and that a patient's own intentions, conscious or not, can determine the direction of the result.

It seemed only by coincidence that I was even in a position to learn from this unfortunate convention of renal failures. During my first rotation as a medical student, in neurosurgery, I befriended a surgical intern, whose next rotation was to be in urology. The illness and subsequent death of a family member required his presence at home, leaving his position vacant. Asked to fill his spot, I was promoted to acting intern for the month, after only four months of clinical training. This was fine with me, but a few eyebrows were raised in the emergency room the first time I showed up in response to a call for a stat urology consult.

Now that I am more fully immersed in Native American spirituality, I recognize that my being made acting intern was no coincidence. I was learning firsthand that most doctors rarely consider the larger, encompassing questions about the body, mind, and spirit that medicine people address. And I was learning this at a young enough age not to dismiss it; a few years later, I might have ignored things that disturbed me in the interest of getting ahead.

The great thrill for most of my teachers was in diagnosis. As one neurology professor said, "Most patients are very boring. What is interesting is what they might have and making sure they don't have it. What is left after that—the treatment and so on—is either boring or difficult. Few diseases respond in the textbook manner to the drugs we offer them. Some diseases respond to no drugs. Invariably, patients never do exactly as they are told. Patients have the pesky habit of doing what they want, regardless of our advice." At Stanford, I learned a term for this phenomenon, too: doctors call it "noncompliance."

Throughout that April day I found myself wondering just how

many treatable cases are revealed by those invasive biopsies, and how many biopsies it would take to justify what we had done to Señor Martinez and what we were preparing to do to his daughter. After all, removing a kidney is no piece of cake. She could develop an infection herself, even die. How many successes justify a loss? Who decides such things? I knew better than to talk to Vickory again. Habra was less than three months from graduating and returning to Riyadh, so I couldn't count on his sympathies, but maybe Friday night after rounds, when the urology department retreated to the Stanford Coffeehouse, I could talk with him over a beer.

As it turned out, I didn't have to wait long to hear the question debated. A little before eight o'clock the next morning, we gathered in the urology conference room for our weekly discussion of transplant candidates. Because this was a teaching hospital, senior physicians sometimes expounded on the more interesting cases. When I slid into my chair across from Dr. Habra and saw that Sr. Martinez was scheduled for discussion, I wondered if anyone would point out that his own doctor had caused his illness. Doctors have a word for that occurrence too, a long, Latinate word that allows us to distance ourselves from the truth of the idea. We doctors call a disease caused by one of our own "iatrogenic." Now I just call it bad medicine.

VICKORY SAILED IN AT 7:59, took a seat at a table at the front of the room, and gave a "You're on" signal to his resident. This businesslike young woman shuffled her pages of notes and then began to tell the gathering of physicians and students about the patient.

"Juan Martinez is a forty-two-year-old, married carpenter from Los Gatos," the resident began. Her hair was black and curly and seemed still damp from her morning shower. Perhaps she had been on call all night at the hospital. "He is status post treatment for sepsis and perinephric abscess with renal failure on the basis of acute tubular necrosis from sepsis." The resident moved crisply through her presentation. She talked about the removal of Martinez's left kidney in San Jose and worked forward from there, never mentioning how he had found his way into the world of nephrologists in the first place. "It has been determined that his renal function will probably not return. His daughter offers him a kidney, and we wish to proceed with transplant."

Vickory asked for questions. There was a brief discussion of the blood urea nitrogen and the creatinine, which serve as markers of renal function. That discussion ended quickly with the conclusion that Martinez's one kidney was not working. Then came a lull, the usual signal to move on to the next case.

I glanced around the room. Dr. Habra was shaking his head at me ever so slightly. But his warning wasn't necessary; I had learned my lesson the previous morning. I would not give Vickory a second chance to mock me. I had given up hoping that anyone else would see anything remarkable about Martinez's case when Robert Upton, the chief of our renal transplant service, spoke up.

"Hey, Dave," he said. Given his status as a transplant surgeon, Upton could call anyone by first name, including Vickory. "What was wrong with this guy before his abscess? Any idea how he got sick?"

"Complication of renal biopsy," Vickory said dryly, closing Martinez's chart.

"But what was wrong with him before that?" Upton asked. "Why was he biopsied?"

"Proteinuria," Vickory said with finality, looking around the room, hoping for other questions.

"Caused by what?" Upton persisted.

While Vickory hesitated, I glanced at Habra; he was sitting forward in his seat as well. Outside our door a cart of breakfast trays clattered by.

Vickory thought an instant more, scowled, and admitted, "We don't know." His resident quickly opened her files and wrote some frantic notes to herself. She had already become skilled at appearing not to notice anything potentially embarrassing to her attending physician.

"You want us to transplant this guy and you don't know what was killing his kidneys in the first place?" Upton said, making a show of being amazed.

It was a legitimate question. Unless the disease that destroyed the original kidneys was identified and controlled, transplantation was pointless because the new kidney could be attacked and destroyed in the same manner as the old one. In Martinez's case, however, the kidneys had not been originally under attack, and Vickory had no choice now but to say so.

"There was nothing wrong with his kidneys," Vickory said impatiently. Seeming to realize where that left him, he lowered his voice and said, "He had protein in his urine. Everything else was fine."

"How much protein?" Upton asked.

"A little," Vickory said quietly. "Consistently one to two plus on urinalysis."

"That's it?" Upton asked incredulously.

"That's it."

Upton let loose his trademark laugh. This abrupt, barking sound was feared throughout the hospital—Upton was not afraid of making enemies. "Ya gotta love this," he said, speaking to the ceiling but clearly addressing the students present. "We'll never be out of a job. When there's not enough real disease out there, we make some."

Vickory glared at Upton, considering a retort. He cleared his throat. In the official hierarchy of the hospital, these two men were equals. But there was a second hierarchy at play, and everybody in the room knew its unofficial and unspoken rules. Upton generated enormous revenue for the hospital and the university. For institutional physicians, money equals power. Vickory said nothing. No doubt he would remember the incident. One day, sitting on some committee or other, he might find a reason to put the scalpel to Upton on another pretext. But that permissible revenge of the academic physician would have to wait.

Everyone had a good laugh at Vickory's expense, leaving the real question of why we do what we do unanswered. The day before, I had seen four men, healthy until our profession stepped in. We could justify what we had done by arguing that the early detection of disease across a population is worth the occasional harm that preventive care inflicts upon an individual. But try telling that to the four individuals in question, or to their families. Why was amusement at Vickory's position the only emotion provoked by the meeting? Why weren't we shocked and outraged at what we had done?

Other questions of importance to me, had I asked them, were even more likely to infuriate my assembled colleagues. Why was Sr. Martinez recovering while the other three men were slowly dying? Martinez wasn't well, but he was well enough to be discussed as a candidate for transplant. What factors had healed his infection? He was a Mexican Catholic. Had he been supported by the power of prayer? Were supernatural forces real and present for him? What about the other men—had anyone prayed for them? Did they believe spirits or guardian angels were helping them?

Together Vickory and Upton knew as much about kidneys as any two people on earth. Surely they had some thoughts worth hearing about intervention versus a wait-and-see approach. And Habra was about as gentle and sensitive a doctor as you could hope to meet; he must have had opinions about the delicate task of treating people whose ill-nesses are due to their physicians. These were the sorts of ideas I was interested in hearing discussed. Instead, we talked of blood and urine and dysfunctional kidneys until precisely nine o'clock, when the conference ended. Notebooks snapped shut, chairs scraped back, and private conversations started as people milled around the door.

I stayed behind a moment after the conference was over. I was impressed that Upton had challenged Vickory and the standard of care as well. But it didn't seem to affect others in the same way; they were more amused by the power dynamic that was expressed than by the ideas behind it. And unfortunately Upton was probably more concerned with letting the students know his station than he was with Martinez's well-being. This was not what I had thought becoming a doctor was all about. I hated to think the profession might one day require such a performance of me. I hoped, if it did, I would have the strength to resist giving one.

I got up to walk to a window. It looked across a concrete courtyard on to another brick-and-cement wing of the building. The window was shut tight. Air was controlled at this institution. My great-grandmother would have been appalled by a building without working windows, shut up tight as a Tupperware container. She would never have attempted a healing in a room shut off from the rich resources of heaven, earth, and sky. She was a gardener as well as a healer. Besides medicinal herbs, she grew tobacco, marigolds and watermelon, beans, squash, tomatoes, and heavily plumed stalks of corn. The composition of her garden was a measure of her mood.

My Cherokee grandfather, Archie, would have been unable to pray in a room in which his tobacco smoke could not rise to the heavens to summon and greet the spirits he communed with. Archie's cigars—or smoke sticks, as he preferred to call them—would have succeeded only in activating the smoke detectors and summoning the fire marshal. Archie would have wondered how people could get well without feeling the healing powers of the sun on their skin.

What a vast difference between the hermetically sealed hospital and the ramshackle Kentucky church where the snake handler's congregation gathered. The brightly lit, sterile rooms of Western medicine couldn't have been further removed from the darkly mysterious sweat lodges where, I had been reading, my Native American ancestors held their healing ceremonies.

The academic world had met my thirst for knowledge throughout high school and college—but it had proven to be as spiritually barren as it was intellectually bracing. Now my spiritual desires, which had never been well addressed by the tidy theologies my mother favored, were demanding my attention. I stood with my back to the window, looking over the empty conference room, listening to the echoes of the hour-long discussion of transplant candidates, waiting while two lessons emerged. Neither had anything to do with kidneys; both, I realized, had been part of my curriculum from my first day at SMCMC.

The first was a lesson about patients. From a modern doctor's perspective, a patient is a bundle of biological matter, a collection of tissues to be rolled in and out of treatment, X-ray, and operating rooms. A doctor needs to know nothing about the soul wrapped in those tissues. In fact, we were taught that the less we knew, the better—the more objective we could be.

I started wondering about Juan Martinez. A forty-two-year-old carpenter from Los Gatos. I bet his parents had come from Mexico when he was still a child. Perhaps they were looking for the good life in America. They traded the long traditions of a life in Mexico for the orange groves of San Jose—now plowed under, replaced by homes, malls, and parking lots. Juan's health had gone the way of the orchards. Until recently Juan was dying; now, for a while, he was not.

We had no idea why Juan had been one of the relatively rare casualties of renal biopsy, or why he had been granted a reprieve. Nor were we particularly interested in finding out. We didn't know anything about his relationship with his wife or his daughter. In fact, if by accident we had seen anything telling when his family visited, or caught some sense of their feelings in their glances and questions, we actively tried to forget it.

We didn't know about his anger at us or how it might affect the course of his disease. About his faith, if he had any. About what he believed had caused his illness. Was it *El Destino,* the fate Mexican-Americans are said to believe in? What did he believe was the meaning of his life? How had this illness altered that? I wondered what he might have told us about his illness and his recovery if we had only listened more and measured less. Or what we might have learned about the three dying patients who shared his room, whose only hope now lay in miracles, and for whom we therefore had no hope.

The second lesson was a vision of ourselves as doctors. We were being taught to do no more than diagnose disease and manage conditions—including those which arose from our own interventions. But we were not to be embarrassed by our own impotence; we were to accept it gracefully. We were learning to deny our ignorance of the mysteries of health and disease. We were well on our way to becoming not just doctors but paragons of "scientific objectivity," holding sacred hard numbers and physical data instead of subjective world views. Only the foreign doctors like Habra could see through the smoke screen of omniscience we used to obscure the things we did not know.

We viewed ourselves as having the only possible answers to health and disease. Didn't royalty from Saudi Arabia fly all the way to California to be treated by our professors? Wouldn't we soon be the colleagues and equals of these "learned" teachers? Our confidence in our world view was not diminished by the death of a patient, so long as we measured the process and documented it thoroughly. Even if we were able to save just one of four patients who came to us with severe kidney infections, we could walk away from the working day believing we had done all there was to do.

I loved science. I still do. Of course, in my college years I had encountered many people who were of the opinion that scientific discoveries precluded the possibility of a spiritual realm. But I didn't agree, and I had inspiring models to follow. Sir John Eccles, a Nobel laureate for his work on adrenaline and its role in the nervous system, was a visiting lecturer at Indiana University while I was an undergraduate there. He believed that science gave proof of God and the soul. Many of my professors thought he was a crackpot; I never missed a lecture.

Two MONTHS AFTER meeting Señor Martinez I was bumping along in the back of a pickup truck toward the Wind River Reservation in Wyoming. I squinted my eyes against the bright sunlight to watch the gentle hills and prairies roll by. I had finished my urology rotation without getting into any more dangerous philosophical discussions, but I had also firmly resolved to pursue the magical world of Native American medicine I had been reading about. I didn't know how exactly to go about pursuing it, or where it would lead me, but I could feel in my heart that I was bound to try.

There weren't many people to whom I could talk about this desire and the conflicts surrounding it. I needed a mentor, someone who could help me discover a path toward spiritual medicine. I was lucky to find the friend I needed. Eddie, an Arapaho-Shoshone medical student, hailed from the Wind River Reservation I was now heading toward.

Like other universities in the early 1970s, Stanford was actively recruiting minority students. Our class of one hundred students included three other Native Americans. Counting the classes ahead, there were nine of us. Most were full-blooded and had grown up on reservations, but a few others were of mixed blood, including a blond Comanche woman. We all hung out together, and I first met Eddie through this informal support group.

All of us had in common cultural values that were at odds with expectations at Stanford. We were more inclined to cooperate than compete. We froze before the rapid-fire question-and-answer sessions on ward rounds, which medical students call "pimping." Our group never tried to make someone look bad on rounds—though others did that to us, behaving viciously one moment, then good-naturedly thumping us on the back when the resident was gone.

Many behavioral habits confused us. We weren't used to people who were unwilling to sit in silence, who sought constant eye contact, who had a general lack of respect for illness, death, and dying. The two Dineh students from northern Arizona had it worst—their sacred laws concerning death and dying were continually being violated. But we all felt a culture gap to some degree, and took comfort in each other's company.

One day, during my third rotation, Eddie sought me out in the pediatrics ward. He told me he would soon be going home to attend a healing ceremony for one of his relatives. I was thrilled and terrified when he invited me to come. Although I very much wanted to participate in a Native American rite, I was afraid to be found lacking, to be rejected for being a half-breed, for not speaking their language, or for committing some awful faux pas during the ceremony.

Native American religion was illegal at the time, having been outlawed by an act of Congress in 1895. Although schoolchildren learn that the Constitution protects freedom of religion, Native Americans were long denied the right to practice theirs. We were forbidden from congregating. We were not allowed to keep sacred objects, including pipes and eagle feathers. Eventually the injustice was recognized, and our right to practice our religions was restored by Congress in 1975. But the old laws were still on the books in 1973 when Eddie's family brought Nelson, a medicine man, down from Lame Deer, Montana, to treat their uncle, Jimmie Left Hand. His chest pains had gotten so bad that Jimmie couldn't meet the demands of his job, driving a delivery truck. The Indian Health Service doctor had diagnosed angina (chest pain caused by an insufficient supply of blood to the heart muscle) and wanted Jimmie to go to a hospital in Caspar for more tests, but Jimmie wanted to try a healing ceremony first.

If the local police discovered the ceremony, Eddie explained, the participants could be jailed and their sacred objects destroyed. These threats were real in Wyoming, where some of the police were fundamentalist Christians intent on routing paganism from the reservation. Other local cops were less diligent, especially those who were Arapaho or Shoshone, who participated in the traditional ceremonies themselves. One interesting character was the local Catholic priest, Father Stone—he attended the clandestine meetings and sat ready to declare them orthodox Catholic rituals should any fundamentalist cops burst in. "The way he figures it, we all pray to the same God anyway," Eddie told me.

We were headed west from Caspar along U.S. 20-26, toward Riverton, a small city in west-central Wyoming at the edge of the reservation. The same highway took tourists to the ramparts of Yellowstone National Park and the Grand Tetons. From Riverton they turned north through Thermopolis. Devil's Tower was in the opposite direction.

Eddie and I leaned against the bales of hay in the back of the truck with his older cousin Kiefer. Eddie or Kiefer would sometimes chant a song as we watched the rocky hills roll by. Sometimes the sound of the rushing wind was too loud for me to make out their words. Kiefer's mother was Kiowa, from Oklahoma. "Kiowa like to make up legends," Kiefer said. "We got here late, only two centuries ago, so we had to work hard to make up as many as the other tribes around here already had." He laughed.

Before making this trip, I had begun struggling to remember my early childhood. Much of it seemed as far away from me as the legends Kiefer was spinning out for my benefit. In fact, I had been using stories to get back episodes from these times, writing out short pieces in an effort to recall long-forgotten memories. On visits home I would grill Archie about my past and his. I would talk to my grandmother Hazel, his wife, while she was cooking corn bread, greens, and bacon. I bought the few books then in print about Native American traditions, especially those of Vinson Brown, and read them avidly. In fact, I was so distracted by these pursuits that I had failed the anatomy section of my National Board exams. While passing overall, I still faced having to study anatomy again all summer long—Stanford students are required to pass each section, not just the exam as a whole.

But the wind in my hair and the late afternoon sun on my face were working to remove my current worries about medical school. Cresting the top of a hill, the truck frightened a herd of pronghorn antelope, which bounded away from the road, leapt over the sharp angles of a rocky hillside, and disappeared behind a stone escarpment. Under scrub sage and tumbleweed the brown earth hid its unlovely past—the bones of settlers and Indians who had slain one another, the carcasses of the buffalo herds massacred after the building of the railroads. For as far as the eye could see, nothing stood taller than two feet except the rocks that marked the graves of some long-forgotten men.

"We have a few trees on the reservation," Eddie promised, winking.

We stopped for a milkshake at Yellowstone Drug in Shoshoni, a two-street town just before Riverton that catered to tourists on their way to the park. At Yellowstone Drug they counted every milkshake they sold. If your receipt number matched the last three digits of the total they had sold so far that year (by July, the total was up over twenty thousand), you won something. We didn't win anything material that day, but while we slurped our shakes Kiefer had the time to tell us a story about Devil's Tower he had heard from his Kiowa grandmother.

"Eight kids were playing there," he said. "Seven sisters and their brother. They came too close to a sacred place. Suddenly the boy was struck mute. He couldn't say a word. He shook all over and got down on all fours. His fingers became claws and fur grew over his skin. Before

long he was a bear. He scared his sisters. They ran from him in terror.
He chased them, thinking he was still a boy, running after his sisters. He
didn't know what was happening to him. He had no way of knowing
yet that he was a bear. Probably he was just as scared as the girls. He
chased them to the stump of a Great Tree, which is now called Devil's
Tower. The Great Tree told the girls they should climb all the way to his
top. The bear tried to follow them. Maybe he was just lonely, or maybe
he was scared because his sisters were running away from something
and he wanted to run away from it too. But however deeply he sank his
claws into the bark, he kept slipping back down the Great Tree. When
the girls reached the top, they kept going. No one knows how or why
they did that. It was probably the magic of that sacred place. The bear
kept trying to get to them, and he scratched the Great Tree's bark on
every side. The seven sisters stayed in the sky. They became the Big
Dipper."

I loved the storytelling, but it also provoked my fears. Fears of rejec-
tion, and of failing to understand things others took for granted. I didn't
really know what Kiefer meant by his story—if he meant anything. Was
it just a kid's tale, or was it a coded message I ought to understand? I
nodded sagely when Kiefer finished, and hoped I looked convincing.

I was afraid, too, of mystical powers in the night that would turn on
me, perhaps kill me. I had been told that we would be going straight into
a sweat lodge. While I had read about lodges, I had never been to one.
Eddie had kidded me the whole way to Caspar about how hot it would
be and how disgraceful it would be if I had to leave. He told me that
future fathers-in-law tested potential sons-in-law by taking them into
the sweat lodge. If they made it through, they could marry the daughter.
If they shamed themselves and their families by fleeing from the heat,
that was the end of the courtship.

I was terrified of how the heat would affect me. I had never even
taken a sauna or gone into a steam room. I preferred the cool fog of the
Pacific Coast to the humid heat of Kentucky, Ohio, and Indiana, where
I had grown up. Also, my childhood fear of the dark still lingered.
When I was very young, Hazel would tell gruesome stories about the
evil spirits and escaped convicts that lurked in the dark of night to eat
little children. During my later childhood, I cringed in terror when my
stepfather asked me to go to the barn after dark by myself. When he
made me go down into the basement at night to put coal into the fur-
nace, I would cover my head with a sweatshirt and peer out of the tiniest
opening, thinking that somehow this would protect me.

Eddie had told me that the sweat lodge was absolutely dark inside.
And hot. Yet the stakes were high. My acceptance hinged on my behav-

ior in that lodge. The closer we got, the more frightened I became. The sweat lodge had taken on an importance beyond anything else I had done or had yet to do. In fact, I felt like my whole life, my soul and my being, would be tried that afternoon in the lodge.

I felt something crawling on my neck and almost jumped out of my skin. It wasn't a bug, though; it was a piece of hay Kiefer was playing with. Eddie and Kiefer were laughing at my nervousness, trying to tease me out of it.

I was worried about being a half-breed, about not looking the way I should. Eddie and Kiefer looked the way most people expect an Indian to look. My own appearance is typical for a Cherokee; I'm often mistaken for a southern European (most usually a Yugoslav, for some reason). Like many members of the related Iroquois tribes, the Cherokee are not a very dark-skinned people. Some Cherokee are even fair-skinned. I'm a little more olive than fair. My skin can turn really brown in the sun, but I hadn't been outside much since starting med school.

"What's the problem?" Eddie asked, interrupting my ruminations.

"Nothing. Well, worrying," I answered distractedly.

"About the sweat lodge."

"That and everything else."

"I'm sorry," he said. "We'd better stop teasing you. Let me make sure you know what will happen."

One of Eddie's uncles was driving the pickup, with his big black Stetson on the seat beside him. Rifles filled the gun rack. Eddie moved closer to me so he could speak over the roar of the wind and the road.

"They've been heating the stones already," he said. "My brother Floyd is the firekeeper. He builds the fire and gets it just right. He prays over it and with it, helps it to burn strong in the four directions, and makes sure it stays sacred. When it's ready, he places the stones onto the fire, piles wood around them, and keeps them covered until it's time for them to come into the lodge. Then he'll carry them in with a pitchfork."

"When we get there, the men will be ready to go in. They've planned to wait for us. Nelson will lead the lodge. We'll all follow him inside. He doesn't do mixed lodges, so if the women were planning to sweat, they'll have already done so. It'll just be the men of my family and Nelson and you, and any old men that Nelson has invited, and any singers he's brought down from Lame Deer to help."

"What about Jimmie Left Hand?" I asked.

"You'll meet him this evening. This afternoon's sweat is to purify those of us who will be there tonight to pray for Jimmie. He's probably too ill to join us in the lodge right now." Eddie bowed his head thoughtfully before continuing. "Nelson will fill his sacred pipe and put it on the altar outside. Then he'll have Floyd bring in the first bunch of stones. Then we'll close the door and he'll start to sing. Like I said, he'll probably have a singer with him to help."

"I don't know any of the songs."

"Sit next to me in the lodge," Eddie said. "Hum along with me. You'll catch some words right away. Kiefer and I will keep singing some like we've been doing, so you won't be hearing these songs for the first time."

"When does he open the door?"

"A day later." Eddie laughed. "Just kidding. After the songs are done for the first round. We usually sing the directions song, and a pipe song, and a prayer song, and maybe an eagle song for the first round. But if you get scared or are too hot, tell him and he'll open the door early."

"Never," I hissed, thinking I'd rather die of heat exhaustion than embarrass myself in front of Eddie, Eddie's family, and Nelson, the great medicine man.

"That's the spirit." Eddie clapped me on the back. "Keep thinking like that and you'll do fine." He wore jeans today, and a denim jacket. Eddie's jet-black hair—short on top and long in the back—danced in the wind. His skin was richly dark despite his year under the fluorescent lights of the hospital. I thought how natural and self-assured he looked here, compared to how nervous and out-of-place he looked in his white lab coat back at school.

"No one back at Stanford would believe what we're doing," I said to Eddie.

"You think anyone on the rez would believe what happens *there*?" We were inside the reservation grounds now, bouncing along a dirt road. The sun was setting over the high peaks of the Continental Divide. Long shadows were growing from the rocky hills around us.

Eddie continued explaining the sweat lodge to me, how it was built, what would happen. "It's supposed to symbolize the whole world," he said. "Also the womb of Mother Earth. Even though it's a half sphere above ground, you're supposed to think of it as a whole sphere going down inside the earth as far as it stands above the earth. The pit in the middle of the lodge is where they put the stones. Think of those as your placenta. You're returning to the womb of Mother Earth. The placenta is there to doctor you and to take away the wastes and the toxins that you no longer need. You're going to sweat them out. The stone people get filled up with the energy of the sun when the wood is burned. Then they give that energy back to you. That is the medicine." He paused a moment. "We cover the lodge with canvas and plastic tarps. Once, we used to cover it with skins, but no one can afford that now."

We passed a small crossroads with a store, a gas station, and a church. Several dilapidated houses were standing by faith alone on either side of the road. Dogs scurried off the highway at the sound of our approach. Old men sat on the store's porch. Shortly afterward we turned onto a very rough dirt road. We must have continued on that road half an hour, bouncing past jackrabbits and scrub sage, washes and hills. "It's more fun to ride out here on a horse," Eddie said, after a particularly rough bump.

When the truck stopped, I could see smoke coming from a fire just over the next ridge. Someone hollered from the top of the ridge in a language I didn't recognize. "Hurry," Eddie said. "They're ready to start."

We ran up the ridge. A short way down the other side sat the most beautiful simple structure I had ever seen, a half sphere covered with a dull green army-surplus canvas. The door faced west, and before it was the fire, glowing bright hot. Eddie's brother stood bare-chested beside it, soaked with sweat, leaning on his pitchfork. Before I knew it, we were standing beside the lodge, shucking our clothes down to our underwear. Eddie's father had towels for both of us. The other men were already inside. I was terribly conscious of my too-white skin. Nevertheless, I hastily pulled off my T-shirt, dropped my jeans, and tied a towel around my waist, just as Eddie was doing. We each draped another towel around our shoulders; I was glad to cover my paleness. Then we bent down and went inside.

Eddie said something as he entered. I mumbled something similar, trying to sound just like him. Twelve men were sitting around the circle. My heart was beating in my throat; my moment of reckoning was at hand. I followed Eddie to the back of the lodge. He spread his towel on the ground and sat on it. I did the same. As soon as we were seated, Nelson yelled something out the door. There was a flurry of sound, and Floyd appeared with a red-hot stone on his pitchfork. He put it down just inside the door. Nelson took an incredibly long, beautiful pipe and touched the pipestone bowl to the stone. He said some words; then two men lifted the stone with deer antlers and placed it in the westernmost part of the pit as Nelson spoke again. He was speaking Northern Cheyenne, which I had heard before only in audiotapes of peyote rituals. He sprinkled sage over the rock. The sage promptly burst into flames. I was already too hot.

Nelson repeated this process six more times as Floyd kept appearing with stones, each one seemingly larger and hotter than the one before it. After the seventh stone had been laid out, Nelson handed Floyd his pipe. Floyd leaned it against a wood frame on the altar. Nelson said something else and Floyd grunted. It was intimidating not to understand a word.

"Ten more stones," Eddie whispered to me, interpreting what had been said. Oh my God, I thought, my heart sinking. I suddenly felt weak and light-headed. I was already overheated and the door hadn't even been closed yet. What is happening to me? I wondered in a panic; then I thought of the boy in Kiefer's story, who had turned into a bear and couldn't understand that either. I found the story oddly comforting as I too felt the rumbling beginnings of a deep inner change, one over which I had no control. A sweat lodge can make you feel as helpless as a baby, dependent on Mother Earth for survival.

Once the seventeen stones were all arranged, Nelson spoke again and Floyd closed the door. It wasn't dark, though—I decided Eddie had only been teasing. The reddish glow from the stones filled the inside of the lodge. I began rocking back and forth. Nelson started shaking a bear-claw rattle. His singer began the Four Directions song and everyone joined in but me. I started humming along as Eddie had suggested, catching a few words here and there. Sweat poured into my eyes. My heart was racing. I could hardly catch my breath. I felt as if I was going to die from the heat. I tried to remember the symptoms of heat exhaustion, but my mind just wouldn't work. I couldn't stay focused on anything. Great, I thought, I'm getting delirious.

The sounds comforted me, however, and carried me along. I wrapped myself in my towel to keep the searing steam from burning my skin. I made a little opening in the towel to breathe through, as I had done years before with my protective sweatshirt. I put my head low to find air, any air, anywhere.

Just when I thought I couldn't take another moment, Nelson called out and the singing stopped. The door opened. I tried to look cool despite my panic. Eddie looked me over. "You know, you're sitting in the hottest spot," he said, laughing. "You're doing good." I groaned. No, I hadn't known. Yes, Eddie had sat me there on purpose.

Nelson chatted with everyone while we cooled off. I must have been a sight—filthy head to toe, from rubbing dirt on my sweaty skin to stop the burning; hair disheveled, hanging stringily down to my shoulders. I couldn't see Nelson all that clearly because the light was poor and I'd left my glasses outside the sweat lodge. Now I saw what Eddie meant— things got darker as the stones cooled. Eddie said something and pointed at me. Nelson looked me over. "Welcome," he said finally, in English.

Before the door closed again, Floyd brought in ten more stones. It got hotter and hotter. This time the song was a prayer song. Suffering greatly, I hummed along. I had made it through one round, I would make it through another. I remembered swimming two miles at a Boy Scout camp. I had thought I would drown before I finished, but here I was today. I remembered running so hard once in high school football practice that I threw up afterward. And I had gotten through that. I used to give every ounce of energy I had during football games, and then find some more when the two-minute warning sounded. I would convince myself that I could do anything for two minutes. The problem was different now, though, as I didn't know how many minutes stretched before me.

We started praying when the song ended. The singer prayed first. Then came the man on his left. Each man prayed in his own language. The sounds were beautiful. Just when I felt I was adjusting to the heat, Nelson poured more water on the rocks; the steam was cooking my nostrils, I was sure. Finally it was my turn to pray. I prayed in English, the only language I knew. I felt I stood out speaking that way. Nevertheless, I tried to pray sincerely and intensely. I tried to remember how Archie had prayed, and I did it that way. Occasionally one of the men grunted or said "Hau." Obviously they understood me, even though I did not understand them. I felt small and insignificant in that lodge just then. I was a nobody among men of power.

Finally Nelson prayed. Suddenly he stopped himself, then continued in English. I was grateful, and embarrassed, too, knowing it was for my benefit. When he finished, the door opened. I felt the heat pouring out. I was ready to collapse, and we were only half done. To my relief, Nelson called for water. He was speaking English now. "Drink this," he said. "It has been blessed. This water is now the blood of Mother Earth, the life of the stone. Drink it and you will be healed."

Slowly Nelson passed a dipper of water to each person. The full dipper traveled clockwise, the empty dipper returned counterclockwise. "It is this way," Nelson told us, "because all fullness travels the way of the sun and emptiness in the opposite manner." I prayed my thanks when the water reached me. Never had I been so grateful for water. Never had it tasted so good. It filled every cell, every pore of my body, with sustenance. The water came around a second time and many men splashed themselves with it, pouring some over their heads. I followed their lead; the shock of the cold water on my hot scalp was intense. It awoke me from my delirium. I was alert again, if absolutely exhausted. Eddie gave me the thumbs-up sign. Ten more stones were brought in, and the ordeal began again.

The third round involved more prayer songs. Then came a quiet passage when Nelson invited us all to cry out to the spirits for a vision. Did I have a vision? Not while I was struggling just to survive. The most I hoped for was to be able to walk out of the lodge later, rather than be carried out. One good thing was, I was too exhausted now to be afraid. I slouched down to the floor. Soon the door opened. "Sit up," Eddie said sharply. "Be alert. The pipe is entering."

I struggled to sit straight. Floyd entered the lodge with the pipe. I tried hard to coordinate my muscles enough to wipe the dirt and sweat off my face and hands, as the other men were doing.

Nelson lit the pipe, and his singer took the first puff. Slowly the pipe went around the circle. The tobacco was both sweet and harsh. I puffed carefully—Eddie had warned me not to let the pipe go out.

"Think of your prayers," Nelson said. "As you smoke and the smoke goes skyward, it goes all the way to the Lodge of the Creator. There your prayers will be heard and answered."

When the pipe had made its way around the circle, Nelson finished the tobacco. He returned the pipe to Floyd, who put it on the altar. "We're almost done," Eddie whispered. "This is the last round." Then Floyd fetched ten more stones and closed the door.

"Rejoice," Nelson said. "Your prayers have already been answered. You have been purified. Now we will celebrate. Each of you take your privilege. Tell us something good. Tell us a story, sing us a song, say another prayer. Whatever you wish to do, that is your privilege." Each man took his turn. One told about a cousin who had been cured of cancer by Nelson. Another told of a relative whose depression had lifted. Another sang a song. When it was my turn, I thanked them all for letting me participate. Then Eddie talked about medical school, and how hard it was for him. He said I had been his friend and made it that much easier. Other men thanked me for that.

There's something, I thought to myself. I had been so wrapped up in what I needed from Eddie, I hadn't thought about what our friendship might hold for him. Perhaps, part of the magic of the sweat lodge was to be found in just this, getting the chance to say something simple but important to a family member or a friend.

Finally it was Nelson's turn. "Open the door," he said. I really rejoiced at that; I had made it through the ordeal without disgracing myself. "I have a story for you."

And the story he told went something like this:

Imagine a young man who has distinguished himself as a great hunter. The coyotes follow him to pick over what he leaves behind. Behind them come crows and vultures. When people are hungry, they count on this young man to find the buffalo on the great plains. He always finds the herds and gets their meat, so the people can survive another winter. He is careful when he hunts to follow the sacred traditions of praying and thanking the buffalo for the gift of their meat for the people to eat.

One August morning, the young man comes to a place by a stream where he knows the buffalo will come to drink. He waits with his bow ready. Butterflies and dragonflies buzz around him excitedly, knowing what is going to happen. He sees a buffalo cow coming toward him, and he draws back his arrow. But before he can let it go, something magical happens. He doesn't know if he fell asleep or if the world turned upside down. A beautiful young woman steps from the weeds to the pebbles at the edge of the stream and takes a drink from a buffalo horn. He stands up and walks toward her. Her hair is wild and tangled. She smells of wild sage and prairie flowers. In less than a moment he knows he loves her. He stands before her unable to speak.

She says, "I come from the buffalo people. My father sent me here because of your good feelings toward all buffalo. The buffalo council knows that you are a good, kind man, so I was sent here to be your wife. So that we can set an example for people of both persuasions—the stand-upright people and the walk-on-all-fours buffalo people—of how to live together in peace and harmony."

They get married and live happily for a time. They have a son and name him Calfboy. But you can imagine how it goes in a small village—people talk. There are some people who don't like this woman because she doesn't comb her hair the right way. She doesn't smell like everyone else or talk like everyone else. She doesn't follow the same customs or eat the same foods. "Where does she come from, anyway?" they ask. "Who does she think she is?"

Pretty soon, people in the village are saying she's an animal and will never be one of them. One day when the young man is out hunting, his relatives get together and tell the woman that she has to leave. They're menacing, so she picks up Calfboy and runs away. When the young man comes back from hunting, he sees his wife and child leaving in the distance and he runs into the village to see what has happened. When he finds out, he's very angry. He sets out right away to bring them back, but they have a head start and are moving quickly.

All day long he follows their trail. When he loses it, the grasshoppers speak to him to tell him which way to go. By evening he reaches a painted tipi. He sees smoke from the cooking fire coming out the top. He sees Calfboy playing outside. When Calfboy sees him, he says, "Come on in, Papa. Mama has dinner ready. She's cooking a good meal." And so the hunter enters the tipi and eats corn and turnips, which is what they would have at that time of year, maybe with wild greens from the trail, flavored with sage and other things like that.

While his wife is feeding him, she says, "I've got to go home to my people. I can't live anymore with your people. You can't follow me because, if you do, my people will kill you. They will be so angry about this whole situation that they'll kill you dead."

And he says, "I don't care if I die. I love you and I'm going to go where you go." Next morning he wakes up and the tipi has disappeared and he is lying there in the grass. He sees a circle of dew around him, so he knows he didn't hallucinate. He sees the tracks of his wife and child leading off and he follows them all day long. Once again at the end of the day he finds the tipi and his son comes out to meet him.

"Mama's going to make it really hard for you to follow us tomorrow, so you won't be killed. She's going to make the rivers run dry. When you're thirsty, look in my tracks and you'll find some water there."

Then his wife comes over. She points out a distant high ridge and says, "My people live over there. You really can't come because they'll be so angry they'll kill you on the spot."

But again he looks at her and says, "It doesn't matter whether I die. Nothing is going to make me turn back. I do this because I love you both." While his wife is asleep that night he buckles his belt through hers, and he wraps her hair around his arm. Still, in the morning he wakes up alone. He sees tracks leading away from where he is, but they are the tracks of a buffalo and a small calf, not a woman and a child. But a flock of ravens comes to tell him that the tracks belong to his family. And they lead up to the high ridge. He follows those tracks across a dry, winding river, and he finds water in Calfboy's tracks, which keeps him going. Finally he gets to the top of the ridge and, from behind a rock, looks out in awe over the whole buffalo nation. There are buffalo everywhere as far as the eye can see.

Calfboy, his son, has been looking out for him. When he spots his father, Calfboy comes running up on all fours and says, "Papa! Go back! They're going to kill you."

The hunter says, "No, son. I came to stay with you. I'm not going anywhere. This is where I belong."

"You'll have to be brave, then," Calfboy warns. "Don't show any fear or my grandfather will kill you. He's the chief of the whole buffalo nation. He's going to ask you to find me and Mama. You'll know it's me because I'll twitch my left ear like a fly is bothering me. You'll know Mama because I'll put a cocklebur on her back. Be alert, Papa, and you'll survive this trial."

And so the hunter comes down off the ridge, and the old buffalo charges him like nothing you ever saw. The old buffalo paws the earth with his hooves and tosses sagebrush with his horns, and still the young man stands his ground. He doesn't flinch. He doesn't move a muscle. He doesn't show any fear. Finally the old buffalo stops and says, "This stand-upright person has a strong heart. He doesn't show any fear. I guess I won't kill him outright."

You can see that his courage saved him. The old buffalo leads him back to the painted tipi in the middle of the buffalo nation. All the buffalo gather to form a circle around them. The little calves are in the inner circle, then the yearlings, then the youngest cows, and all the way out to the oldest bulls, in circles according to age. And the old buffalo says, "If you're so smart, if you're such a good man, show me who your son is."

And so the young man walks around and around until he finally sees a young buffalo with a twitch in his left ear. He says, "This is my son." And all the buffalo are really surprised.

"What a wonderful person," they say. "This guy must be really smart."

The old buffalo says, "Okay, stand-upright person, if you think you're so smart, find your wife for me."

And so the man walks around and around again and finally sees the cocklebur. He says, "This is my wife," as he pats her on the head. The buffalo are amazed. A tear falls from his wife's eye. The old buffalo announces that because this stand-upright person loves his family so much and because he is willing to die for them, they will make him one of the buffalo. And they will have a big ceremony to do this.

The old buffalo says to everyone, "Make a circle around the tipi. We're all going to join in with our thoughts and make him a buffalo." And so they take off all the young man's clothes and cover him with a buffalo robe with horns and hooves attached. Then they put him inside the tipi and tie the door shut. For three days and three nights the buffalo surround the tipi and fill the air with their grunts and bellowings. They sing songs in the buffalo language while they paw at the earth. On the fourth day the oldest buffalo make a sudden rush and push the tipi over. They roll the young man over and over until he's covered with dirt. They squeeze the breath out of his body and breathe new breath into his lungs. They lick him and rub him until all of his human smell is gone. When this is over he tries to stand up, but he can't stand up straight anymore. Finally he struggles to his feet on all fours like a newborn calf. And when they hear him grunting and talking in the buffalo language, everybody makes a big shout and they work even harder, turning him over and over in the grass until he is truly one of them. At last he can stand strong on all four feet.

It was this day that made the buffalo a friend of the human being. Because that brave young man loved his family so much that he was willing to become a buffalo, the buffalo agreed that they would give their flesh to the humans so that little children and unborn babies would have meat to eat to survive the winter. A covenant was created between the people and the buffalo nation.

"That's an ancient story which is considered sacred," Nelson said. "The elders say a story has a spirit of its own. They say that when you retell a story you release the power of its spirit."

Why did Nelson tell this particular story and not another? Medicine people use stories like mirrors, to catch an image of our hearts and minds for us to reflect upon. A story teaches and pleases all at once. At the time I didn't think to question or analyze the story; I was simply caught in its spell. Now I see how, for the sake of love, the hunter in the story is willing to transform himself into something entirely new, something he can't begin to comprehend. He's willing to die to be reborn. This is the essence of what healing requires. Healing will not happen unless you're willing to die for it. If you're not willing to reach into your own depths, at least as deep as your life-threatening problems, then you will not earn the power you need to change them.

The story Nelson told gets to the essence of healing, which is perhaps why he told it. But why tell this story of healing to the men assembled in the sweat lodge, when it was Jimmie Left Hand we had all gathered to heal? Were we being prepared to help him, to be strong ourselves, so we could lend Jimmie our strength? It worked for me. Nelson's story provided a context, a stimulus, and a catalyst for what was going to happen. I was fascinated, even mesmerized, by Nelson. I was ready to open my heart to him because he was so genuine, warm, and caring.

Maybe Nelson didn't choose this story consciously. Maybe it just occurred to him when it came to be his turn. I don't know what the story meant to the other men present. I don't know exactly what the story meant to Eddie, and whether it helped bring peace to him about his struggles at Stanford. I know that the story struck home for me. For not only is it a story about healing and transformation; it is a story about an individual caught between two worlds. And it is a story about a man with a special gift, who discovers why he has been given it—why he is here.

"We're done," Nelson said. "Follow me out." He went first. The rest of us formed a chain behind him. I was behind Eddie. When I finally made it outside, I collapsed to the ground. I did not have the strength to walk another step.

Eddie knelt before me, smiling. "You're stronger than you think. That much is clear about you." I was glad he thought so, but I couldn't have answered if I tried.

"See you tonight, boys," Nelson said, walking past us.

CHAPTER TWO

Where Did You Come From?

EDDIE LAY down beside me in the grass outside the lodge. Despite all his teasing beforehand, now he was as exhausted as I was. The old men were spry, though, almost bounding out of the lodge, then dressing quickly to return to their families and the evening meal. Eddie and I were limp and flabby compared with them. While our education was successfully cramming our minds with information, it was sapping our bodies of strength.

The exhaustion was purgative, however. It cleansed us both of all the hatred, sorrow, pain, and anguish we had stored in our hearts. The sweat affected our souls without needing permission from our waking consciousness. I felt a sense of camaraderie with all things around me, even the old dying tree with a gaping hole in its trunk that stood near the sweat lodge.

The tipi ceremony was to begin at sundown. As Eddie and I lay wordlessly recovering from the sweat lodge, I tried to puzzle out why the Wind River Reservation reminded me of where I come from in Kentucky. With all the physical differences between the places, I supposed Nelson's similarity to Archie was the principal link. Both men brought an underlying kindness to bear on their pursuits; both were able to size you up entirely with a glance. Like Archie, Nelson made you feel immediately at ease, by his obvious personal integrity.

Archie was a half-breed like me. He shared my shame at this. The orphanage that took him in as an infant knew only enough to register him a "half-breed Cherokee Injun." They did not know his birthday, so they set it for tax day, April 15.

My grandmother Hazel, also Cherokee, married Archie after my mother graduated from high school. She and Archie lived with us in Kentucky (as did Hazel's own mother, the healer, until she died).

Our little mountain town rested in the foothills of Lake Cumberland, near the Tennessee border. There were other Cherokee about, all descended from escapees of the Trail of Tears—Andrew Jackson's infamous forced relocation of the Cherokee Nation from lands he had decided were valuable in Georgia and Tennessee. President George Washington had officially recognized the Cherokee Nation a little less than a half century before Jackson rigged up a "legal" pretext to march my ancestors off to barren lands in Oklahoma. Many died along the way; some escaped. Besides the one in Oklahoma, there is today another Cherokee reservation in the mountains of North Carolina, an area to which a sizable number of tribesmen fled. (That reservation is a little more than two hours by car from where I grew up.) And there are enclaves of Cherokee descendants in little mountain communities like mine all along the Trail, mostly north and south of Tennessee (Jackson's home state), started by those individuals who managed to escape, settle, and establish families.

Because Mother and Hazel both worked outside the house, my great-grandmother often took care of me during the day. Or Archie sometimes would take me to work with him at Delmos's Chevrolet garage. I loved this whitewashed, cinder-block building at the edge of town, partly because of the Model T Ford perched on top of its flat blacktop roof. Archie would never explain to me how that Ford got up there, no matter how much I begged him. I imagine he knew the mystery would stay with me longer than its mundane explanation.

Archie was a mechanic at the garage. When things were slow he'd sit outside with me on the mounds of fresh sand they used to clean up oil spills. He'd light a smoke stick, blow smoke skyward to the spirits, and talk to me and them about whatever was on his mind. Then he would pray—in the same matter-of-fact, conversational tone. Even if he did all the praying, it would make both of us feel better. He'd pray to Jesus or the Great Spirit, or to whoever was listening. "God doesn't care what name you use," Archie told me, "so long as your prayers come from your heart."

Sometimes Delmos would waddle by and overhear us. "You can't believe anything Archie says," he'd tease. His manner was mocking but affectionate. Archie tolerated Delmos. He'd smile and nod until Delmos left, then continue with his prayers. Eventually work would draw Archie back to his world of hydraulic lifts and thick, black oil. He'd leave me to build roads and quarries in the sand with my trucks and earth-mover toys.

Archie didn't have formal instruction in any tradition. He respected Jesus, who looked, in the picture Hazel kept over their bed, a lot like a Cherokee. Later, when as a teenager I grew my hair long, Archie would defend me: "If Jesus wore his hair long, why shouldn't Lewis?" By then I had realized Hazel's picture was only one artist's conception of the man, but Hazel and Archie didn't think so. Even as a rebellious adolescent I had sense enough not to press that issue.

Archie lived the golden rule, always trying to give more to others than they asked of him. "That way, I'm never in another man's debt," he explained. He'd had to work to make a living since age five—starting with carrying water to the Louisville boardinghouse where the orphanage placed him. To me, it sounded more like slavery than adoption. But he never complained. I think he was grateful to have been given an opportunity to earn his keep and prove himself worthy. When he was twelve, he started boxing professionally in Louisville until he got knocked out by someone bigger (and probably a whole lot meaner). He briefly lost his vision, and decided to give up fighting when it returned.

Archie's car broke down in our little town one year when he was on his way to see the Grand Ole Opry in Nashville. Delmos had to order parts for the old Model T Ford Archie was driving. Delmos warned hi n that it would take a while, so Archie found a place to stay and even started working for Delmos. Then Archie met my grandmother. She quickly became more interesting to him than the Grand Ole Opry had ever been. The Model T somehow found its way up onto the roof, and Archie got Delmos to help him buy a new Chevy. "A Chevy mechanic has no business drivin' a Ford," Archie argued. "Gives customers the wrong idea."

Hazel loved Jesus and talked to him frequently. She once confided in me that she respected a spirit who could sacrifice so much for people. Like most Native Americans, Hazel believed that if you physically suffer for the people you love, it can heal and protect them. She thought of the crucifixion in that manner. She herself lived to take on the pain of her loved ones (myself included) so that we could suffer less.

Hazel liked to attend one or another of the local clapboard churches on a Sunday evening—if mainly to hear the faithful singing gospel hymns. Crickets chirped outside while the surrounding fields filled with the brilliant flashes of lightning bugs. Whenever she took me, she would cup her hands over my ears when the preacher started to talk about hell.

Archie wouldn't go to Christian churches at all, because, like Hazel, he didn't believe in hell. "A loving God could never be mean enough to create a place like hell," he'd say. "Those Baptists are just tryin' to scare people into actin' like them. There's enough hell on earth without there bein' any call for it elsewhere."

He did take me to see a relative of mine baptized by one of Hazel's preachers. Archie wore his best green mechanic's uniform that day, with the Chevrolet emblem emblazoned over the pocket. He always kept a tire-pressure gauge in the pocket next to an ink pen. I held his hand for comfort as we watched a distant cousin, whose relation to me I didn't quite understand, get dunked in the chilly waters of Lake Cumberland by a fat, bald, and sweaty preacher. I could see the sunlight dancing on the spray off Cumberland Falls.

My mother spent most of her life trying to shrug off her Native American ancestry. She ignored my great-grandmother's activities, and dismissed her as a foolish old woman. Like many of her generation, Mother turned herself inside out in order to conform. By disavowing all things ethnic, exotic, or unscientific, she sought to reap the "good life" promised in the 1950s to all hardworking Americans, as long as they were white. To her credit, she was struggling to better our lives. When I was three years old, she managed to graduate from Berea College, an amazing feat for an impoverished half-breed woman of the time—especially considering that her own mother had quit school in the third grade to work on my great-grandmother's farm.

Hazel and Archie had a faith that was simple and direct. Their heritage surfaced in the Christian beliefs they developed for themselves, but with only occasional contact with the traditions of the reservation Cherokee, the Native American spirituality my grandparents passed on to me was as idiosyncratic as their Christianity. I was not taught Native American spirituality per se. The principles of it were simply there, embedded in Hazel and Archie's daily life (along with steady doses of my great-grandmother's stronger, but Christian-flavored, paganism).

I didn't appreciate the strength or value of the Native American influence on my grandparents' Christianity until I made a more formal study of it as a young adult. Because it was so richly imbued with Native American philosophy, beliefs, and values, my grandparents' belief system seemed to hold what modern Christianity did not—a salve for my occasional bouts of adolescent existential despair. When I cried in my room at night from loneliness, the words of Hazel and Archie and my great-grandmother were far more comforting than any preacher's Sunday sermons.

My despair was born partly of shame. Even though my mother had managed to marry before I was born, talk ran freely in my small town. I was born too soon to have been conceived on the wedding night. I knew people whispered when I left a room, but I wasn't sure why. The whispers confused and hurt me. And I overheard Mother telling Hazel how much better and easier her life would have been if I had never been born. I grew up feeling so ashamed, I didn't deserve to breathe. And so I scarcely could: childhood asthma kept me in and out of the oxygen tent in the small community hospital that was only a few blocks from our house.

Mother would come all the way home from college at Berea when I was hospitalized. As much as I wanted her to come, I was terrified to upset her. I imagined disappearing, so as to no longer number among her burdens. When I thought the man my mother married had abandoned us, I decided I must have chased him away. Hazel said he was a womanizer, but since I didn't know what that meant it was no comfort.

Only as an adult did I understand the truth behind the rumors that had affected my childhood so deeply. One made Archie out to be my father; another reported that I was the product of my mother's affair with an Air Force pilot. One truth is certain: Louis Frank McKinley, my father of record, is not actually my father. Hazel told me that my real father was a Lakota Sioux from the Pine Ridge Agency, but that she was sworn to secrecy and could say no more.

My mother did marry Louis, though, and he was an airman from our hometown. A true gentleman, he married my mother to end her shame at being pregnant out of wedlock. Such considerate behavior was perhaps more common in the 1950s than it is today. He may even have loved my mother; I do not know. He was stationed in El Paso when I was conceived, and my mother visited him there once before I was born. They never lived together and eventually divorced. Today he is the dog-catcher in my old hometown.

Maybe this explains why I am drawn to pursuing Native American culture and spirituality—my journey stems in part from a quest for my father, a quest that remains unsatisfied. In one way the small-town gossips were right: Archie was my true father, regardless of whose blood runs in my veins.

BELIEVE IT OR NOT, Eddie and I eventually got cold. Our flushed, pink faces turned white as the temperature dropped. We were wet and almost naked, and the wind was brisk. The sun was low on the horizon, where buzzards were making frantic circles. Were they following the hunter from Nelson's story?

"How ya doing, Eddie?" I asked, sitting up to rub the dried dirt off my face. Eddie was already sitting, face slick with mud and sweat, eyes closed.

"Dehydrated," he said. He opened one eye, looked at me, and grinned.

I was shivering. He stood and offered me his hand—a good thing, or my legs would have grown roots and I would never have budged again. "Are the lodges always that hot?"

"Twice as hot for half-breeds." Eddie smiled generously, having named my fear for me. He put his hand on my shoulder, maybe sensing the panic that returned as I remembered the overpowering waves of heat and steam. "It had to be that hot 'cause you needed so much extra purification."

"I've never belonged anywhere, Eddie," I blurted out. "And I don't belong here."

"You belong here now," Eddie said seriously. "You earned your place, and respect too. Those old men made it plenty hot to test you. And you passed the test. Hell, *I* almost had to leave. But you sat there and suffered with us, and showed them what you're made of. Showed them that you care about Jimmie even though you don't know him, and that you're willing to suffer for him."

"Maybe," I stammered.

"No 'Maybe,' " Eddie responded, his voice strong and sincere. "You sat there like a warrior. I would be proud to call you my brother. And my grandfather to call you grandson."

"Okay," I said, smiling but not convinced.

"Be careful," said Eddie. "It's an insult to turn down an honor someone gives you." He winked and I relaxed. We pulled our jeans back on, over the dried mud on our legs. We put on our T-shirts and jackets, and laced up our old sneakers. The pickup truck had left and we were expected to walk back; only old men rode. We were alone with the sage and the jackrabbits, finding our energy returning with every step. Eddie pinched my arm.

"Hey," I yelled, swinging at him.

"Catch me," he dared, already starting to run. His feet stirred up the fine clay dust. He was rapidly outdistancing me and I had no choice but to run after him, since I had no idea where we were. I never caught him, but as I ran, the pounding of my feet on the ground drove away my fear. In the gathering dusk, the incessant busyness of SMCMC seemed wonderfully distant. Back in that world, our fellow students and professors were hustling from bed to bed to wrap up their afternoon rounds. I thought of the few minutes we spent with each patient, cutting short their stories as soon as we laid hands on the few isolated facts we believed were critical to our diagnosis.

Somewhere up ahead Nelson would be preparing for the tipi ceremony. If he worked at all like my great-grandmother, he would have spent much of the day listening to his patient, asking about his family, about his behavior and beliefs, trying to understand the connections between the man's life and his illness. He would be meeting with all the family members to tell them what was expected of them during the ceremony and afterward. For him and everyone else who was gathering, spirits were not metaphors. Prayer was not a way to trick someone's body into healing. A spiritual healing works because spirits are real. They must be approached slowly, respectfully, just as you would approach any other intelligent being with whom you seek a relationship.

I remembered once hiding quietly behind our red couch while my great-grandmother "doctored" someone. She listened carefully to all the details of the man's illness. She asked him many questions, then told him a long story. When the story ended she burned herbs and smoked tobacco. For a long time she rocked back and forth, chanting in a low voice. Suddenly she dropped her tobacco and touched the man's head. "You know why you are ill," she said.

The man began to cry. I was too young to understand much of the man's reply, but it was about something he had done wrong, something hurtful he had done to another person. My great-grandmother stood above him that winter morning, her braided hair dangling over her shoulder, placing sacred water upon his brow, bent over the way she did when she was cooking at the stove.

"You must make amends," my great-grandmother said. "You must seek forgiveness before the Creator will forgive you. You must show that you are serious." The man cried more. He mumbled things I didn't understand. When he stopped crying, my great-grandmother lit an herb and burned it in her great iron skillet. I liked the smell; she used the herb frequently. She took her feather and waved it so the smoke traveled all over the man. Then she sang another song and blessed him.

"Come back when you have made amends," she said. "Then we will pray again."

The man did come back. She sat with him; I could see only their silhouettes at the south window, where the sun entered in the winter. He came back several times. Eventually my great-grandmother took him into the special room where I was not allowed and sang some more. I listened at the door, hearing distant whispers and the movement of feet across the floor.

Later, I heard my mother talking about how the man had been crazy. He had been buying more things than he could afford and talking all the time. He got himself in trouble with the law. Then his wife left him. That made him really depressed, and he stopped leaving his house. Mother heard he tried to kill himself, and after that he had to spend some time in a hospital in Lexington.

Now everyone agreed he was getting better. He got out of bed every morning and went to work on time. Where once he had been mean to his daughters, now he was solicitous. He started going to church again on Sundays. He stopped drinking. His wife even came back to him. At the time, of course, I didn't understand what all this meant, except that he was better. Looking back, I imagine this man would have been diagnosed as having a bipolar disorder (then called manic depression). I accepted without question that my great-grandmother's appeal to higher powers had played a part in his recovery.

EDDIE TOPPED a rise and stood tall, catching the meager light shining from a cluster of squat, flat-roofed houses. The bushes before them swayed in the wind. If the collection of simple plywood cabins where Eddie had grown up was modest, the Wyoming darkness that surrounded the little settlement was magnificent. The night was clear. Overhead the moonless sky was so dark the stars burned like bright tiny pinholes in a vast black fabric—a study in contrasts city dwellers are never privileged to see.

Sometime after dark, Eddie's father led us up a hillside away from the cabins. A steady wind from the east rustled around our legs, carrying the sounds of the wings and feet of night foragers emerging from their lairs. A coyote howled nearby. The foothills that had looked so empty in the fading light now seemed full of invisible life. Portals to other worlds open in the darkness—worlds most modern people are too sophisticated or too frightened to imagine. Science prospers in the light of libraries and laboratories, but when the doors close and the light is extinguished, science is gone and ancient magic reigns.

I was not so sophisticated as I had thought. As I followed Eddie and his father along the crest of the hill, my old fear of the dark returned with a vengeance—only this time my raw senses could feel unseen powers moving in the darkness beyond us. We walked without light of any kind. I followed Eddie by listening for his footsteps. I felt humbled and terrified by my awakening ability to sense the presence of spirits. Then I became aware of drums beating in the night. In a few minutes we descended into a ravine, and the drumming became louder. Out of nowhere loomed a brightly lit tipi in a clearing beside a stream. Shadows of the people seated inside flickered on the tipi's walls as we approached.

Eddie's father pulled back the door flap. We entered silently, Eddie making sure to lead me. I was his responsibility, and I knew he would tell me what I needed to do. We circled clockwise (sunwise, by Nelson's reckoning) and sat on blankets. The fire burned brightly inside a circle of stones near the center of the tipi, casting its red-orange glow on people's expectant faces.

I squeezed next to Eddie. I studied the faces around the fire— twenty men and ten women. There was a middle-aged Shoshone drummer with a headband wrapped around his forehead; his long black hair fell to his waist. Two singers of indeterminate age sat on either side of him. A tight-lipped young man with long braids tended the fire, sweat glistening on his forehead. He raked the coals occasionally, moving them slowly, carefully, toward some definite pattern. A balding European man sat beside one of the singers. Dressed in jeans and cowboy boots and wearing a priest's collar, he was Father Stone, our guardian against the armies of religious orthodoxy.

Eddie pointed out the patient, sitting with his gray-haired wife behind Nelson. Although it was only an hour or so after sunset, Jimmie Left Hand already looked exhausted. On the other side of Jimmie sat Nelson's helper, whom I recognized from the sweat lodge, and who was weaving from side to side to the drum's cadence. His face was as creased as a folded and refolded road map. Even with his eyes closed, he looked alert and powerful, just like Nelson. "Before the white man came, the Shoshone-Arapaho and Northern Cheyenne were enemies," Eddie whispered. "Now they are healing one another, walking 'the good red road' together. From wisdom, which is the way of the north, to compassion and kindness, the way of the south. Healing is healing, Nelson says. The spirits don't belong to any particular tribe."

It was hard to hear him over the drums and the voices of the singers. The beat and the volume were overpowering. I had read that drumming was trance-inducing, but I had never experienced its power directly myself.

The light of the fire was the Light of God, permeating my being. I felt the spirit of Christ, as I understood him, entering my mind. I felt him calm my thoughts, creating a modicum of the inner peace I desired. In an ecstasy born of the drumming, I heard wordless mysteries, felt the boundless love of the Christ spirit, caught a glimpse of the compassion of the angels. Though she never read Rilke, Hazel shared the same insight as he: that one moment of an angel's full compassion would kill us. That much love would be a shock to the human nervous system. I felt such a shock building within. It built, and built, and sparked—but didn't kill me. Instead, it cleared my head of thoughts. For a moment I saw, without thinking, without a personality to judge what I was seeing. The Christ spirit had hooked me like a fish from the lake. I saw him standing beside the White Buffalo Woman, son and daughter aspects of the Creator. I later thought of Thomas Aquinas, who never said or wrote another word after his experience of divine presence at the Mass of Naples in 1293. When you are touched by God, there is nothing you can say. There is only wonder and joy.

Time stopped. The absolute stillness was disorienting, and my mind refused to find its bearings within the compass of the tipi. The beat ended and a new drummer began a different rhythm. I wanted to move, but my muscles were blocked and would not respond. Nelson began chanting in Cheyenne. The drumming and chanting continued at a feverish pitch until Nelson motioned abruptly for it to stop. He began a series of singsong prayers, then took Jimmie's open palms and studied them in the glow of the fire. In English, he told Jimmie that his family loved him. That all of us had gathered around the fire to care for him, that he must calm himself and trust in the power of the Creator, that the spirits would come. He would be healed. Nelson asked for another prayer song and the drumming resumed.

The fire had grown low. The taciturn firekeeper laid more wood onto the fire. Shadows danced as people began stirring and the fire-keeper continued to work his silent artistry. The pattern he was working toward was becoming clear: he was shaping the glowing embers into a thunderbird, a healing spirit animal.

The singers stopped. The drummer's insistent rhythm had summoned the spirits. The sudden quiet left an unbearable tension within the tipi. Nelson cried out, thanking the grandmothers and the grandfathers for coming to save Jimmie's life, for giving an old man the chance to be born again. He plunged his feather fan into the water and shook it over the fire. Far away, I tried to bring myself back from my trance. Nelson lifted Jimmie to his feet and fanned him with the eagle feathers, enveloping Jimmie's body in cedar smoke. Nelson continued to chant. His eagle feathers punctuated the chant with a loud, snapping noise as they brushed past Jimmie's body, sometimes flicking his face, spreading droplets of sacred water over his plaid shirt. The pungent odor of cedar carried our prayers up through the smoke hole and across the Milky Road to the Lodge of the Creator. I rubbed my eyes with my fist. The singing again filled the tipi with high-pitched voices and a superhuman energy.

Though the early stages of the ceremony had brought a joy to my heart that I hadn't known in years, now a dark energy was gathering. I stared at the smoke hole. I wished I could escape through it. I sensed the presence of evil. I was as frightened as I had been as a child, waiting on my bed for my stepfather to come and give me the evening's whipping. Inexplicable lights danced in the darkness of the tipi's heights. I felt the strong, primitive fear of the churning darkness, of the approach of irrational and uncontrollable forces. But I had learned in the sweat lodge that fighting fear only made it worse. The way forward lay in surrendering.

Nelson blew a shrill blast on his eagle-bone whistle. The jolt loosened something in me and I closed my eyes, feeling the darkness dissipating. The whistle blew again, carrying me into the tipi's shadows with its vibration. A cool blast of wind moved through the tipi, even though the tipi flap was closed. My ears hurt. I closed my eyes. Feathers brushed my face and droplets of water hit my cheeks. It was not raining outside and I was not in range of Nelson's fan. When I opened my eyes I saw dancing blue lights. I smelled the odor of Archie's cigars. I felt Archie's presence so strongly that I opened my eyes to look for him, thinking he was sitting beside me.

Archie was alive and well, living in Ohio—I'd gotten a postcard from him two days earlier. I'd never heard that the spirit of a living being could travel across the country to a ceremony. But there he was: Archie was with us in the tipi, along with other spirits who appeared as bursts of light and sparks in the shadows. Eddie was chuckling nervously. "Does it smell to you like dog?" he asked. One man's cigar is another man's dog. Perhaps another aspect of the Creator had been revealed to Eddie.

I caught Nelson staring at me with an intensity that puzzled me until I realized he was looking at something above or behind me. Perhaps he was seeing the presence Eddie and I were feeling. The eagle-bone blast must have loosened something in Jimmie, too, because he had fallen back into his wife's arms. He was sobbing. The drumming and singing stopped again. Nelson spoke urgently into the energy-charged silence.

"The grandfathers have come," he told the crowd. "The ancestors are here. They say your prayers will make Jimmie well. Pray for him now, right now. Everyone!" Nelson commanded. "Pray out loud for Jimmie! His soul has been ripped away from him and your prayers will bring it back." I hesitated, unsure of the right way to pray. Nelson stared at me across the remains of the fire. "Pray as your grandfather taught you to pray," he said.

How could Nelson possibly have known what I was thinking, let alone how Archie and I had prayed together? But I felt Archie's presence and remembered his having said that the spirits don't care how you pray as long as you mean it. So I began to pray as best I knew how, speaking softly in English amid the other languages.

Nelson turned to his singers. "Sing the song they sing while the people pray," he said. The singers resumed their high-pitched chanting.

The drums were even louder than before. Nelson prayed in Cheyenne, and across the tipi I heard a man praying in English to Holy Mary, Mother of God.

Sometime before dawn the prayers ended. Eddie's father passed around sacred pipes, and we smoked and thanked the grandfathers for having come and the Creator for having heard us. I took four long puffs on the pipe, following Eddie's instructions to blow smoke in each of the four directions, touching my left shoulder with the stem of the pipe before passing it to my left. When the pipes had been smoked and their vapors were still curling up toward the smoke hole, Nelson said that the grandfathers had told him that Jimmie's soul would reenter his body and he would be well. Nelson told Jimmie he would give him medicine to take. Eddie whispered, "Nelson has a suitcase full of plants back at the cabin. Wouldn't you love to know what they are, and what they're for?"

Eddie's family gave Nelson blankets and herbs and tobacco and other gifts, and people spoke of their love for Jimmie, who sat basking in the sunlight falling through the now-open door flap of the tipi. Nelson led another round of prayer in thanks for Jimmie's healing, and in remembrance of relatives passed on. I silently thanked the spirits for sending some part of Archie to me during the night. Several women left the tipi to get food, along with water and sage tea. Once everyone had been served, we ate.

When Eddie and I left the tipi an hour or so later, we found Nelson waiting outside. "So you're going to be doctors," he said, looking us over.

"Maybe so," Eddie answered shyly.

After having experienced Nelson's power in the ceremony, I was likewise loath to admit that I was studying to be a doctor. But Nelson nodded approvingly at us and said, "We need good doctors." He spoke briefly to Eddie in a language I guessed was Arapaho and then said to me in English, "Remember to honor Coyote and your grandfather. Coyote does exactly what he was created to do. He is faithful that way. You must be, too."

I told him I would be, and then gathered my courage to ask what he had seen over my shoulder when the grandfathers arrived. Nelson just spread his hands in a gesture that swept over the foothills and across the continent, covering the entire world. "Everything has a purpose," he said.

Later that morning, while Eddie napped in the sun beside the cabin, I walked back up into the hills. I hadn't paid much attention to the path we took after the ceremony, but now I tried to retrace our steps. I hiked for about an hour in the area where I thought the tipi was, but couldn't find a trace of it. After a while I gave up and sat down on a hilltop with a good view of the mountains, thinking about what Nelson had said. As for honoring Archie, that came naturally. I had brought along a cigar with me, and I sat down and smoked it in tribute to my grandfather and his manner of prayer. But Coyote?

I'd read enough Native American cosmology to know something about Coyote and his trouble-making role in creation. To what purpose was I supposed to put his stories? According to Nelson, everything had a purpose. That covered a lot of territory, but I was impressed enough with the old medicine man to consider the idea. I thought of one of the first stories I had ever heard about Coyote, and his trip to the Land Above. This story wasn't one I'd read; it was told to me by a Pima Indian friend from Stanford. And it went something like this:

One evening Coyote came across Buzzard, who was telling a story about the time he flew to the Land Above. Very slowly and deliberately, in the way that buzzards tell stories, Buzzard told every detail about flying up, way up into the clouds, higher than he'd ever flown before, so high that he didn't know how he would get back down. But once up there, he found an opening in the sky that looked like the mouth of a cave.

Coyote was so excited, he couldn't help but interrupt. "Tell it faster, Brother Buzzard," he said. "What happened next?" Everyone was annoyed with Coyote because interrupting a story is such bad manners, not to mention sometimes sacrilegious. True to form, Coyote didn't realize how rude he was being. He couldn't contain his excitement about a new place that he'd never been. Maybe he'd go right away himself—forget about his chores, his wife, and his children.

Standing by the side of the fire in the dark night, Buzzard told about his fear and trepidation as he carefully snuck through the opening in the sky. Once through it he discovered a whole other world. There were people singing and dancing. There were plants and animals, many of which he had never seen before. It was exciting, but he feared the hole in the sky would close up and he wouldn't be able to get back to his own kind. Coyote interrupted again. "Skip to the end, Buzzard. Because you've got to take me there, tonight. You've got to show me this place."

Beating his naked chest, Buzzard defied Coyote's bad manners. More slowly than usual he told about how, with fear pounding in his heart, he ran as fast as he could to the opening and jumped through it, back into the sky of this world, where his wings caught an updraft of wind that allowed him to coast down to the fireside, to where he was now telling his story. All the animals knew Buzzard spoke the truth, because buzzards do not lie.

After the story ended, Coyote slinked up to Buzzard and asked again to be taken to the Land Above. Buzzard wasn't too sure that he wanted to go back. And he certainly didn't want to take Coyote, but he didn't know how to say no without being rude.

Buzzard knew all coyotes love games of chance. They love to gamble and play tricks on others. Buzzard said he'd only take Coyote to the Land Above if Coyote would promise not to gamble with the Sky People. But Coyote was already counting on cleaning up with the Sky People. Because they wouldn't be familiar with his games, he'd have the expert's advantage, and they wouldn't suspect his sophisticated tricks. So when Buzzard demanded a promise, Coyote answered, "Oh, sure, fine," the way people do when they aren't really listening.

Buzzard prayed to Wind, asking to be lifted up and carried to the Land Above. Wind came and took them swiftly above the clouds and through the opening in the sky to the Land Above. Coyote clung tightly to Buzzard's back, shivering with fear at the great height and trying not to look down. After a while, he could not even open his shivering eyes.

When they arrived and Coyote climbed off his back, Buzzard admonished him to be back at the cave entrance by sunset. Buzzard said this was imperative because he could not stay aloft at such a height in the cold. He needed the last bit of the sun's rays to carry them safely back down. Coyote nodded, but he wasn't listening. He was adding up all the money he was about to win from the Sky People.

Coyote had a wonderful time. He tried to trick all the people in the sky with his games, but they were too sharp for him. He had met his match. And the Sky People had their own games of chance, which fascinated him so much that he didn't notice the time passing—until suddenly he woke up and it was dark. He had fallen asleep and missed the rendezvous! Suddenly he remembered what Buzzard had said about flying home before dark. He was stuck in the sky and didn't know what to do.

Coyote ran lickety-split to the opening in the sky, but Buzzard had already left. Coyote looked down and couldn't even see the ground because it was so far down. He cried bitter tears at not having heeded Buzzard's warning. Coyote did not want to live forever with the Sky People. He wanted desperately to go back to the earth, where his tricks worked at least some of the time. In his frenzy, he figured that his only course was to jump. Terrified as he was, he backed up and ran toward the opening. Then he stopped. Three more times he ran and three more times he stopped short, panting with fear. On the fifth try he tripped over a stone and fell a long, long way down.

Two days later a bag of bones hit the ground with a thud. It was Coyote, landing on the earth. He had been so high that without wings it had taken Wind that many days to set him down.

Coyote's burial was prepared and his bones were placed on the hillside *in the proper manner in a sacred place. Prayers were said. Complaining about Coyote's tricks had been fashionable, but no one wanted to be rid of the trickster forever. The animals asked the Great Spirit to pick up Coyote's bones and give him life again somewhere else. When the prayers and songs ended, the animals returned to their homes, sadly humming the last song to themselves. After all, what would life be without coyotes? Someone has to challenge rules that have no reason or meaning.*

That night the Great Spirit answered their prayers. The Great Spirit took Coyote's bones and spread them all over the earth. Every bone, every fragment of bone, became a coyote. The animals woke up to an annoying clamor just before first light — what was it this time? On every distant hill was a little coyote, howling at the moon, imploring it to stay awake. And the next evening every distant hill had a little coyote on it, howling at the moon to come out and play.

I sat there on the hilltop, remembering what it was like to be a child, to believe in my great-grandmother's Cherokee stories. I dreamed at night of the animals and heroes of those stories. I loved my stuffed animals and filled them with the spirits from her tales. Education had distanced me from the spirits of my childhood, but they returned to me with emotional immediacy in a Wyoming tipi.

What triggered their return and my emotion? Was it the appearance of Archie's spirit, which Eddie had noticed too? Or was it the clairvoyant words Nelson spoke? I didn't really care, because for me there was no question but that what had happened was real. I started running along the hilltop, trying to remember everything—all the things I hadn't thought of for so long. I felt like an ancient animal, racing along the deer trails, feeling ecstatic in the sunlight. I thought of the young boy turned into a bear, running in an effort to make sense of what had happened to him. I was thrilled to have rejoined the world of spirits, of ceremony, of the world I had come from.

ONE COLD WINTER'S EVENING before going to her room, my great-grandmother announced she would die that night. Earlier that day she had been carrying wood as usual to the black iron cookstove and cooking greens in her cast-iron skillet. Although she was old, she was not infirm. The family was stunned by her casual announcement. When Mother called it superstitious nonsense, Great-Grandmother did not argue or insist. She simply told us she loved us and said good-bye. Hazel took her seriously and began to cry. "Oh, stop!" was my mother's response to them both.

Great-Grandmother kissed Mother's forehead and headed to her room. I waited a few minutes and then sneaked off to watch from her doorway. She nodded at me, to acknowledge my presence. She lit a candle on her bedside table, turned out the electric lights, and knelt to sing her death song. Her long, soft gray hair lay on her shoulders like one of the mohair afghans she used to crochet. When the song ended she gave thanks for her long life, asked the Great Spirit to take her, and climbed into bed to die. I went to my room and cried.

The next morning, the trees outside coated with ice from a freezing rain, Mother found Great-Grandmother's lifeless body tucked neatly in the bed. You would think that her premonition would have forced my mother to give more credence to my great-grandmother's beliefs. If it did, my mother never showed it. But the death did release the hold of that Kentucky land upon us. Mother was free to make her overdue pilgrimage to Ohio, the land of plenty, the Canaan of the 1950s for the underemployed of our state. How common this was could be seen any Friday in the traffic jams on the bridges over the Ohio River, as masses of displaced Kentuckians made the weekend trek back to visit the relatives they had left behind.

My mother eventually found a job teaching English at Shawnee High School and rented the top floor of a nearby farmer's house. She helped Archie land a job as a janitor at the high school where she would be teaching. Even with their two jobs, it seemed we couldn't get by—until shortly after moving into the house, when my mother announced her plans to marry our landlord, who lived downstairs. I had barely met him during those two months before their engagement. At first, I was excited at the prospect of finally having a father. Frank married my mother at Christmastime in the Methodist church where he was an elder.

His family held three consecutive farms along a rarely traveled stretch of the state highway that led to Rising Sun, Indiana. Frank sold and serviced milking parlors and equipment, and raised corn, hay, and hogs on the side. Brother Bruce was a dairy farmer. Grandfather helped the two boys run their spreads, staying fit by laboring hard from dawn to dusk. Frank turned out to be a strict and stern taskmaster, just like his father. He would have loved living in the early 1800s, when the work of turning the wild Ohio foothills into docile farmland had just started. But in the 1960s Frank had to content himself with working a piece of land already under cultivation for more than a century. He made his money on the milking equipment and supplies, but he loved gabbing with other farmers about farming, and in the evenings he'd plow or cultivate or plant. There was always work to be done—we would bale hay, pick corn, harvest soybeans. On weekends, there were fences, barns, and silos to repair, hogs to take to market, and cattle to butcher. Farming is all-consuming whether it generates a profit or not.

When they married, my stepfather asked my mother to give away everything she owned. But he was stuck with me, like the weeds in his football-field-sized potato patch, which he set me to toil over for hours. Frank expected me to be a big help to him with the farming, just as he had been to his father. But farming was not my passion; science was. I read physical chemistry texts in the truck while I drove around with him on weekends, writing up orders for milking supplies, cleaning pulsators (the devices in milking lines that generate vacuum pulses to suck milk from the cows), or helping with the occasional milking-parlor installation he'd contracted. I enjoyed driving the big corn picker in the distant fields, amid the constant drumming of ears of corn tumbling into the wagon I pulled behind me. Quails and foxes scared up from the hedgerows ran out of the way of the roaring diesel. The powerful floodlights let me work long after dark, alone in a world of tall corn and animals.

I don't remember what started Frank and me fighting. Mother stayed out of our arguments. She was too busy having babies, one after another on an almost annual basis, to pay attention to the troubles between Frank and me. I would mow our large lawn, and Frank would go out and mow it again, as if I hadn't done anything. I watched him from my upstairs window, weeping as he redid my work. I was bitter and lonely. One of the few excuses I found for getting out of farmwork was schoolwork. I thought if I excelled in school, Frank would look foolish demanding that I go out to the barn before my homework was finished. Education became my salvation.

When my mother married, Archie and Hazel moved to a small apartment above a bar in downtown Shawnee. I missed them terribly when they left and felt deserted by them. They solved that by having me over to their apartment for frequent visits. I spent many happy hours there playing with my toy soldiers while Hazel cooked and cleaned and told me stories. On Sundays, she took me to the Presbyterian church across the street. Sometimes I went with Archie to work. I liked the strange smells in his janitor's room, the huge, circular locker-room sink where twenty people could wash their hands at once, even the gritty, powdered soap I've only known schools to use.

I was nine years old when Frank decided that my problem was that I had been spoiled. "Spare the rod and spoil the child," he recited. Truly I had never been spanked, except for the time my startled mother slapped me after I tried to dart across a busy street. Frank decided to end my insolence with nightly whippings. He'd have me put on my pajamas and wait upstairs on the edge of my bed. Listening as he mounted the stairs and yanked his sinister belt through his pant loops was always worse than the whipping I got. I reluctantly told Archie once what was happening. I didn't think any good would come of it, as I didn't expect he'd be able to help me. But one rainy evening Archie showed up in our kitchen. When Frank came in, Archie silently picked him up by the front of his shirt, raised him six inches off the floor, pinned him against a door, and promised to kill him if he ever laid hands on me again. My boxer grandfather towered over Frank's five-foot-three-inch frame. Archie's threat saved me from further whippings, but it also started a cold war between Frank and me that has never thawed.

I felt a spiritual hunger in those years that nothing could satisfy. We went to Frank's Methodist church in Shawnee, Ohio, but I found the services dry and stultifying. At age eleven I took Billy Graham's Bible Study Correspondence Course. When that was finished, I decided to read the Bible from cover to cover. I still have that book with the notes I wrote in the margins. The Bible led me to Søren Kierkegaard; I read every book of his during my twelfth year. Then I read Paul Tillich. These men taught me about faith. It was Kierkegaard who coined the phrase "leap of faith"; Tillich made his reputation addressing the problem of doubt in the modern world.

Billy Graham was fine with Frank, but when I moved on to philosophy, I was in suspicious territory. What he didn't understand he ridiculed. He would holler until he was red in the face about the atheistic, Communist books I was reading, to no avail. Since I had Archie as my protector, I could read Karl Marx in front of Frank just to get to him. Neither Marx nor Lenin really interested me, but their names on the spines of books drove Frank bonkers. I found Buddhism and Zen more promising philosophies, but was drawn to them primarily because of the antics of some of the ancient Zen masters. The wild spontaneity I valued I have since found is also one of Native America's particular gifts to the spiritual world.

At thirteen I put my faith in existentialism and hitchhiking—the latter an odd artifact of Boy Scouting. While working on a physics merit badge, I traveled to the University of Cincinnati main campus, where I met a professor who was interested in being my mentor. I started spending every Saturday at his laboratory helping him do a study of the morphology of splashes. (I now think he was working on an aspect of chaos theory.) We used high-speed photography and laser lights to record what happened during the splash of a steel ball into a pan of water. Later I helped him study the behavior of electricity at extremely low temperatures.

I loved being at a college and pretending to belong. I loved the tree-lined paths, I loved the fat, lazy squirrels, I loved the restaurants and the libraries and the bookstores. One day, when my mother wouldn't drive me, I hitchhiked. That led to the insight that I could probably hitchhike anywhere, so one momentous spring break, with false bravado, I held out my thumb and headed for Boston. My excuse was wanting to visit Harvard. When I needed to sleep, I would find a college dormitory and drape a book over my lap so as to appear to have fallen asleep studying. Nobody ever bothered me. Sometimes I was befriended by students, and that would often land me a spare bed in a dorm or a fraternity. I hitchhiked throughout most of the Northeast—from Toronto to Syracuse, Rochester, Albany, and Boston, down to New York and Philadelphia, and back to Cincinnati. Once my mother, in a desperately generous mood, bought me a plane ticket to Boston. I got off in Philadelphia, the first stop, cashed in the ticket, spent the weekend at the University of Pennsylvania, and continued to Boston by thumb.

The University of Cincinnati had a branch campus—about twenty-five miles from Frank's farm. I decided to enroll for evening classes, acting as if I was entitled, which appeared to make it so. Soon I was spending two long evenings per week there. I discovered I could enroll in any course I wished, as long as I ignored the prerequisites. Of course this practice put the onus on me to work extra hard to make up what I hadn't already learned. One of my first courses, appropriately enough, was the psychology of adolescence, Psych 211c. I don't think I gained any insight into how to be one, but I earned an A and I entertained the teacher, especially when she discovered I was fourteen. And it was a lot more fun than staying at home.

Around this time I remember Archie telling me a story about how the Creator calls us to do his work. We'd been fishing in the pond on Frank's farm for a while when Archie laid down his fishing pole and lit up a cigar. There was nothing to catch in that pond but small perch, and we always threw them back, but Archie liked to fish because it relaxed him. We sat on the bank while he smoked. Archie had his green janitor's uniform on, which he wore even when he wasn't at work. For no particular reason, I started humming "Amazing Grace."

Archie joined me in humming, then in singing the song for a while. He asked, "Did you know that song is the national anthem of the Cherokee people?" I didn't. "It was made famous from being sung on the Trail of Tears, from Tennessee to Oklahoma."

It was November and the frogs were gone. The algae had died and the pond looked almost clean. A fence kept the cows outside in the field, which kept the pond from being clogged with manure. A pipe brought water from the pond hundreds of feet back to the farmhouse to supply all the toilets, and our toilets always smelled of algae because of it. But my stepfather thrived on that kind of economy.

"Do you know who wrote that song?" asked Archie.

"No."

Archie took a long pull on his smoke stick before continuing. "Well then, I'll tell you. Once upon a time there was an English sea captain. He had a boat fulla slaves he was carryin' from Africa to the United States. I guess that makes it some time before the Civil War. Well, they ran into a terrible storm. The captain was sure his boat was gonna sink. He thought, 'Am I seein' my last day on earth?' The boat rocked left and right, up and down, almost turnin' over in answer to his question. Then he did somethin' he'd never done before. He got down on his knees and he prayed to the Creator. He begged for forgiveness. He said, 'Creator, I know I've sinned by sellin' these poor people into slavery. Forgive me. If you have to take my life tonight, then take it, but spare theirs, and please forgive me. And if you should spare *me,* I promise I'll never do it again. I'll turn this boat around and take these people home and I'll never sail a slavin' ship again.'

"Well, the story is that the storm suddenly quieted down. Pretty soon the waves were calm. And what do you think, Lewis—did the man ignore his message? Did he doubt what had happened, once the storm stopped? He might have. A lot of people *would* have. But he didn't. He didn't up and decide it had all been some big coincidence. No sir. He turned that boat around. He ordered his crew to sail back to Africa. And they almost mutinied when he gave his orders, but when he explained how he had saved their lives, even that band of cutthroat slavers knew they were hearin' the God's honest truth. So they stayed on with him and they turned that boat around and they took those people back to Africa. And he went back to England and wrote this song.

"When you get the call," Archie continued, "I hope you listen like that captain did. That would make me a lot more proud of you, no matter what, than anythin' else I can think of." Then he took several more long puffs on his cigar, blew the smoke toward the Creator, and said, "Amen," almost as an afterthought. He dug a small hole beside the pond and placed the remaining tobacco inside it, then covered the hole carefully. He picked up his fishing pole and stood up. As he started back toward the gate in the fence, I stayed a moment looking into the dark water of the pond, watching my reflection, and then ran to catch up with Archie. Thinking back, I wonder what he had seen that day that caused him to tell me the story.

I WANTED MY grandfather to be proud of me, so I promised I would listen for my call, just as I promised Nelson I'd be faithful. Before coming to the reservation, I would have said that my call had come when I decided to become a doctor. Now I understood that this was just one in a series of messages. Just as important was the "wake-up call" in the renal room at SMCMC. I was being alerted to avoid complacency, to avoid the seduction of success in conventional medicine, and to continue to strive for a vision of what real healing could be. I sat thinking for a long time on Eddie's Wyoming hilltop while watching the afternoon shadows stretch across the hillsides. When the sun finally set and the sky was darkening, I returned to the cabin, tired and grungier than when I had left, but happy.

When it was time to go, Eddie's father shook my hand. "Come again," he said. Kiefer was driving the pickup this time. I tossed my bag into the back and climbed over the gate. Kiefer's girlfriend got into the cab and Eddie rode in the back with me. We drove north toward Riverton and then back down the long, straight road toward Caspar. We stopped again at Yellowstone Drug in Shoshoni. We still didn't win anything, but the milkshakes were good, and we picked up some free bumper stickers to take back with us to Stanford. The sun came out from the clouds as we passed through Moneta and the turnoff to Lost Cabin. I sat back and watched the bare hills roll by, wondering what Archie was doing just then, and whether he could see me when he prayed.

Riding through Powder River, Wyoming, population 10 or so, past the lone gas station and general store, I began to realize what kind of doctor I wanted to be. I wanted to walk both roads, the Anglo and the Indian, though I realized that I ran the risk of being rejected by both cultures. I could stay out of trouble by acting as if both views had their place—one in hospitals and the other on reservations—but at that moment I was too much in love with the world to do that. Through the sweat lodge, the tipi ceremony, and my morning run along the hilltop, the whole world had spoken to me. The earth had swept through me and left me changed. I would no longer accept the view that people are only the incidental occupants of a set of organs.

Eddie and I flew back to Stanford from Caspar. I returned to Professor's Rounds, in which the chairman of the department, an expert on pediatric blood diseases, heard us present cases before discussing our diagnosis and treatment plans. Again I sat through months of conferences in which we all honed our abilities to please the chairman and to measure our patients' declines and demises. These months were harder because the patients were children.

One day in July, during a lull in pediatrics, I wandered over to the renal room of the ICU. Dr. Habra had gone back to Riyadh. I didn't really expect to see April's four proteinuria patients still in the hospital. Indeed, Dr. Jackson's bed was empty. Brasher's bed was occupied by a woman, as was Brown's. Martinez's bed now held a very sickly Hispanic man who was sleeping flat on his back. His face was pasty and bloated, and his expression, even in sleep, was terminally weary. I started to pass by and then noticed the sickly man's muscular arms. On one was a heart-shaped tattoo. I tried to remember whether Señor Martinez had had a tattoo. The Hispanic man's eyes opened and he caught me staring. I gave a slight smile and he nodded, the sort of recognition a bed-bound patient would give any passing doctor who might or might not be coming to see him. I left quickly, as if I had somewhere else to go. Almost three months had passed since I'd met Sr. Martinez, and now I couldn't be sure whether the man in the bed was the forty-two-year-old carpenter or some other middle-aged man dying of renal failure. I could have checked at the nurses' station on my way out, but I didn't. If this was Martinez, I didn't want to know.

CHAPTER THREE

Who Are You?

I ARRIVED in Madison, Wisconsin, in June 1975. Having just finished med school, I was set to begin a combined residency in family practice and psychiatry. After the various rotations at Stanford, it seemed to me these specialties would provide me the best opportunities for becoming a physician-healer. I was looking forward to this next step in my journey toward credibility and skill.

Family practice was an emerging, open-ended specialty at the time; its practitioners tried to take a more holistic view of patients. Psychiatrists likewise recognized that people were more than just cells and organs. I had some experience with both specialties at Stanford. The associate dean there worked hard to provide a nurturing experience for his students. He made certain you followed traumatic rotations with gentler ones. After my stints in neurosurgery, urology, and pediatrics, I had a peaceful interlude in a rural family practice at Point Reyes Station, near the national seashore, where I was introduced to acupuncture and home birth methods. Back again at Stanford I worked in psychiatry, pediatric cardiology, pediatric hematology, immunology, and pathology before finishing with a final rotation in internal medicine.

The career-track students, who competed for internships at the nation's ten most prestigious hospitals, took no easy rotations. I was never driven by that kind of vertical ambition, as I called it, that drive to get to the top of the pile. I took a more horizontal course. I was interested in developing a career that would integrate my many interests, and in so doing maybe even change the face of modern medicine.

The University of Wisconsin in Madison was not on the list of the nation's very best hospitals, but it was certainly quite a good place. I chose it partly because of a promise that I could work toward my two chosen certifications at once, reducing the seven years they would take sequentially (four for psychiatry, three for family practice) to only five. And I hoped to be able to work with native healers in Wisconsin. During my last year at Stanford I had studied informally with two Cherokee medicine men in northern California, and I planned now to follow that spiritual path, albeit in fits and starts.

I rented a small house outside of Madison; the house was dwarfed by enormous oak trees out front and surrounded by fields of waving green corn. The landlord must have wondered who this hippie doctor was when he first saw me—I wore my hair in a ponytail that reached almost to my waist. I think the fact that I was married convinced him that I was conventional enough to be trusted.

I had met my wife four years earlier, when I was seventeen and she was twenty-one. Rather than go home one summer during college, I had arranged to spend the vacation at Stanford's Hopkins Marine Biology Station in Pacific Grove, California. I was looking for passengers to share the driving expenses. A friend of mine knew a girl, Ellen, who happened to need a ride out west—she would be taking summer courses at the University of California at Santa Cruz. Ellen and I spent the long drive getting acquainted with each other's plans and dreams. We were both still young enough to have more of the latter than the former.

Since neither of us knew anyone else in California, we spent most of our free time together. We got along well and agreed to share an apartment when we got back to Bloomington. I was amazed that any woman would want to live with me. I recall the signature gag of a character on "Laugh-In": "Blow in my ear and I'll follow you anywhere." That's pretty much all Ellen had to do to win me. One of the problems with moving so quickly through high school and college was that I always lagged behind on the dating scene.

Not that I looked or acted like a kid. As long as the people I was around didn't already know how young I was, things were fine. For two summers I worked as a camp counselor at a Boy Scout camp east of Cincinnati. The first summer I was a nature counselor; the second summer I asked to be a lifeguard, thinking I'd be more attractive to women. Wishful thinking perhaps, but when I asked a pretty girl out, for the first time I was accepted. I came home one Friday night to buy a new sports jacket. I told my mother what it was for, and she promptly called the girl's mother to say I wasn't allowed on dates because I was only thirteen. Everyone at camp had thought I was seventeen, including my sixteen-year-old date.

That wasn't my last date, but it was the last one my mother heard about—until I came home from college one day, asking to borrow some money to make a down payment on a Toyota Land Cruiser. At the time they cost $2,700, and I had money from a student loan to cover the balance. When my mother agreed, I casually pulled out another paper for her to sign—I needed her permission to get married. She halfheartedly objected but finally gave in. The lease had fallen through on the apartment Ellen and I had found for ourselves two days before classes started. The only housing left was earmarked for married students. We tried to bluff our way into a place, but given our different last names, a marriage license was demanded. So we set out to get one.

If I make our decision sound a little casual, it's because it was. Ellen argued that getting married was no big deal: we could always get divorced, and it was the quickest way to get what we wanted. And this was the 1970s—along with protesting the war, my generation was challenging all the accepted rules of society. I don't think Ellen thought of our marriage as a permanent arrangement any more than I did. While still at Indiana, we were even a little embarrassed about it. For a long time we didn't tell anyone but the student-housing people that we were married. More roommates than newlyweds, we lived separate lives, taking different courses, socializing with different sets of friends. We did travel together a good deal. On semester breaks Ellen and I would take mini-vacations, with the Land Cruiser doubling as transport and accommodation.

What neither of us anticipated is how powerfully the psyche responds to the shapes and forms of ideas. It's not all that different from the healing I witnessed in Wyoming—Nelson told Jimmie he was well, Jimmie believed him, and it was so. So watch out before you go telling people you're married. There is truth to the proverb "As you say it is, so it shall be." Ellen and I graduated from Indiana in January of 1973, me with a degree in biophysics, her with one in psychology and dance. Ellen felt the pull of California, and so we left together for the West Coast.

When I started school, Ellen made some passing comments about wanting a baby. I was upset when Ellen told me she was pregnant. I did not feel like a part of the decision. I knew what a job being a parent would be and I didn't feel ready to be a father. My own lost father still weighed heavily on my mind. I worried about how I could afford a child and school, though friends assured me that the school's financial aid package would expand to cover a child.

Ellen wanted to have the baby at home with midwives. We discovered the Santa Cruz Birth Center. As a physician I wanted to know home birth was safe. Encouraged by Dr. Donner at Stanford—a guru in the natural childbirth movement—I embarked on a study of home birth and its emotional effects on mothers and babies. Ellen's timely interest in the topic drew her into the work. We became partners on the study and on several related studies that followed.

As luck would have it, when I received my schedule for the school year that August of 1973, my last rotation before the baby's birth was to be OB-GYN. Then I would be off for three weeks for Christmas break, then three weeks of research. My OB-GYN evaluation read that I performed well, but nevertheless, had allowed my wife to have a home birth. In reality, Ellen had told me I could go to the hospital when she went into labor and she would stay home and have the baby. It was her awareness of how hospitals degraded and humiliated women in labor that led us to a home birth.

Our first study on home birth outcomes was published soon after our daughter was born. The birth was a wonderful experience. And our investigation of natural childbirth created vocations for Ellen and me, generating work we are both still engaged in more than twenty years later. But powerful as both were, neither the birth nor the work brought Ellen and me closer together as a couple. We spent years trying to create the feeling of being happily married, but the feeling never lasted for long, and never for both of us at the same time.

Almost as soon as I finished at Stanford, Ellen and I bundled our daughter into the Land Cruiser and towed our belongings in a U-Haul trailer to Wisconsin. I thought of Eddie's family and Jimmie Left Hand as we crossed the Rockies just south of the Wind River Reservation. Eddie had told me that Jimmie's doctor, refusing to believe angina could just disappear, subjected Jimmie to a painful round of tests before concluding that Jimmie had never really been sick in the first place. I congratulated myself for having found a Lutheran hospital for my residency, where the doctors would be more open-minded than Jimmie's had been. I assumed the group of holistically inclined physicians who had founded the family practice program at Lutheran Hospital in Madison would, as a matter of policy, respect the connection between a patient's spiritual life and physical health. I thought of Father Stone, and hoped I would find others like him where I was headed.

As I watched the country roll by hour after hour, I felt a gathering sense of relief. The trials of medical school were behind me. The days of being an impotent observer were over. Not far ahead was a hospital whose family practice training program was dedicated to exploring how social, emotional, and physical factors worked together to determine people's health. I would put into practice my belief that scientific medicine was compatible with, and even complementary to, religion and shamanism. In time I would find a faculty position somewhere, where I would train other young doctors to view themselves as healers.

My ultimate goal was to change the way medicine is practiced. Twenty years later, that sounds like a brash plan for a young med school grad. But I didn't think I was being immodest. The type of healing I wanted to bring into medicine was not my invention; I would only be passing on a tradition that had been developed over centuries—and which I was only beginning to study seriously. As a legitimate doctor, I saw myself as a possible conduit through which ancient knowledge could pass into a modern world. I did not have to be clever or persuasive or powerful. I did not have to invent anything. I had only to be faithful, and willing to stir things up a little, like Coyote. The shaman's spiritual approach healed people in tipis and churches. People would see that it could work in hospitals and clinics, too, if only someone could find the right place to introduce it—and I was sure the right place would be the family practice clinic at Lutheran.

For the first year of my internship, my time at this teaching clinic would be limited to one half day per week. I was also to spend a half day at the crisis intervention center for my psychiatry residency. The rest of the time I would be serving a standard internship with three-month rotations in internal medicine, obstetrics, pediatrics, and shorter tours of surgery and psychiatry.

My first two rotations taught me more than I wanted to know about how modern medicine views death and birth. I learned the first lesson at the bedside of Mrs. Hannah, a frail ninety-four-year-old woman I met on my internal medicine rotation. Her mind was intact, but her body was failing, organ by organ. She'd been hospitalized with exhaustion, shortness of breath, low blood pressure, faintness, dizziness, incontinence, indigestion, and insomnia. She had been in the hospital for two weeks while her physician, Dr. Floyd, the chief of internal medicine, was "working her up." Working her over was more like it. Anyone could see she was dying. But we had to know *why* she was dying, and so we were consigned to investigate her every organ, force our way into the hidden passageways of her body, even tie her arms to the bedrails when our procedures were too painful to pass unresisted.

I grew up around enough old people to know when someone is dying, and Mrs. Hannah had all the signs—a pallid complexion, a paucity of movement, a reluctance to take food or drink. There is, however, no entry for "Dying" in the *International Classification of Diseases*. Dr. Floyd's charges were told to look for diseases, whether we could treat them or not, and we were supposed to keep her alive during the search. We put an IV into her arm to provide fluids, a tube into her stomach to provide food, and another tube into her bladder to drain her wastes away.

I was incensed at what I perceived to be a lack of respect for Mrs. Hannah, and for dying. Several classmates agreed with me but shook their heads and steamed blindly ahead. I felt compelled to protest. By nature I am one of those fools who tries to stop a street fight or argue with an arbitrary traffic cop. These tendencies didn't improve my popularity. I left one slightly troublesome reputation behind in California; Mrs. Hannah was the start of a new one in Wisconsin. For I was the lackey expected to detail for her each morning what tortures the new day held in store—X-rays, tomograms, upper and lower GIs, and scans that required radioactive elements to be injected and concentrated in certain organs.

Despite our diligence, the source of Mrs. Hannah's problem eluded us. Dr. Floyd was sure she had cancer, and that we just hadn't found it yet. Damned if we wouldn't find one eventually, or make one for her. Day after day we cheated her from death. Somewhere toward the end of the fourth week, Floyd decided that she needed a barium enema. I asked why we didn't just let her die.

"That's a swell idea," he said. "Do you want to go tell her family that's the best we can offer?"

"Sure," I said. "Her daughter's coming in this afternoon. Shall I go discuss it with Mrs. Hannah?"

"Don't even think about it," he said, wincing as if he had a migraine. "Write the order for the barium enema."

So we gave her one, and no one was surprised when it revealed nothing. It did lower her blood pressure precipitously and knock her fluids and electrolytes out of balance. For a day Mrs. Hannah hovered close to death. She had the misfortune to survive. We nursed her back to a kind of health again, where at least she was strong enough to withstand the new tests Dr. Floyd wanted to do.

As the days rolled on, I found myself spending more time with Mrs. Hannah, at first out of a need to apologize for what we were doing. But then she began to ask me questions, slowly drawing out my life story. All the while she told me hers. Sometimes she would even joke about the futility of the endless testing. In the presence of my colleagues, she gave curt responses to our continual questions about her deteriorating body. But to me, after we had gotten to know each other, Mrs. Hannah admitted that she knew she was dying. She asked me for all the details of my great-grandmother's death, and wished she had the power to choose her own moment to die.

Mrs. Hannah wasn't worried about dying. She was a devout Catholic, forced into the Lutheran hospital because of a lack of beds at the nearby Catholic Hospital. She believed she was on the verge of passing on to another existence. Here on earth, even her children's children were grown and healthy, and she didn't feel she was leaving anything important undone. As she told stories of her youth and her life, Mrs. Hannah revealed how proud she was that she had never moved out of the parish where she was born. "Ninety-four years is a long time," she boasted. "I've outlived one husband and three priests. One baptized me. Another saw me married, and baptized my children. A third baptized my grandchildren. Now there's a fourth hovering around, waiting to give me the last rites."

I let her know that she didn't have to accept our treatments. She had the right to refuse them.

"No," she said. "An old woman doesn't have any rights. If I say no, they'll just tie me down and do it anyway, or get a judge to order it done. Besides, they're just doing their job. They're only doing what they think is right."

"But doing their job doesn't mean going against your wishes," I said. "I could talk to them."

"No," she insisted. "I don't want to cause any trouble."

"But they should respect your wishes. It's not right."

"Of course it's all right." She was smiling sweetly now, and closing her eyes, drifting off to sleep. At moments such as these, I felt a peacefulness in her company I had only read of people feeling in the presence of saints.

I INTERRUPTED PRIEST number four's visits to Mrs. Hannah more than once, when I accompanied Dr. Floyd on his rounds. One afternoon the priest pressed his card into my hand and told me to page him when I had some free time. I never did, but a few days later he was waiting for me when I came to see Mrs. Hannah. Her bed was empty.

"She's not . . ."

"Oh no," he reassured me quietly. "She's down in Nuclear Medicine for another scan. She told me you'd be coming around about now, so she asked me to wait for you and talk to you."

"To me?" I asked, puzzled.

"Sure," he answered easily. "She says you're taking her dying hard. I'm Father Pat Mahoney." He offered me his hand. "I'm the hospital chaplain. Sometimes I talk to the interns about their fear of death."

"The interns?"

"They're usually more frightened than the patients. Many of them have never faced death before."

"How many patients have?" I said, then immediately regretted my sarcasm. Though Mrs. Hannah and I had joked about his hovering, Father Mahoney's concern was unexpectedly welcome. "What really bothers me," I said, "is how we torture Mrs. Hannah to keep her alive when she's so obviously ready to die."

"It's hard to be an intern," Father Mahoney reflected as I sat down in the other chair in the room. "You bear the burden of decisions that others make."

"I just want to do what's right for people," I said. "Sometimes that seems almost impossible."

"I know," he said. "I sit even further on the outskirts of medicine than you. I help patients pick up the pieces after their doctors are through. Doctors bring bad news and clear out, then I help their patients to grieve. The families of the dying ask me to sit with them while the doctors make their curt announcements that so-and-so has just passed away, and they cry with me after the doctors leave. I know what you're going through. I know something about the brutality of medicine."

"But what can we do?" I asked.

"We can hold on to our faith, no matter what," he said. "Mrs. Hannah thinks you're a very special person." I blushed. I was embarrassed. "You're special because you care," Father Mahoney said, giving me a piercing stare. "Very few doctors do. No one else has ever come to see her like you have, and she's noticed. And so have I."

"Don't tell anyone," I said, with a short laugh. "I'm trying not to ruin my reputation in my first month here."

"I understand," he said. "I really do. I'd like to be a help to you, if you need it. Mrs. Hannah will die, as we both know, and it'll be harder on you than her. So please, come see me anytime."

The next afternoon, when the daily diagnostic assaults were over, I sat with Mrs. Hannah in her room. She asked me to close the curtains. Clutching her rosary in her frail hands, she asked me to say the Lord's Prayer with her. Then she trudged through a string of Hail Marys, fingering each bead as carefully as if it alone held the key to her soul's salvation. I sat silently by her bed, praying too, for forgiveness for my part in what we were doing to the poor woman. I promised God that when I was in a position to make the decisions, I wouldn't torture dying old people.

When Mrs. Hannah finished reciting her memorized prayers, she continued in a high, quavering voice to ask God to watch over the people of her parish, her friends and neighbors, her children and grandchildren. Then she asked for forgiveness for herself. The effort of praying exhausted her, and she lapsed into a long silence, so long I thought she had fallen asleep. But when I stirred in my chair, she sighed and asked God to bring her home.

It struck me how similar Mrs. Hannah's prayers were to my great-grandmother's long, meandering supplications, with the members of our family always mentioned early on, and always with her own needs addressed only at the end.

I LEARNED MANY useful skills during the internship, such as how to make a hole between a person's ribs and insert a chest tube to reexpand a collapsed lung, and how to thread a catheter through the jugular vein into the heart to monitor pressure and give fluids. I learned how to manage a heart attack so as to minimize damage to the heart muscle, and how to use a defibrillator to restart one that had stopped beating. I learned how to patch up people shattered in car wrecks, and how to manage bullet wounds to the chest.

Lifesaving techniques such as these are among the glories of scientific medicine. Modern methods of managing trauma are largely without parallel in traditional medicines (as, of course, are some of the modern trauma associated with automatic weapons and car accidents). Our techniques are certainly powerful, and when you master them, you feel powerful yourself. It wasn't hard to see how a surgeon like Dr. Floyd could become intoxicated with the feeling of power, deciding it originated from him, not from the interventions he had learned. It was also easy to see the inhumane result of this delusion. We never did learn what Mrs. Hannah's problem was. She was still living on tubes and IVs on my last day of internal medicine.

As bad as doctors can be at helping people approach the end of their lives, my next rotation, in obstetrics, showed how much worse we often are at helping lives begin. In rural Kentucky, birth had been a reasonably normal process that sometimes took place at home. My mother was born at home, although she would have been better off at the hospital. Hazel was poorly nourished, and she delivered early—my mother weighed only two pounds, two ounces at birth. The local doctor came to the house and sadly informed Hazel that my mother would not live, but Hazel would not accept that prognosis. To keep her warm, Hazel placed the baby in a shoebox on the kitchen stove. Every day the doctor came to the kitchen door and entered the house warily, dreading what he would find, and every day he found a baby who was a little larger, a little more robust, a little more ready for life. Eventually the doctor stopped coming around, a tacit acknowledgment that my grandmother—not he—was the expert on the subject of this particular baby. Hazel told me proudly that the doctor hadn't charged her a thing. After all, he told her, she had ended up teaching him a thing or two.

The obstetrics culture at Lutheran was structured instead around the belief that mothers only get in the way of the birthing process. Dr. Jason, a six-foot-six-inch giant with a thick, Ulysses S. Grant beard, was the embodiment of the idea. The nurses on the OB floor said the sound of Dr. Jason's heavy footsteps coming down the hall had scared more than one mother into pushing out her baby. Dr. Jason was generally considered to be Lutheran's expert on labor and delivery. His only serious competition was Dr. Poirot, a short, wiry man with a neatly trimmed beard the color of rusted nails. Like Jason, Poirot was in his mid-forties. He made up for being physically unimposing by being the fastest-moving obstetrician east of the Mississippi. The nurses had a prize set aside for anyone—patient or staff—who could keep Poirot in conversation for more than thirty seconds. It was still unclaimed when I left Wisconsin.

I'd already published two articles on home and midwife-assisted births, and I had come east to Lutheran with a third, this one study unfinished. To complete it I needed a large pool of hospital births as a data set to compare to my California home birth figures, matching women from one set to women in the other by age, pregnancy risk status, number of prior pregnancies and deliveries, and socioeconomic status. I started exploring the birth records from Lutheran to find the data I needed. Finding appropriate matches would take a good long time, and I already had too much to do, but interns were encouraged to do research and the records were available. Fearing criticism of the time-consuming task, I didn't talk much about my study. I did talk fervently about the benefits of home birth—and when the obstetricians heard secondhand about that, I had one strike against me. When they learned I was also meeting informally with the local midwives, I was two strikes down, before many of them had even met me.

Most of the obstetricians at Lutheran viewed midwives as the enemy. The official stance hadn't changed much since the Flexner Report of 1905, which characterized midwives as dirty, ignorant immigrants. My superiors let me know in no uncertain terms that I should not be promoting childbirth outside the confines of the hospital. Too zealous to listen, I countered their arguments with studies from around the globe on the benefits of midwives and home birth. Doctors' opinions would be swayed by the most current research, I naïvely thought. My opinions drew the sharpest criticism from Dr. Jason. His forbidding demeanor kept me from asking him about the Cesareans he routinely performed for reasons that seemed mostly to relate to his own convenience.

Like many doctors in 1975, Jason held his patients to Freedman's curve, which tells how many centimeters per hour the cervix dilates in a "normal" labor. Today, more than twenty years later, some doctors (and even some midwives) still impose the infamous curve on their patients, ignoring the fact that the curve is an average: by definition, most patients will labor either faster or slower than the average (just as only 3 percent of women deliver on their due date). Jason was of the opinion that all *his* patients should progress *faster* than Freedman's curve. He punished slow mothers either with intravenous drips of Pitocin, a hormone used to strengthen contractions and speed up labor, or Cesarean sections. Poirot agreed with him that the only good labor was a fast labor.

They actually had arguments about how much time in labor was "permissible" for a baby. This was the justification for whatever they thought or did, that it was good for the baby, whether or not the available scientific evidence contradicted their positions. More important than how much time the woman spent in labor was how much time the doctor spent at the hospital. Hours wasted with a laboring mother meant hours, and money, lost seeing patients. Both doctors had reputations for giving women Cesareans at dawn so they would be able to keep morning office hours. (A 1988 study in the *New England Journal of Medicine* proved that Jason and Poirot weren't alone in doing this.)

I counted their Cesareans in the OB log book. Jason's rate was 48 percent, a close second to Poirot's 49 percent, both well above the hospital rate of 13 percent. At the time, the national rate was well under 10 percent; it has since risen to about 25 percent. Today, as in 1975, doctors are encouraged to do Cesareans rather than avoid them. Although even the Centers for Disease Control agree with natural childbirth advocates that 25 percent is far too high a rate, in practice doctors are rarely faulted for doing one unnecessarily. It is safer, from a malpractice point of view, to lose a baby or a mother to a Cesarean (since you appear to have done everything possible) than to choose not to do one, even though the mother is much more likely to die from the operation than from any other kind of delivery. It is hardly surprising that many obstetricians now take a "better safe than sue-able" approach.

One cold October morning at 6 A.M., well before dawn, I came for my twenty-four-hour shift on the obstetrics floor and found the night nurses preparing for *two* sections. Jason was to perform one, Poirot the other. Both of the women had been admitted during the night. Neither had been laboring particularly long, and neither's baby was in distress, but for Jason and Poirot, it was a simple decision. Dawn was approaching, dilation was incomplete, office hours would arrive before babies— hence the Cesareans.

Inside I was fuming, but I had already tried rational discourse. I had spoken to Jason of the evidence against routine Cesareans that I had collected at the Stanford Medical Library. I had given Jason papers that he would never bother to read, and received only his scorn in return. Well, not only scorn—he also made a few nasty comments about me to the residency director. This translated to "Mess with me, and I'll give you more trouble than you can handle." So I held my tongue, watching him endlessly repeat a practice I considered *mal*practice, as I still do.

Since Jason and Poirot shared identical views on obstetrics, they had to cultivate other ways to compete. On that morning, while scrubbing for surgery, they hit on wagering $100 to see who could do the faster Cesarean. An operating room nurse was assigned to time each surgery, beginning with the incision and ending with the last suture. It was my fate to be on Dr. Jason's team, operating on a Mrs. Atkins. I wanted to run away and hide. I couldn't believe that this was happening. This was just about as bad as the time I witnessed one of the Stanford OBs give a woman an episiotomy *after* she delivered, so as not to deprive her husband of the pleasure of a tightened-up vagina.

I finished scrubbing my hands and backed through the OR door with water dripping off my elbows. The nurses were busy prepping and draping Mrs. Atkins. The anesthesiologist applied the mask. Blue-suited, masked nurses were moving throughout the room, deftly skirting the sterile areas as they set the stage for this great contest.

"Give her a general," Jason roared, looming over Mrs. Atkins, flexing his fingers. "And do it quick. You hear me? Now!" he shouted. "Now!" He frightened the anesthesiologist into a crash induction. Regional anesthesia would have left the mother conscious and better able to bond with her baby, but general anesthesia is quicker, and there was money at stake. The anesthesiologist turned up the halothane anesthetic and added barbiturates to the woman's IV. "Start the clock," Jason said with relish, shaking his scalpel at the timekeeping nurse. "I'm cutting the skin." The mother jumped and let out a scream. "Put her out, damn you!" Jason shouted at the anesthesiologist. "She's not gonna remember anything anyway."

I heard the anesthesiologist muttering under his mask, "Screw this whole fucking place," pressing ahead anyway with his crash induction. He verbalized my feelings of nausea and disgust as Jason plunged ahead. "Clamp," he called, having already opened the woman down to her bladder. I sighed and redirected my attention to the work. He was ready for me to retract the bladder so he could cut down to the uterus.

Assisting at other Cesareans, I had opened the uterus, removed either the baby or the placenta, or closed the incisions. But this was my first time helping Jason, and he quickly decided that the most helpful thing I could do was to stay out of his way. I was happy to step aside. In a frenzy, Jason cut the baby out, passed it to the pediatrician, tore the placenta off the uterine wall, and set about sewing up Mrs. Atkins's uterus almost before the baby had drawn its first breath. Finishing off the last suture, he tossed his needle holder and tissue forceps onto a stainless steel tray and raised his hands like a rodeo cowboy who has just tied up a calf.

"Seventeen minutes!" proclaimed the timekeeper. "It's a new record for a Cesarean."

"That should be good enough to beat Poirot!" Jason said gleefully. And it was. Poirot had encountered numerous minor difficulties that he wouldn't discuss afterward in the locker room, except to complain that his patient's tissue was unfairly crappy for a woman of twenty-four. His operation had extended well over twenty minutes. Poirot paid up his $100 and left without changing. Of course, both men had made far more than $100 in the OR that day. While the cash exchanged in the bet was a pittance, it was a powerful symbol of supremacy. Jason sat at least another seventeen minutes in front of his locker, bragging to anyone who would listen about his new record, counting and recounting his twenties. He speculated that his new record might be a standard that would last "as long as the game is played. I'm the Babe Ruth of obstetrics," he crowed, "the Mickey Mantle of the OR."

FATHER MAHONEY approached me that afternoon in the cafeteria as I was struggling to eat some lunch. "She died last night," he said quietly. I looked up at him stunned. I had been miles away from Mrs. Hannah, caught up in the miseries of Jason's brutal wager. Then, as I really heard Father Mahoney's words, the sadness sank deep into me. I hadn't been to see her for several weeks; I felt ashamed that her death had come and gone, unnoticed by me.

"She was grateful for her suffering to end," Father Mahoney said. "And she was grateful for your help and your visits."

I looked down at the floor, not wanting to acknowledge how quickly the problems of obstetrics had taken over my attention. "I haven't seen her in ages," I stammered.

"I know," Father Mahoney said gently. "She knew how busy you were, once you moved on to obstetrics."

"But I shouldn't have forgotten her."

"You didn't forget her," Father Mahoney said. "And she'll never forget you. She told me to tell you that, and to tell you that she would be sure to commend you to the angels and the saints."

"Then she died well?"

"As well as she could."

"You were there?" I asked hopefully. As if his presence would make up for my absence.

"I was there," he said, nodding, "and she's finally at peace, as she wished." He put his hand on my shoulder. "Don't be afraid to come see me just because you're not Catholic. These moments of people dying and being born, taking their first breaths and last breaths—these determine what kind of doctor you'll be. You have the makings of a good doctor, so long as you don't let your training destroy the depth of your feelings."

My name was being broadcast over and over on the loudspeaker; I didn't know how long that had gone on, but just then we both became aware of it. "I know you have to answer that page, so I'll be going." Father Mahoney rose, patted my hand, and left. I ran to the phone.

"Dr. Mehl? This is Linda, the charge nurse. It's Mrs. Atkins. She hasn't put out any urine through her Foley since she returned from the OR."

"I'll be right there." I walked the hundred yards to the postpartum ward, wondering what I would find. Some nurses make mistakes, forgetting, for instance, to unclamp the tube. But Linda sounded both experienced and worried. When I saw her, I placed her—she'd been pointed out to me before by an appreciative intern. She was about my mother's age, and she took pleasure in looking after the residents. She handed me Mrs. Atkins's chart from the rack at the nurses' station as we walked toward her room.

Mrs. Atkins's urine-collection bag was genuinely empty, and the clamp was genuinely loose. Since there was nothing restricting the flow of urine from the bladder to the bag, one of two things had gone wrong. Either her kidneys had stopped working and she was in renal failure— or Dr. Jason had managed to tie off both ureters as he was sewing up his incision (ureters are the tubes that connect kidneys to bladder). Given the speed of the morning's operation, I assumed the latter had happened. I checked our new mother's vital signs on the nurse's chart and found no indication of shock. "Did she ever—"

"No indication of kidney problems before her surgery, Doctor," Linda answered, anticipating my question. While we still had to rule out acute tubular necrosis as a cause of the kidney failure, both Linda and I knew the likeliest answer.

"Am I the poor jerk who has to call Dr. Jason and tell him what he's done?"

"Better you than me," she replied with a laugh, "since he's been known to shoot the messenger when he doesn't like the message."

This, from a doctor supposedly dedicated to *Primum non nocere*— "Above all, do no harm"! This internship was going to drive me into therapy, I thought to myself, where at least I'd have somewhere to voice all the shameful secrets I was having to keep. I wished I had the courage to confront Jason. But I wanted to finish the internship, so I bit my tongue and prepared for the onslaught of the good doctor's rage.

I had to beg, then demand that his receptionist interrupt his office hours. She finally fetched him after warning me severely that he would not be happy, and that I'd better be really sure that this was important. "Tell him it's about Mrs. Atkins. He gave her a Cesarean this morning," I said, "and she's not putting out any urine."

"Who?" Dr. Jason asked when he got on the line.

"Mrs. Atkins," I repeated.

I imagined Dr. Jason shaking uncontrollably with rage, sitting behind a big desk in the conference room of his office, his face fire-engine red. He was silent, however.

"Your record-breaking Cesarean," I reminded him. *My* cheeks were flushed, if his weren't.

"Oh, shit," Dr. Jason said, in his panic forgetting to berate me. "Get an IVP," he said, "stat." IVP stands for intravenous pyelogram, a test in which we inject a radio-opaque dye into a vein and then X-ray the abdomen to document the passage of the dye through the kidneys, ureters, and bladder.

Two hours later I was going over the films with the radiologist. He looked at me and back at the films; then he raised his eyebrows. I tried to return his cynical smile, but my mouth felt uncoordinated, tight at the corners. This is a nightmare, I thought to myself as I looked at the films and saw where the ureters were tied. They were ballooning like fat sausages above the ligatures. The calyces of the kidneys were thick and dilated. We were going to have to go back into surgery to undo the damage. Imagining Dr. Jason's apoplectic face, I wished I could just get into my car and go home.

That afternoon, when Dr. Jason's office hours were over, we reopened Mrs. Atkins. This operation took longer than seventeen minutes. Jason, unable to find where he'd tied off the ureters, had to call in a urologist. Jason had obviously recovered from the shock of his mistake, since he ran through his usual repertoire of off-color jokes while we waited. The nurses did a good job laughing and appearing to love his jokes this time as much as they had the last time they'd heard them.

"What's wrong?" asked the urologist, Dr. Richardson, as he entered the OR. Richardson was a quiet man from New Mexico famous for his Stetson hat. In Wisconsin, where standard headgear was a Frank Deere baseball cap, his hat was as unexpected as his cowboy boots.

"Her ureters were accidentally tied off," Dr. Jason said. "And I can't

86 • LEWIS MEHL-MADRONA

find where to untie them." Jason then stepped aside, without ever directly asking the urologist for his help.

"Any idea how this happened?" Richardson asked. I looked away, playing with the hemostat in my hand. Jason's jocular air had vanished. Richardson took Jason's shrug for an answer and went to work. While Jason stood uselessly by, Richardson located and removed the offending sutures. He asked a nurse to check the Foley catheter bag to see if it was now collecting urine. It had already begun to fill, so Richardson nodded his approval and told the nurse to call X-ray to send up a portable machine to make sure the blockage was gone.

"This was Dr. Jason's record-breaking seventeen-minute Cesarean, you know," called out the anesthesiologist. "Do you think we should add *this* surgery onto the seventeen minutes, or—"

"What do we need X-rays for?" Dr. Jason barked, mainly to interrupt the man. "We've got urine."

"Wait a minute," Richardson said, "this was a what?"

"The all-time hospital-record-breaking seventeen-minute section," piped up the anesthesiologist, now fiddling with the gas meters on his machine. "He and Poirot made a bet to see who could get through it the fastest."

"You did *what?*" Richardson hissed at Jason, as if he couldn't believe his ears.

"Just fix the goddamn ureters," Jason boomed, "and there won't be any trouble here." Everyone froze and waited while the portable X-ray machine was rolled into the OR. Then, as the technician moved it into position over Mrs. Atkins, Richardson spoke slowly and deliberately.

"Why don't you just kill the next one? I bet you could do that in ten minutes."

Jason stood tall, all six and a half feet of him shaking with fury; his florid complexion made him look almost psychotic. While this pillar of the Lutheran medical community sputtered and shook, Richardson turned and headed for the door. Pausing at the entrance, he said, "Don't forget to check the X-ray before you close; make sure both ureters are working."

"You're way out of line, Dr. Richardson!" Jason thundered.

"*I'm* out of line?" Richardson said, incredulous.

"You can't come in here and slander other doctors, at least not in *my* OR," Jason shouted, quivering like a volcano set to erupt. Richardson remained calm, which redoubled Jason's rage. "You'll never set foot again in any OR in this hospital," he threatened, moving menacingly away from the operating table and toward Richardson. "I will make your life hell."

"Oh, but you already have," Richardson said softly. "And think of what you've done for hers. Make sure you check her X-ray," he repeated, "and call me back if you need more help."

I broke scrub quickly, tossing my unused gloves into the trash basket. I was not a player in this drama now; Jason, already up to his elbows in Mrs. Atkins, didn't even notice my leaving. I was running after Richardson, the brave man who had stood up to Dr. Jason, wanting to speak to him, to thank him. Having caught up to Richardson, I told him how amazed I was at what he'd said.

The wry comments of the anesthesiologist were one thing—a surgeon will put up with a lot from one, because once you cross an anesthesiologist, all the members of the department may well find themselves too busy to ever assist your operations again, pretty much shutting you down. But Richardson was Jason's colleague. I remembered Vickory declining Upton's challenge back at SMCMC—and those two had been equals. This time, the physician under attack was politically much more powerful than his assailant. In addition to being the chief of obstetrics, Jason was president-elect of the hospital's medical staff.

"Jason is a reckless fool surrounded by reckless fools," Richardson said now, shrugging off my praise. He pulled his scrub top over his head. On went the Western shirt, the bolo tie, the silver belt buckle, and the cowboy boots. He walked over to the coffee machine and poured a steaming cup. He handed the Styrofoam cup to me and poured himself another.

"Still, you were courageous to stand up to him."

"Neither courageous," he said, "nor stupid. I'm quitting my practice here and moving back to New Mexico. Don't even think of crossing a man like Jason unless you have somewhere else to go. I sympathize, though. Interns eat and swallow shit. That's the nature of the beast."

"But he shouldn't be allowed to get away with this, should he?"

"I wouldn't recommend your making any trouble," Richardson warned. He opened the door to the corridor and disappeared.

I bent my face over the coffee's steam, thinking how out of character it was for an attending to offer an intern coffee. When I left the room, the sun was setting over the Wisconsin marshes. By now more patients would be waiting to be examined in Labor and Delivery. I had another twelve hours left on my shift, and I had to make the best of it. Richardson was right; I wasn't in a position to say anything. I opened the swinging doors to L & D and marched inside.

One week later Mrs. Atkins left the hospital with a healthy baby. No one ever complained about her seventeen-minute Cesarean. No malpractice lawyers ever subpoenaed records. She probably had her next baby with Dr. Jason. Over the years I've learned that doctors rarely get sued—no matter how bad a job they do—as long as they manage to send the patient home healthy. I knew some doctors at Lutheran who *were* being sued, and ironically most of them had done a very good job with patients whose bad luck it was to have illnesses we didn't (and don't) really know how to treat. Malpractice suits usually stem from bad outcomes rather than bad doctoring. Mrs. Atkins should have been furious with us. As it was, she actually sent us a letter thanking us for the good care she received, and for finding a specialist who could fix her so quickly when complications set in.

I HAD ONE private ritual I never tired of during those years in Wisconsin. It was one I shared with my young daughter. I would bundle her up, strap her into her carrier, and walk around the block with her. The walk was no small undertaking. Given the farm country where we lived, our block was five miles around.

These walks gave me a good two hours alone with my child, and gave me also her innocent, delighted reactions to the farms and woods our promenade took us past. In cold weather—and in Wisconsin the weather was cold more often than not—I bundled my daughter up until she seemed more a ball of yarn than a child. In very cold weather we would stop in a local-yokel's bar three quarters of the way home. The place was called the Deerfield Tavern, and I would always order a cup of hot chocolate for the two of us to share. After warming up we'd continue on home.

I used to meet my friend Alex at the Deerfield. Alex was a psychiatry resident at the university's hospital who lived on a farm near mine. We had met by chance at the tavern's Friday night fish fry. The Scandinavians thereabouts liked to take some fish, let them go a little off, then fry 'em up. To them it was a delicacy. Alex had more of a taste for the rotten fish than I did, but the beers were cheap, and the pool table was pretty much ours for the taking, so we continued meeting at the Deerfield to unwind. After Mrs. Atkins's Cesarean I told Alex this latest horror story.

"Wow, I can see why you'd be upset," Alex said, leaning over to line up his shot. "I mean, once you opened her up the second time, you had to forfeit the record. When are you ever gonna get close to seventeen minutes again?"

I laughed at Alex's misrepresentation of my distress. He was doing it intentionally, to get me to loosen up. "Really though, this is nothing to laugh about," I told him. "How can I just stand by and let this happen?"

"You take this shit way too seriously. You'll never survive internship if you get so upset over every abuse of power you come across. Can't you just do what you're told and forget about it?"

"Be a good German and ignore the plight of the Jews? Drive the truck to the concentration camp and forget about where it's going?"

"Ouch." He stood up, frowning, without taking his shot. "Lewis, there's no comparison."

"That's what it feels like to me. That's what I want you to understand."

"For you this little obstetrical drama is as bad as the gas chambers."

"Or the genocide my people suffered from the smallpox-infested blankets the U.S. Cavalry gave them," I said.

Alex looked more closely at me. Then he leaned over the table and took his shot. He missed, scratching the cue ball into the side pocket.

"Nice shot," I said.

"Thanks." Alex grinned sheepishly and stood up. His expression grew more serious. "I'm sorry. I didn't realize how much this upset you. You have every right to be just as angry as you want to be."

"Now the other interns are starting to complain to me. One guy said, 'This missionary zeal of yours makes it harder on the rest of us. We've all been labeled troublemakers because of you. Can't you just shut up and let us finish this damn internship in peace?' "

"And does this surprise you?" Alex said in a Viennese accent, mimicking his analysis of our conversation. I laughed as I recognized his Freud imitation. But I appreciated being able to talk out some of my conflicts with Alex. And he had his own problems from his psychiatry residency to share with me.

My wife was less helpful to talk to (another thing Alex and I often discussed). She was as busy as I was, caring for our daughter and preparing for her own career as a psychologist. Her observations seemed to me to be perceptive but rarely offered with much sympathy. Ellen was understandably upset by how much time I had to spend at the hospital. Doing two internships at once was proving harder than I had anticipated, since both departments were pressing me to spend extra hours in their service. To unwind, aside from spending a couple of hours once a weekend at the Deerfield, I escaped to my books on Native American peoples and their traditions.

I think Ellen was surprised at the way the interest I took had developed from a little exploratory reading into a consuming passion. My personality when I was seventeen, when I met and wed Ellen, probably gave little indication that I would come to study my heritage so seriously. I had been somewhat oblivious to the value of my past when we met, though I had been proud to be part Native American, and had taken Ellen to a Thanksgiving Day demonstration at Plymouth Rock. We still laugh about the ruddy-faced Irish cop who hollered at us to get back on the boat and go back where we came from.

Alex lent me a friendly ear, listening with great interest to my stories of the healing ceremonies I'd witnessed in Wyoming and California. He was also a half-breed of a sort: half Mexican and half Jewish. His unusual heritage always guaranteed a unique perspective. He had mystified his classmates in medical school by choosing to live in a trailer on a dry wash outside of Tucson. He was as interested in farming as psychiatry, so he understood my own extracurricular pursuits. He was among the few people I spoke to of my desire to find a shaman to study with, and among the even fewer number who did not find my desire absurd.

MY ONE MORNING a week at the family practice clinic was a disappointment. While many of the staff physicians did differ philosophically from mechanical doctors like Jason and Poirot, they didn't practice very differently. They didn't have the time or the knowledge to take the holistic approach they espoused. What doctors do most in America—and what the doctors did at the clinic—is write prescriptions. They do not practice hypnosis or arrange healing ceremonies. Even psychotherapy or behavior therapy is too far out for most doctors, regardless of the impact that studies have shown these treatments can have on a patient's health.

The Wisconsin management experts had decreed that residents should see four patients an hour. At first, no one was terribly concerned when I didn't meet my quota. Still, it was expected that I would come up to speed as time went on, and Dr. Barbour, the clinic director, began to hint that I should see more patients. He told me I spent too much time with people; I was too interested in their psychology. "You'll never make a living working like this," he said, "so get used to it now."

The logic was simple and unassailable: More patients meant more procedures. More procedures meant more billing. More billing meant a solid economic foundation—the kind of foundation we needed to sustain our clinic. One spinal tap, at $250, equaled two hours' worth of office visits. Only by doing such procedures, the argument went, could we afford to practice the kind of medicine we wanted—but the truth was that we were too busy doing procedures even to try another kind of medicine. We were locked into our assembly-line approach, ordering endless diagnostic tests, scribbling prescriptions, and hurrying off to the next appointment. Although this hectic routine made many of my fellow residents feel important, it depressed me. I wanted to practice my idea of good medicine and chafed against any restrictions on my developing personal style. I wanted to discover, develop, and deepen the qualities that were uniquely mine.

Despite my lifelong insecurities, I have always believed I have a mission on earth. I have lost my way often enough. I have suffered from low self-esteem, but I believed, even as an intern, that I had something to offer, something that drove my urge to become a doctor. I believed spirituality could soften and humanize medicine. I saw Native American spirituality as a tradition I might be able to partake in and then share with others. Other spiritual disciplines also have much to offer, of course, but they have less to do with me.

I was too driven by my sense of destiny to see merit in any accountant's argument. I believed that doctors must transcend business concerns to minister to the sick, and I paid no attention to our practice management lectures. But nearly all our billings were paid by insurance, and health insurance was and is designed primarily to cover procedures and short office visits. (There have been some efforts to change this, but the business of medicine remains procedure-driven and discourages longer appointments and counseling time. Now, the experts actually encourage doctors to do as *little* as possible for each patient they see— they call it managed care.) Luckily, although I didn't always accept the counsel of Dr. Barbour, not all patients need or want healing, and some need procedures, so I still managed to get enough accomplished to meet the requirements of my residency.

Then there were patients for whom I developed a more personalized course of treatment. One of these early patients was Doug, a forty-year-old psychologist who lived outside town with his pregnant wife, Lisa, a stewardess for Eastern Airlines. I met them at a potluck dinner sponsored by the group of home birth midwives I was informally advising. Doug stood out because there were so few Hispanics in Wisconsin. Doug and I talked over the tabouli bowl about his ulcerative colitis, a puzzling and painful digestive disorder that involves inflammation of the colon's mucous membranes, resulting in chronic diarrhea and lower abdominal pain. Doug's doctors had prescribed steroid enemas and a drug called azulfidine, then the standard therapy. These measures provided minimal relief and not-so-minimal side effects. Doug was desperate to find an alternative therapy, so I offered to see him at the family practice clinic. He called the next morning for an appointment.

Doug's history and physical took more than an hour. Extravagant as that was, I managed to clear out another hour to learn more about the events that preceded his colitis. I soon discovered that, like many of us, Doug was a living contradiction. He found it much more difficult to relax than I had imagined he would. At social events and meetings of the local home birth support group, he seemed a pretty laid-back fellow, but when I talked to him in the office he whined and complained, angry that he was sick, nervous, and anxious, angry too that he had to work so hard to support Lisa.

His public mask was of a hip and enlightened therapist. Privately he was rigid and stubborn—"uptight," in the jargon of the time. The conflict between who he was and who he wanted to be was embodied in his work as a therapist. Although he lived in his mind and found emotions difficult, he practiced his own unique kind of therapy which pushed his clients to get in touch with their feelings and to powerfully express them. He had studied in California with Stan Grof and had built on that foundation in developing his own personal style.

Not long before Doug became sick, one of his clients appeared after hours on the front steps of Doug's office near the State Capitol. The man pinned a note to his shirt, put a gun to his temple, and shot himself. In the note, removed later from his body, the man laid his death at Doug's feet, because Doug hadn't helped him enough. He wrote that his tears were melting him; his pain was turning him into a gaseous substance. He wanted to die while there was enough of him left still solid enough to kill.

The suicide was big news. Doug began to suspect everyone he knew of talking about him and his failure behind his back. His colleagues and his wife assured him he was not to blame for the suicide, but Doug felt responsible. He accused those who said differently of patronizing him. He wanted to quit seeing clients but felt trapped in his job, as he was not qualified to do anything else. He was relieved in a way to develop colitis, as it gave him a physical (and therefore legitimate) reason to stay home from work. He was slowly withdrawing from life, riddled with doubt, and sinking deeper into debt.

For a while, Lisa had picked up the slack in their finances by increasing her flight schedule, allowing Doug to spend most of his time at home caring for his illness. Now, Doug told me, Lisa's pregnancy was disrupting that arrangement. She wanted to cut back her hours and was asking Doug to work more. He felt his colitis made this impossible. Although she tried to be sympathetic, Lisa was beginning to resent Doug's illness. It was Lisa, Doug reported bitterly, who had pushed him into taking drugs so that he could "function better"—her euphemism for returning full-time to the job he now hated.

I kept scheduling Doug for one-hour meetings, knowing that his colitis was worsened by emotional factors. Dr. Barbour believed in the relationship between mind and body, and agreed that there probably was "an emotional component" to Doug's illness, but wasn't very hopeful that we could use that knowledge to help Doug. "Send him to a psychiatrist if he needs that kind of help, but don't tie up valuable clinic time," he told me. "You have a tendency to try to do the impossible." When I persisted, he shrugged and agreed to let me continue seeing Doug, whom he thereafter referred to dryly as my "healing project."

"Thank you. You won't regret it," I promised.

I began treatments with a combination of acupuncture and hypnosis. "Where did you learn acupuncture?" Doug asked, yawning on the office exam table while several small, thirty-gauge needles were sticking out of his skin. Acupuncture made him sleepy. I inserted the last needle.

"I took a six-week elective in acupuncture during medical school. Then I did acupuncture one morning each week at Stanford's general medical clinic for the next year."

"Funny you thinking Wisconsin would be more progressive and liberal than California," Doug added thoughtfully, "since I made the same mistake before you. I should never have left south Florida. I should've stayed in Coral Gables or moved north to Palm Beach. Of course then I could never write my book about killing dairy farmers with primal therapy. Hey, you should write a book—*Hypnosis and Bucky Badger,*" he joked, referring to the local university's omnipresent mascot.

"Maybe we ought to get you well before we write any books."

I wasn't sure acupuncture would work for Doug. I was casting about for something that might shift Doug's awareness, but lacking both knowledge and experience, I didn't have a firm therapeutic plan. My only certainty was that with personalized care Doug would improve. And we did slowly wean him off his medications. Progress was slow, but it encouraged Dr. Barbour. He was the one who had made it possible for me to practice acupuncture in the clinic. Although he didn't believe acupuncture worked, except by the placebo effect, he valued his trainees' independence and was willing to let them try new things.

While Doug thought of himself as being in touch with his feelings, I was getting to know the control-freak side of him. In my developing understanding of healing and psychotherapy, I was beginning to see how Doug's rigidity, fear, and stubbornness were slowing our progress. Doug genuinely wanted everyone to be happy, but he wanted to be the one to *make* them happy. His patient's suicide had demonstrated how little control he actually had.

Back then, I couldn't understand why Doug insisted on feeling responsible for the suicide. Now that I know more about psychotherapeutic options, I think Doug's style of therapy was probably not the best choice for the patient in question, and may well have made him worse.

Doug had probably been fighting with the patient for control of their sessions. Otherwise, why would the man have left this world with such a big "fuck you," shooting himself on the steps of Doug's building? Doug may also have minimized the psychotic nature of his client's troubles. No one would ever know whether the man's suicide note was metaphorical or a reflection of what he saw as concrete reality.

Doug's colitis was his body's way of synthesizing these raging internal conflicts. Working with him taught me how sickness can proceed on several levels at once. I could measure biomedically what was going wrong. I could tell from talking to Doug the tremendous emotional conflicts he was going through. I knew his relationships were off-kilter, from brief conversations with Lisa. At every level, the physical, the mental, and the interpersonal, the man was ill.

In some ways Doug's illness was helpful, even restorative and nurturing. It ameliorated his feelings of blame and guilt by moving the theater for their expression inside his own body. Each level's complaint was also an offer, a key. The problem was, I wasn't sure where to look for the locks that corresponded; that was beyond my ability at the time. It would have been futile to just *tell* Doug that he had the power to heal himself. In fact, he didn't—not until his awareness somehow changed. He couldn't be anything but who he was. And for now, he was most comfortable being sick.

Doug could have found power in recognizing how little power he had. Doug would have loved such a Zen-like conception. He would have turned the idea over and over in his mind, considering its endless possibilities. But the message would never have made him jump, never moved him forward like spurs catching a horse's flank, never reached the hidden caverns of his heart.

So we kept up the acupuncture and hypnosis, and his intestines healed slowly. He made little or no progress toward exorcising his client's ghost or adjusting his picture of himself as a failed therapist. Somehow we needed to find a way to engage Doug more fundamentally than I was able to do.

"I FOUND him for you."

It was Alex calling me, in the middle of one of my endless obstetrics shifts. "Found who? What time is it?"

"Ten P.M. human time. Your shaman. This old farmer told me about this crazy Indian hereabouts. Named Paul. This farmer never trusted him, until Paul healed his daughter. Wanna meet him?"

Because Alex fancied himself a farmer, he'd drive all the way to Sun Prairie or Blue Mound when he heard a tractor was on sale, then spend his time chatting with the farmer who owned it, since the tractor always cost more than he could pay. Or almost always. He did finally locate an affordable tractor, but unconsciously he made sure it was so broken down that he would have to spend all his time chatting with farmers about how to get it running again. He never actually got his tractor to work often enough to justify his time and money, but he did get it painted the correct, impeccable Frank Deere green. And he also managed to get himself covered with the same sweet and wretched scents of hay and manure as his farmer buddies.

It was on a visit to Black Earth, looking for parts, that Alex heard about Paul. "I can take you to meet him," he offered again.

"But *you* haven't met him yet," I protested. Alex's perpetual optimism worked to balance my gloomier disposition. He bumbled into all kinds of crazy situations and could always talk his way back out of them.

One week later we were in Alex's truck, wobbling our way toward Black Earth. Every few miles Alex glanced at his scribbled directions. "Turn north two miles, then west four miles to the end of the road," he muttered. The end of the road was strewn with the wreckage of derelict farm machinery; some of it could have fetched a good price from an antique dealer. Paul's rambling old farmhouse sat a few hundred yards from the rusted machines. There were fields of corn on one side of the house, a forest and stream on the other.

"You know, Lewis," Alex whispered conspiratorially, "Paul uses peyote in his ceremonies." A flock of Canadian geese was flying south. We watched the V-shaped formation pass overhead until it was as small as a speck in the sky. "Let's see if this old coot's at home." Alex turned off his engine.

"You mean you didn't check to see?"

"He said he was going to be. But you never know with these medicine men. Maybe he's disappeared and we'll have to find him. You know, stalk him through the woods."

"You've been reading too many adventure books." But come to think of it, the front of the house did have an unwelcoming face. Alex hesitated, undecided as to how to approach. As we sat, the door of the house opened and a man strode out toward us. "At least he didn't disappear on us," I said to Alex, opening my door and hopping out of the truck.

Slowly we walked toward the man, who had crossed the soft black dirt of his front yard to stand before us. It was Paul, but his face was friendly and he was chubby—hardly the formidable, stony-faced, hardened mystic I was expecting.

I was to spend many days with Paul. He was a Chippewa medicine man who practiced the peyote religion. Later I discovered that Paul's version of the peyote religion was a highly idiosyncratic blend, concocted by merging ancient Chippewa beliefs with elements of the newer tradition of the Native American Church. This latter is itself a hybrid, of Christianity and Native American spirituality. Members of the church sing their songs in Cheyenne and follow very specific rituals and procedures—many of which Paul altered to suit his own purposes. But though Paul drew as he saw fit from any tradition he encountered, he had a reputation for healing people. And he was willing to teach Alex and me what he knew.

Although I wasn't comfortable with using hallucinogens for healing, I was intrigued with Paul and his talk about peyote's medicinal powers. Alex said he had heard people came from all over Wisconsin for Paul's healing ceremonies and the herbs he administered. Paul confirmed this, warning us about peyote.

"Peyote is like a wild animal," Paul said. "It doesn't attack you, but it approaches from a distance and observes you without showing itself. The more you drink, the more it trusts you, and the more it trusts you, the more it is willing to draw near and show you its secrets."

I asked Paul what the secrets were, but he said he couldn't tell me. "Why not?" I asked.

"Words fail when you try to talk about peyote's secrets," he said. "Anything you say sounds simple-minded."

"Why?" I asked. "What is there that you can't say with words?"

Paul laughed. "Think about that question a minute," he suggested.

I still didn't like the thought of using mind-altering drugs, and I was especially reluctant to let a wild animal loose inside my head. Still, I wanted to learn what Paul knew, so two weeks later, with a harvest moon swollen against the sky, I tried his peyote paste during a tipi ceremony. It tasted terrible and I ate only a little, so maybe it knew I didn't trust it. At any rate, it apparently didn't trust me, because all it did was make me sick. For a while I thought the only thing that was going to be revealed was my dinner. In the end I kept it down, although a number of the other supplicants didn't fare as well. I wasn't exactly inspired by a drug when the best I could say about it was "It didn't make me throw up."

As the ceremony was winding down, Paul assured me that there was more to learn from peyote. I would experience its secrets the next time if I would only take more medicine. "You must trust that you will get what you need, when you ask for it sincerely. I have a story for you." He settled down and bade me sit beside him. Alex, curious, came over to join us.

There was a time when the people were starving. Two young men were out hunting, but day followed day and they never found a thing.

Then one day they saw a beautiful woman in a white dress standing before them. One of the men knew right away this was a sacred being and fell on his knees before her in the snow. The other man had bad thoughts in his heart and started running toward her. He figured that since they were out here alone and no one would know, he could have his way with her. His friend yelled at him to stop because any fool would know that a mortal woman doesn't suddenly appear in the middle of nowhere in a beautiful white dress, but the man wouldn't listen. Just before he reached her, she held out her hand. A cloud appeared and enclosed the man, and his bones fell to the ground with only his tattered clothes around them. His friend was frightened, naturally, and started slowly moving backward.

"Stop," called out the young woman. "Your heart is pure and your intentions are good. You have nothing to fear. Go home and tell your people that I will come tomorrow and they should prepare a feast with their last remaining food. I will bring them what they need so that they will never go hungry again."

Out of respect, the man did not answer her but did just as he was told. The people of his village listened with some fear, for he brought with him the bones of his friend. They worried about using up all their stores of food but decided they had no choice, and went about preparing a feast.

The next morning, the woman walked into the village and into the lodge of the leader. She spoke with the elders of the tribe for quite some time, and when they emerged, a pact had been reached. The oldest of the elders carried a bundle.

The woman spoke. "I have brought you a gift from the Creator so you will never go hungry again. It is the Sacred Pipe. The stem comes from a buffalo bone. The bowl is the blood of the earth, which has been made into stone. When you put the two together and place the tobacco inside and pray in the manner I have shown your elders, then the Creator will hear you and your prayers will be answered."

The woman walked out of the village and turned around four times sunwise. A cloud descended over her. When the cloud lifted, there stood a white buffalo calf who ran off in the snow. The villagers feasted all day in her honor.

"People don't just get everything they ask for," I protested.

"Don't they? What about your friend, the one with the ulcers. Isn't that exactly what he asked for?"

"Well, what if I asked for a million dollars," Alex joked. "Would I get that?"

"Is that what you want?" Paul asked his simple question in such a penetrating fashion that Alex stopped kidding and started thinking.

"*I* want to learn to be a healer," I said, still trying to pursue what I was interested in. "Do you think I have it in me?"

Paul looked at me a moment. There was a warmth in his eyes and a compassion in his manner that I had noticed before in the company of Archie and Nelson. Then Paul answered, with a healer's gentle sincerity, "Why are you asking me? Am I the expert? What do you think?"

"He's already a healer," Alex offered. "If an insecure one."

"Healing is messy and confusing. Look at the births you are witnessing, Lewis—healing is like that. There is commotion. Disorder. Mess. But from this chaos comes new life, new being. A new spirit and body are thrust into the world. Before you can become a healer, you must make friends with chaos. Next time, try the peyote."

I was no longer expecting to find any holistic thinkers at Lutheran or the family practice clinic. But at least the winter was the only thing harsh about life in Madison, where urban problems seemed almost not to exist. Driving into town during the frigid winter mornings, I felt pretty good about where I was and what I was doing. As an intern, I might be ordered to run unnecessary procedures, but the time at Lutheran was passing, if not passing smoothly. And whatever my problems with the institutional medical machine, I had found a healer who was beginning to teach me a kind of medicine I wasn't ever going to learn in a hospital.

CHAPTER FOUR

Healing Stories

ONE NIGHT after Doug had been in my care for several months, a new opportunity presented itself. It took the form such opportunities often take—a health crisis. Doug had a seizure. It was a spontaneous complication of his colitis. The only physical finding we had was the presence of a blood clot in his arm, which caused it to swell up and throb painfully. I saw him that night in the emergency room at Lutheran and diagnosed two potentially serious conditions: thrombophlebitis (inflammation of a vein in conjunction with a blood clot) and cellulitis (an infection of the skin). I called my attending and we admitted Doug for intravenous antibiotics, heparin, and Dilantin to prevent any further seizures. At midnight, when the IV was in place and his drugs were running, I pulled up a chair and sat next to his bed.

The hospital was as quiet and as close to dark as hospitals ever get. Those few minutes we sat in silence, Doug looked dazed, weak, and pitiful. The medications would serve to relieve the swelling and redness in his arm, but I was frustrated that his colitis wasn't responding better to treatment. As long as his bowels were in rebellion, one thing after another could go wrong, and sooner or later it would be something I wouldn't know how to treat.

Doug lay so still I thought he might have drifted off to sleep, but after a while he sighed and said, "It's back to drugs." He sounded miserable, as if he had failed some important test. The veins on his neck stood out like gnarled tree trunks. His face was distorted, his nose flattened, his mouth and cheeks twisted into a hideous, agonizing leer.

"For a while," I told him. "But not forever." I was learning from Paul that a healer must maintain a vision of a healthy future for the client—especially when nobody else can or will. Doug's muscles bunched and quivered, and his legs and arms shook sometimes, making me fear that he might have another seizure. "The antibiotics will stop the cellulitis, and the heparin will dissolve any new blood clots and prevent the one you have from moving to your lungs or heart," I said with more confidence than I felt.

"Which will keep me alive long enough for something else awful to happen," Doug said, over the sound of his beeping IV pumps. "I'm whining. I'm sorry." The skin on his arms was pale and so taut it almost seemed his muscles or bones would break through it. The reddened patches of the infection took on an ugly, blackish hue in the subdued light.

"I don't blame you for being frustrated, because it frustrates me, too. We don't know why you had a seizure, or why you're having these complications now. You seemed to be getting better, however slowly."

"Too slowly," Doug said bitterly, "and now I'm getting worse, maybe even dying. I'd do anything to get better." Doug's body contracted in violent spasms as he started to sob.

I hesitated for a moment, wondering if I should say what I was tempted to—that maybe there was more we could do, that maybe a healer could help. I had no idea what to do next myself for Doug, except call upon Paul and the supernatural. I suspect all doctors sometimes feel as lost as I felt then. What do you do when a dangerously sick person turns to you for help, and you've already tried everything you know? I couldn't ask the attending, for it was clear when we admitted Doug that he knew as little as I did about curing colitis. Colitis is exactly the kind of chronic disease medicine men can sometimes help, taking patients beyond the limits of modern physicians. But scared interns aren't supposed to call in medicine men for consultations. And I might lose my position if Doug spoke to the wrong person about the idea. For once I decided to keep myself out of trouble, and keep my mouth shut.

Doug closed his eyes. Tears were coursing down his cheeks. I was hoping Doug would fall asleep soon so I could go home, but when I started to get up, the chair squeaked. Doug opened his eyes and fixed me with a stare. I pursed my lips and tried to look as if I knew what I was doing, though I was thinking, Oh God, now what?

Another thing I was learning from watching Paul work was how to employ stories as healing tools. I once told Paul how spellbound I was by my great-grandmother's stories. He pointed out the word I chose—spellbound—was no accident. Stories can function as a kind of hypnosis. They help prepare people's minds to accept healing. My great-grandmother never called what she did hypnosis, but doctors use the term to describe various techniques of delivering unnoticed suggestions to a patient's unconscious, and that's exactly what she and Paul used stories to do.

I was happy to discover that storytelling hypnosis can be used in hospitals without raising any eyebrows. It's close enough to the familiar technique of visualization to pass unnoticed. When I introduced it carefully, few doctors paid attention, and fewer patients found what I was doing strange. For most patients, the only strange thing was that I was sitting with them long enough to tell a story.

Since I couldn't think of anything else to do, I decided to tell Doug a story. Paul had recently told me a good Miwok creation story, and I thought that whether or not it did Doug any good, it would at least pass the time and ease my own fear and anxiety.

"I'm going to tell you a bedtime story. Maybe you'll be able go to sleep afterward." I settled into my storytelling voice.

Everything wasn't always as it is now.

Doug rolled his eyes and groaned.

"Look, I'm going to do this, so get comfortable. It's not like you're busy with work or anything," I reminded him. "Pretend you're a child on Christmas morning, listening to your grandfather tell a story. Sometime when you were really happy."

"Thanksgiving was always my favorite holiday."

"Thanksgiving it is."

We forget, you know, that things weren't always the way they are now. Wherever we are, whatever we have, sometimes that seems like all there is. But everything began somewhere. Lisa's pregnancy began somewhere, your illness began somewhere. Even the earth began somewhere—just as a healing has to begin somewhere.

"Yours has already begun, by the way, even though you think you've fallen off a cliff."

"If you say so," Doug said. "Go ahead. Tell me about beginnings."

In the beginning, there was Coyote. She was lonely, the way we are all lonely sometimes. Whatever else there was around, it was small and distant and hard to see. And the earth was as cold, dark, and boring as a winter blizzard. With nothing much to see, there certainly wasn't anything fun to do. Coyote was very bored. And then she met Silver Fox, who was also very bored. So they were very, very bored together. But as any bored person knows, it's much better to be very, very bored with a friend than to be very bored alone.

So after the two were bored together for a while, Coyote had an idea. She said, "Let's make something."

"Sure," said Silver Fox. "But how do you make something?"

"I think you have to sing it," said Coyote. "Close your eyes very tight and sing along with me: 'I want to see something. I want to see something. I want to see something.' "

The sheet covering Doug's body and the polished floor beneath his bed were as white and sterile as the world Coyote found herself in. As I continued the story, a nurse came to the door, looked for a few moments at the bizarre spectacle of a doctor telling a rambling animal story to a patient, then crept soundlessly away.

Coyote and Silver Fox closed their eyes very tight and sang together. They sang, "I want to see something. I want to see something. I want to see something." While they sang, each imagined what they wanted to see. Coyote closed her eyes tight and imagined seeing something to eat. Silver Fox closed her eyes even tighter and imagined seeing something majestic and uplifting. They sang and sang, and they danced and danced. Then they sang and danced some more, until they were exhausted, and then they got up and did it again. Finally, utterly and totally fatigued, they fell into a deep slumber. They slept and slept and slept, and when they awoke, lo and behold, there before them was a beautiful white-topped mountain with an elk standing proudly near its pinnacle.

"Beautiful," sighed Silver Fox.

"Food," gasped Coyote.

They spent the whole day gazing at the food on the beautiful mountain. They really enjoyed that day, the first day anything worth seeing had ever been seen.

I paused, wrapping my white lab coat around me for warmth. Hospitals get cold after midnight. Doug lay still, not responding, breathing slowly, but remaining alert and interested. So I told him in great detail about the second day, when Coyote and Silver Fox dreamed up water, and the third day, when they dreamed up the other animals. I told him how they spent the fourth day admiring their creation and then dreamed up the sun to show it off better. Then they slept a while; the sun unexpectedly awoke them with its warmth on the fifth day. They played in the sunlight, and when they napped, they dreamed up the plants.

They were so exhausted they slept through the whole sixth day, sun or no, which is when all the bad things crept into the world.

Then on the seventh day, Coyote and Silver Fox were so happy with their creation that Coyote resolved to do something really special. "I'm really gonna outdo myself this time," Coyote proudly proclaimed. "I'm gonna make something smarter than I am."

"That shouldn't be hard," said Silver Fox, who by now was getting tired of Coyote's bragging. "Go ahead and make something smarter than you." So Coyote scrunched up her brow and frowned a tight little frown, and she sang and sang and sang and she danced and danced and danced, and then she stepped on a big thorn and howled and something remarkable happened. People were born—naked and sort of ugly, even compared with a coyote. Silver Fox regretted that day almost immediately, because she knew anything smarter than Coyote was likely to cause trouble.

And on the eighth day and all the rest of the days thereafter, Coyote and Silver Fox stopped creating. They hadn't exhausted all the possibilities, but they were too busy with another job. From the eighth day on, Coyote and Silver Fox had their hands full trying—without a lot of success—to keep those pesky people out of trouble.

Forty-five minutes had passed and Doug hadn't said a word. He'd listened carefully and allowed himself to be drawn in. Now he seemed to be sleeping. Somewhere around the third day I'd begun to understand what meaning this story held for me at this particular moment. I hoped Doug's unconscious was discovering the same meaning I was—that creation is always possible. That if you're willing to sing and dance long enough, you can create anything, even health. And as Coyote found by stepping on a big thorn, sometimes the most interesting discoveries follow—maybe even require—pain.

When I finished, Doug's eyes were closed, and he was deeply relaxed. So I gave him suggestions to drift off into a deep sleep. I told him I would be slipping out to go home and get some sleep myself, and then I would see him again in the morning.

I ARRIVED EARLY the next morning, still tired. I'd stayed in the hospital too late to get a full night's sleep, given my forty-minute commute. I grabbed a cup of coffee from the cafeteria and went upstairs to see Doug. He was wide awake and drinking his liquid breakfast. He watched eagerly as I crossed toward him.

"Okay," Doug said. "So what did the story mean?"

I played coy with him. "It doesn't have one meaning. It means whatever it means to you."

"Don't try to pull that shit with me," Doug said. "Tell me what the story meant."

"If I tell you what it means, maybe it won't mean that anymore."

"What kind of bullshit is that?"

"I guess it's shaman bullshit," I said. "It's part of the rules. When you tell a story, only the listener is allowed to say what it means."

"Who says?" Doug demanded. "Who makes these rules?"

"Medicine men I've hung out with. People who do healing."

"Nobody does that around here."

"Actually, there are some people who do."

"What is it they do?" Doug asked. "And where do they do it? How come I haven't ever heard about them before?"

There was a lump in my throat now. Which one of us was Coyote here? Telling Doug about Paul could get me in a heap of trouble if it backfired, but Doug had come this far with me and this was all I had left to offer.

"Paul is the man I know," I said. "He's Chippewa and he does very powerful healing ceremonies. People with all kinds of problems come to him for help. You know, given the status quo around here, I probably can't recommend him to you."

"Oh, great."

"But if you happened to call my friend Alex, the psychiatry resident from the university, the one I brought to the home birth meeting?—I bet he could recommend Paul to you. And I wouldn't be in any position to say anything about that."

"And would giving me Alex's number be an okay thing to do?"

"I don't see why not."

"A medicine man, huh?" Doug thought that over while I wrote out Alex's phone number.

"I guess so," I said, "although he wouldn't say so if you asked him. But I've been out to his house and seen what he does and it is impressive."

A red-haired nurse poked her head through the door, saying, "It's time for your antibiotic." Then she disappeared.

"A medicine man named Paul." Doug shook his head, but he was looking happy, even hopeful. "And you think he can treat colitis?"

"I think he can help you." I was glad he didn't ask me why I thought that, because I couldn't back up my hunch with a rational reason.

"So that's what the story was about," Doug said.

"What?"

"About what just happened."

"Sure," I said, trying not to look too confused. "Absolutely." I left the room, so Doug could start to interpret the story as he liked. This is the marvel of a story. Something new had happened between us, through the telling, that was entirely unpredictable. Something true. Maybe Doug would be pesky again soon, pesky and well, like the people Coyote created. For the spirit of the story had infected Doug—the spirit of transformation, which is much deeper and more profound than any intellectual interpretation. Maybe that's why shamans have their rule. Explaining a story can only limit what it can do.

THE NEXT MORNING it was back to my rotation in obstetrics, where I learned that an unnecessary Cesarean isn't the only way to bungle a birth. Like Jason and Poirot, most of the obstetricians at Lutheran had problems with any delivery that didn't go according to the textbook. And, unfortunately, not all the babies born at Lutheran were willing to be born in a textbook manner. Breech babies were considered particularly uncooperative.

Mrs. Baylor was a young, first-time mother in late pregnancy. Her attending physician, Dr. Coombs, wanted to induce labor because he thought she might be overdue. I did Mrs. Baylor's admission history and physical and discovered she was not at all sure when she'd had her last period. When I called Dr. Coombs to tell him she had arrived, I mentioned that uncertainty, adding, "Maybe we should do an ultrasound to make sure of the size of the baby. We wouldn't want to induce a preemie."

Ultrasound wasn't commonly done then, but in this case I thought it would be a good safeguard. Premature babies have underdeveloped lungs; lacking the chemical surfactant, they cannot maintain the membrane tension necessary to keep the alveoli of the lungs from collapsing with each breath. Respiratory distress inevitably follows. But Dr. Coombs brushed me off, anxious to get back to the patients crowding his office. "Totally unnecessary," he said. "She's plenty big. Any fool could tell that. Except maybe an intern." He laughed. I didn't.

I did add, carefully, "She's big, but I was worried that I felt two heads." Dr. Coombs called me an idiot, then told me to stop screwing around and get the labor started. I shrugged, feeling embarrassed and worried, and hung up the already dead phone.

The first lesson of internship is that the attending physician is always right. Attendings are far too busy to waste time considering the opinions of interns. In those days I was a slow learner, so I argued sometimes. Or tried to, and ended up in more trouble than it was worth. Or got the phone hung up on me.

"Linda," I said to my favorite charge nurse, "what do I win if I'm right, and she has twins?"

"You'll be lucky to escape with your skin," she laughed, a gentleness in her voice, a warmth. I wrote out an order for an intravenous drip of Pitocin. But Linda was already getting it ready. "You want to start with two drops per minute, don't you, Doctor," Linda said.

"Of course I do. Whatever you say."

Linda smiled as she wheeled the equipment toward the door, knowing I knew she didn't need my help to do her job. "It's a good thing you have your mother around to keep you out of trouble," Linda said as she disappeared through the door frame, leaving her laughter behind her.

We had to raise the dose several times, but by dinnertime Mrs. Baylor was having the strong contractions Coombs wanted. I stayed with Mrs. Baylor most of the night. After my success with Doug, I wanted to experiment more with stories, to see where they could be useful. I tried telling Mrs. Baylor a story to help her cope with her pain.

To put Mrs. Baylor at ease, I said I didn't have anything else to do for a while. I introduced the story by saying I wanted to entertain her and help her relax before the hard part of labor began. Then, having chosen a story from her own culture that included the metaphor of birth, I told it to her, taking care to embed within it images of successful and normal delivery. I told Mrs. Baylor the story about the Jews being "delivered" safely out of Egypt. Of course, she already knew the story, but I embellished it with timely details about, for example, the young nation's difficult but ultimately successful journey through the narrow passageway God had created in the waters.

Near dawn, by happy coincidence, came the cry of a newborn baby from down the hall, prompting me to remind Mrs. Baylor that this would be her reward at the end of her all-night labor. Dr. Coombs came soon after and was aghast to find his patient laboring without medication. He stormed out of the room, yelling for Demerol, loud as a muezzin calling the faithful to prayer. He also called in an anesthesiologist to give her an epidural (a spinal anesthetic). Mrs. Baylor protested weakly, saying she didn't need medication, but Dr. Coombs ignored her. Linda told me later that Coombs sedated virtually all his patients because it made them easier to manage—less able to complain or demand his time.

"Give her the epidural," he told the anesthesiologist when he arrived, "and I'll be back after morning office hours. She won't deliver before noon," he announced confidently.

An epidural paralyzes the lower body and eliminates bodily sensations. In doing so, it also eliminates the powerful emotions associated with birth and does away with the laboring mother's need for human contact. Recent animal studies have shown that it interferes with the mother's ability to bond with her baby. In humans, epidurals are associated with a higher incidence of postpartum depression.

I left the room once the epidural had been given; my presence was no longer needed. Feeling defeated, I lay down on a cot in the physicians' room to take a nap. My efforts to help Mrs. Baylor during the night now seemed pointless. She had been laboring successfully, occasionally twisting and turning in pain, but fully conscious and excited about seeing her baby. Now, as the hour of birth approached, she was lying stupefied in bed, watching a morning quiz show on television. I was angry, and crushed. Working with Mrs. Baylor throughout the night was for my benefit as much as hers. I had something to prove to the doctors at Lutheran, but Dr. Coombs hadn't let me see it through. I lay still on the cot, finally drifting into a weary, discouraged sleep.

Linda woke me an hour later. Mrs. Baylor's water had broken and two little feet protruded from her vagina. I took one last look through the windows at the forested hills in the park across the street, praying for deliverance. Then I rushed after the nurse and found the situation just as described. The waters were tinged with greenish-brown meconium (a newborn's first feces). Meconium in the waters is not unusual in a breech birth, because the baby's abdomen is squeezed on its passage through the birth canal. There is some risk of the baby aspirating (breathing in) the feces. The risk is small when only small amounts are present, as was the case here. My heart was beating furiously as I stared at the baby's feet, knowing that Dr. Coombs might not make it to the delivery. Pausing to take a deep breath, I remembered the breech births I had witnessed during my acting internship with Dr. Donner in medical school.

"Take your time," I said aloud as the baby's legs began to show. Linda was hurrying to get a gurney to take Mrs. Baylor to the delivery room when the patient let out a sudden roar, and the legs descended further to reveal a baby's behind. I hastily looked around the labor room for a pair of gloves, remembering what my mentor had taught, that the key to a successful breech delivery was not to rush it. "Calm down," I reminded myself, rubbing the sweat off my palms onto the legs of my white scrub suit. Keeping a watchful eye on the baby's color, I wrapped a towel around the little boy's bottom to keep him warm while he worked his head through his mother's cervix. Entrapment of the head is the big risk in a breech delivery, and you cannot believe how relieved I was when that baby's eyes finally appeared and he looked at me, just before his whole head cleared the vagina. As I picked him up, he seemed to tilt his head to listen. I realized I was still mumbling to myself to stay calm;

these were the first sounds the baby heard as I handed him to a nurse to be bathed and weighed in the next room.

My reverie was cracked by the sudden curse of Dr. Coombs bursting into the room. "Why didn't you call me earlier?" he demanded. He had thrown on a scrub suit over his shirt and tie. He frowned as he stared at Mrs. Baylor.

"You said she wouldn't deliver before noon," I reminded him.

"She wasn't supposed to," he said, frowning distractedly. I looked to see what he was staring at. Another pair of feet!

While Linda tried to get Mrs. Baylor onto the gurney she had fetched, another nurse appeared in the hallway with a small but healthy-looking boy. "Four pounds, two ounces!" she called. Dr. Coombs took another look at the feet protruding out of Mrs. Baylor, cursed again, and began his procedure for breech delivery—namely, yanking the baby out before it could cause any trouble. He pulled hard on the infant's wet feet and gained a new purchase on the legs. He pulled a second time, hard again, until we could see the baby's scrotum. But the cervix responded to this tugging by clamping down on the baby's head. Dr. Coombs cursed under his breath. I don't know if he had ever been in such a fix before. In desperation, he tugged harder. The baby's thin neck stretched as taut as a bowstring, but the cervix held the head in place, and the baby began turning a terrible shade of purplish blue, its feet soon as dark as the withered winter leaves outside. Despite the doctor's tugging, the boy would not slide through the passageway his brother had negotiated on his own minutes earlier.

The pediatric staff assembled at the doorway to the labor room looked as scared as I felt. Dr. Coombs gave a last Herculean tug and yelled for general anesthesia. He stopped pulling, and Linda finally transferred Mrs. Baylor to the gurney, sprinting her down the hallway toward the delivery room, while we all ran behind.

"Well, how about a delivery," the anesthesiologist joked, his words dying in his throat as he saw what was happening. He spun around and threw himself into preparing a crash induction. While the mother was being knocked out, a snarling Dr. Coombs burrowed into her with his forceps. She went unconscious, and he clamped onto a head. Out came a limp, unmoving baby. The pediatricians went to work.

The soft voices of the pediatrics team, as they worked to resuscitate the little boy, drifted over to me. Dr. Coombs was letting me repair the episiotomy. One of the pediatricians was pointing upward, probably toward the neonatal intensive care unit, and talking quickly. As we were finishing our work, the baby disappeared in its warmer.

Minutes later a nurse called in, "The second baby is three pounds, eleven ounces." Dr. Coombs scowled irritably, getting slowly to his feet off the stool, and brushing imaginary dirt off the arms of his sterile gown. My head ached, my mouth tasted bitterly acidic, and my gloves were sticky with a mixture of blood and meconium. I felt as if I had a bad hangover.

Mrs. Baylor's two babies together weighed almost eight pounds, which explained why Coombs had thought she was ready for delivery. The firstborn boy's lungs were not mature, but he did well in the nursery and was discharged several weeks later. He was to be a normal, healthy infant. His brother was not so fortunate. His lungs were also underdeveloped; in addition, I was told, the neurological problems he sustained from oxygen deprivation during his traumatic birth would probably result in permanent brain damage and maybe seizures, retardation, or cerebral palsy. The neonatologist commented privately about how strange it is that we save babies to suffer, when perhaps they should be allowed to die.

Doug left the hospital five days later. "I'm going to call Paul," he said as I sat at his bedside writing his discharge papers. "I never thought of doing anything like it before. But something about it is strangely appealing. Exotic even."

Doug followed through and did meet with Paul. I accompanied him to several meetings, and eventually Paul was ready to perform a ceremony for Doug.

"It's my debut night," Doug kidded nervously to the friends and family members who had gathered to join in the proceedings at Paul's farm. Ellen did not come.

Paul carried his suitcase of ceremonial supplies out of his house, and I helped him lug that and other supplies back behind the barn to the tipi, set far back in the pasture where no one could see it from the road. The sun was fading in the west, already hidden behind the trees. One of Paul's helpers was carrying an armful of wood from the woodpile by the barn to an impressive stack he was building by the tipi. Another nephew was stepping inside the tipi, ready to start the fire. Unfortunately, in my enthusiasm to learn ceremony, I was away from my daughter. I was filled with sadness in that moment—that my life was so busy that I didn't spend enough time at home, that I was not with my wife and daughter. I resolved to take a long walk with my daughter that weekend, around our four-mile-long block. At age twenty-two, I still felt I could have everything I wanted.

Putting aside my thoughts, I helped carry wood, water, and supplies for the ceremony, which began several hours before midnight and lasted well past dawn. Paul and his helpers filled the long night with singing, drumming, prayers, and peyote. Doug frowned as he drank the bitter peyote tea. But each time the tea was passed around, Doug drank more. He passed repeatedly through the stages of nausea and relief that peyote brings, vomiting discreetly into the towel he kept in front of him. Sometime in the middle of the night, with the fragrant odors of cedar filling the tipi, Paul majestically stopped the songs and gestured for Doug to stand with him. Doug, between bouts of nausea, stood next to Paul. The way Doug was bobbing and weaving, he was lucky to have been able to climb to his feet at all.

"Doug has sponsored this meeting," Paul said. Doug struggled to stand proud and tall in his brilliantly colored Mexican blanket. "He has done this because he has a wife and a baby, and we have come to pray for his healing so he can take care of them and be a good husband. He is not here for himself, and he asks nothing for himself. He asks for healing only because of his wife and baby, who need his help. He wants to be well. He wants to be able to work and to support his family." Paul spoke loudly over the snapping fire, with flames reaching almost to Doug's rugged face.

The black-red coals in the center of the tipi seemed to glow brighter each time Paul spoke. Lisa sat quietly on the ground beside Doug, holding on to his leg. Paul had insisted that Lisa not take any peyote because of her pregnancy. Even if she hadn't been pregnant, I doubt that she would have tried it. She'd been skeptical of the healing ceremony when we first discussed it, and she'd gone along only because she was as desperate as Doug. Now she sat wide-eyed, watching the healer with her husband.

Paul began to fan Doug with his eagle feathers. He had explained to me that he used those feathers to brush away bad energy. While he fanned up and down Doug's arms and legs, Paul and his singers chanted. Doug swayed to their rhythm, his shadow covering Lisa, then revealing her, then covering her again. His eyes were open but looked as if they were focused on something far away. His face was radiant.

He gazed up into the heights of the tipi, where the sparks danced like a flurry of snowflakes. I watched with awe as this highly educated, solidly middle-class, and thoroughly intellectual psychotherapist gave himself over to a healing process he couldn't begin to understand. Paul did not ask Doug to use either of his favorite tools, insight or explanation. Instead, Paul asked only that Doug pray and have faith in the ceremony, and that he be willing to become a different person. Paul had already told him how to do that in their prior meetings.

"Doug is a counselor," Paul told the people sitting round the fire.

"His job is helping people, and now it is our job to help him, and pray for him." A pool of yellowing smoke hung in the air above Paul. "Now," he told Doug, "the grandfathers have arrived and have spoken to me, saying that you will be well if you will do what you tell others to do. You must walk your talk. You're the only one who knows how to do that, and the grandfathers say that you have the power to do so."

Doug nodded, and from far off he said, "I can do that. I can walk my talk."

"It might be easier," Paul suggested, slapping Doug on the back, "if you talked less." Doug almost fell forward with the force of Paul's blow. Doug smiled broadly. He opened his mouth to answer but stopped himself, then smiled again.

The wind picked up outside the tipi and blew with a kind of shriek. I thought I could hear the voices of the ancestors beyond the walls of the tipi. They were riding the wind and singing to us all. Doug turned toward me and smiled broadly, his face looking incongruously drawn and wispy, and I wondered if he could also hear them. He looked up at the dark hole in the top of the tipi and gasped, as if he could see the starstrewn sky above or the spirits that rode on its winds.

When I'd helped arrange Doug's healing ceremony, I was thinking that Doug needed a shift in perspective, but I didn't truly understand what order of transformation was needed. And Doug wasn't the only one who needed to transform that night. Attending a healing ceremony is more like going to church than assisting in surgery—the supplicant is usually not the only one affected. The spirits who came to Paul's Wisconsin tipi gave me two visions, one to show me I was on my true path, the other to show me where I had strayed from it.

I had sipped only enough peyote tea to be polite. Both my visions came, I think, more from the ceremony than the peyote. The first vision is hard to put into words, as Paul had warned they can be. The insight was nothing you wouldn't find echoed in Coyote stories, Christian scriptures, the teachings of philosophers, even the daily quote on the newspaper's comics page. But the ceremony made this simple, fundamental truth resonate as never before. I saw that we create our own world—as surely as Coyote and Silver Fox created theirs in the story I'd told Doug. That there is, in the physical world, no objective reality. That if we refuse to believe in healing, healing does not exist. If we sing and dance only of molecules and drugs, then molecules determine our fate and drugs will be our only hope. What we believe in is what comes true, and if we believed in Doug's healing, then it, too, would come true. What we sing and dance is what will be.

In my reading I had already encountered ideas like these, as I'm sure

Doug had, too. But that night in the tipi offered not an intellectual appreciation of the idea but rather a deep and emotional understanding of it. Only at that same emotional level can we use it to heal ourselves. And most important, I glimpsed the limitations of the individual in this process. Many New Age versions of the idea that we create our own reality place too much emphasis on the power of the one. At the ceremony for Doug, I was sensing that it was the shared visions of the many that form the world as we know it. That need for the group to hold a shared vision was why we were there in the tipi. Our shared vision, our prayers, were needed as a kind of scaffolding to support Doug's healing.

If I'd had only that one vision, the experience in Paul's tipi, despite its drama, would have been just an affirmation of lessons I'd already begun to learn. I had been correct in my assessment of Doug's problem: the dominant culture's worship of power and self-importance had taken hold of Doug, had stoked his unhappiness and finally his illness. And yes, I had been right in thinking that a healer could take Doug farther down the path toward wellness than a physician. I must have been feeling a bit smug that night, because the spirit's second gift was not exactly gentle.

"Think you're pretty smart, eh?" a Coyote-like spirit asked me. "What would Jennie say?"

When I first met Jennie, a thirty-six-year-old woman pregnant with her first child, she was planning a home birth with one of the local midwives. Jennie also wanted to see a doctor, so she came to Lutheran, where I saw her in the family practice clinic.

Jennie was a worrier who came for prenatal visits with more questions than anyone could answer. I tried to calm her fears through visualization—a technique in which you talk a person through an imagined experience that may or may not be realistic, to offer them new perspectives on both conscious and unconscious levels. I helped Jennie visualize her upcoming birth experience. Knowing that she liked gardening and walking in the woods, I chose images from nature to reassure her and teach her that she already instinctively knew how to give birth. But after each session, her fears would return. Each week she found a different complication to ask about. Each week I would tell her there were no signs of any complications, and that her body seemed perfectly capable of giving birth.

"How do *you* know my body can give birth?" she asked during a visit late in her pregnancy. "What makes you so sure? I don't like to exercise. I don't even like to sweat, so what makes you think I can make it through labor?"

I was annoyed—even exasperated—by Jennie's constant doubts. I was as brusque in my own way as Dr. Jason when I told her something he'd probably never think to say: that the body is part of nature and nature knows how to give birth. "It's a natural process. Eons of evolution have gone into making your body ready for this."

Several days later, her body seemed ready to go. For two days Jennie labored at home. But she didn't progress past four centimeters of cervical dilation, which meant she had not yet entered what is called active or hard labor. Her midwife called me to find out what to do next. She had already tried everything that I suggested: She had given Jennie a shower. She had gotten her out of bed and had her walk around while she sent Jennie's husband away to sleep. She had worked to help Jennie welcome labor. But she felt that Jennie was so afraid of it that she was forcing her body to hold back. Worried about how long this had gone on and about the possibility that her client was getting dehydrated and exhausted, I suggested that the midwife bring Jennie to the hospital. "If nothing has changed by the time she arrives," I said, "we can give her Pitocin. But sometimes just coming to the hospital will start a mother going when secretly she's afraid of laboring at home."

After she got to the hospital, I waited until the nurses called me to come see Jennie and her entourage, giving her some time to relax and perhaps begin to contract. The situation was worse than I had suspected. Jennie was in tears, shouting, "I want a C-section right now!" There was no call for one yet, since she'd yet to reach hard labor. She *was* dehydrated and exhausted. She believed she had been in labor for four or five days, but her midwife assured me that her early labor had been forty-eight hours at most. I convinced Jennie that we had to try Pitocin first to speed up her labor and make the contractions stronger. This was true even if she did end up needing a Cesarean. "Strong contractions will mature your baby's lungs," I said. "And I know you want your baby to have strong lungs so it can breathe well."

I spent the night with Jennie, attempting to give her hypnotic instructions to ease into the pain, and to sleep between contractions when her attention was no longer needed. Her labor would go faster and more easily, I suggested, if she would dream about how much she looked forward to seeing her baby in her arms. By dawn, fully dilated at last, she began some ineffectual attempts at pushing. Her midwife and I continued to urge her to coordinate with her body more fully. The baby's head was slowly descending. She was still pushing at 9 A.M. when Dr. Tobias, my attending, showed up.

The first thing she did was ask Dr. Tobias for a Cesarean. She cried about how little she had slept in the last five days. Tobias told her he could get the baby out with forceps. He told her this would actually get her over her misery more quickly than a Cesarean, so she agreed, and Tobias had me call the anesthesiologist to place an epidural. I had little experience with forceps and would not have thought to try it myself, but I had great faith in this particular doctor's abilities. He had delivered thousands of babies in rural Wisconsin. If he said he could do it, that was enough for me.

Well before 10 A.M. Jennie was up in the stirrups in the delivery room and the rest of us were gowned and gloved. The anesthesiologist had placed the spinal block and Jennie felt no urge to push at all. Then, as Dr. Tobias took the forceps from the nurse, I was confident that all would be well. The morning sun shone brightly through the room—a good omen, I thought. Tobias put the cold, ugly blades into Jennie's senseless vagina. It was a hard pull. Despite Tobias's experience, he was struggling and sweating. He groaned and put his foot up on the delivery table for leverage, pulling so hard that Jennie shrieked. Tobias yanked, and finally a baby boy came into the world.

Jennie didn't have enough strength left to hold her son and wasn't interested in anything but sleep. Tobias handed the boy to Jennie's husband, Warren. There were forceps marks on the baby's face. This is common and not necessarily serious. But Warren was worried that something wasn't quite right, and he was correct. The baby's facial muscles were droopy on one side. Forceps delivery can cause facial paralysis and weakness, but even a little function is an excellent prognostic sign that full function will return. Still, Warren was naturally concerned that his son had come into the world with anything less than perfect health.

The difficult labor had taken its toll on Jennie, too. Inspection showed that she had developed a vaginal hematoma (a swelling caused by an internal bruise). For the next few days she complained of severe pain, which did not improve even as the bruise went away. As the weeks went by and her pain persisted, Jennie gradually forgot that she had begun by believing in home birth and became more and more convinced that we had mishandled her labor. The head of obstetrics at Lutheran agreed. In his review of the case, he criticized Tobias—the attending physician and therefore legally responsible—for not having performed a Cesarean.

Confident that we had done the right thing in saving Jennie and her baby from a Cesarean, I helped Dr. Tobias answer the complaint. I righteously cited the literature on bonding, decreased maternal mortality, and a lower incidence of child abuse following vaginal deliveries. Unlike many of the hospital's doctors, Tobias didn't completely disagree with my views—but he was angry with me for mentioning them, as it only made things worse for him politically. I seemed to alienate him when my intent was to be supportive.

A few months after the baby's birth, Warren and Jennie moved to Hawaii. Not long before Doug's healing ceremony Jennie sent me a card saying her pain was so severe that she could not have sex. She said I was to blame for denying her the Cesarean that would have spared her the trauma of birth, and she made other personal criticisms that left me upset.

So, what would Jennie say? I sat in Paul's tipi and tried to answer the sarcastic spirit's question as honestly as I could. Jennie, I thought, had come to me an angry and unhappy woman. And even if we had given her a Cesarean and it had gone smoothly, which it might not have, she would probably have been angry about something else. C-sections are major surgery; like any major surgery, they can be complicated by infection, pulmonary embolism, hemorrhage, and problems with anesthesia. Problems unique to sections include the increased association with maternal mortality and child abuse I've mentioned, and with postpartum depression. All things considered, I still believed strongly that even a difficult natural birth is less risky than a Cesarean.

But had I considered all things? Like Doug, Jennie was a living contradiction. She had sought out a midwife for a home birth, but from the beginning had displayed a stubborn lack of faith in her own ability to have a baby. I was convinced that her impulse to try natural birth was right for her, but in the unflinchingly honest atmosphere of the peyote ceremony, I had to admit that my convictions had more to do with my own beliefs than with Jennie's.

Jennie needed more than the usual hand-holding and reassurance. She had come to me because she needed a major transformation before giving birth. I had not bothered to seek out what really prevented her from having a normal labor. I had accepted the beliefs of my midwife friends uncritically, that all women can easily give birth naturally.

Jennie was a woman who needed intensive help to give birth. I've met a number of women like her since. Many things—prior sexual abuse, a traumatic infancy, degrading family beliefs about birthing or being a woman—affect a woman's experience of her pregnancy. The ceremony was teaching me that Jennie had been asking for help as best she could, and I had missed her sincere request for healing—I wasn't yet sophisticated enough to notice that she had made one. The clue should have been my annoyance with Jennie, my irritation, my anger, which should have alerted me to the fact that my usual methods weren't working. My negative feelings toward Jennie had stemmed from my own frustration at not being very successful in helping her.

My response had been more like cheerleading than healing. I had the illusion that if I filled Jennie full of positive images, helped her visualize normal birth, and talked about the perfection of nature, she would give birth like anyone else. Unfortunately, Jennie was participating in the larger group vision that birth is abnormal and unnatural. And a group vision is almost always stronger than any one individual's. I had been blinded by my arrogant faith in the natural process, even for those who had no such faith.

Some of my blindness was born of ego. In the tipi I suddenly recalled having come to Wisconsin believing I could go a year without performing a section on any of my own patients. I remembered thinking a Cesarean-free birthing record would establish the legitimacy of the alternative birthing techniques that interested me, since others would be curious about how I had managed this feat. Although I hadn't been conscious of this while Jennie was laboring, it was clear to me now that I had been determined not to let Jennie's self-doubts stand in the way of my plans. I knew she could deliver vaginally despite what she thought, so I had pigheadedly ignored the signs that all was not clear for a normal delivery. My failure became Jennie's failure.

In recognizing that, I saw the similarities between myself and Doug. He believed that if he was any good, he should be able to *make* his patients well. I saw the folly of his beliefs, but how different were mine? Was my stubborn insistence on natural birth so different from Jason's and Poirot's insistence that labor should end before office hours? I wanted to think so, but right then I wasn't quite so sure. I said a quiet prayer asking the Creator to forgive my arrogance and guide me back onto a more humble path. I promised to help the next Jennie who came to me.

When I finished my prayer I looked at Doug luxuriating in the glow of the shaman's fire and asked myself what I would do if he relapsed soon after the ceremony. Would I accept his lingering illness any better than he had accepted his client's suicide? Any better than I had accepted Jennie's wanting a Cesarean? I'd already shown that I was capable of seeing what I wanted to see instead of what was actually there—in short, that I could act just like the doctors I criticized. Could I reform? Could I become a healer like Paul?

Doug was a different man after his night in the tipi. On the drive home he told me he knew when the prayers first started that he would get better, but it was the feathering that actually transformed him. "Before last night, I would have told you that feathering is a symbolic act," he said. "But when Paul fanned me, I could actually feel bad energy being swept away. When he was done, I could feel that something was physically different about me." And something *must* have been physically different, because his colitis rapidly improved as we continued to use acupuncture and hypnosis during his clinic visits. By the time the baby was born, his intestines were healthy and he was back at work—where, he told me, he was listening more and talking less.

Jennie and her baby both recovered. I answered her angry note as openly as I could, and we continued to correspond on and off for some time. The baby's facial paralysis was gone by the end of his first two months. Jennie suffered for several years with vaginal problems that baffled her Hawaiian gynecologists. One doctor diagnosed depression, but Jennie angrily threw away the medications he gave her. Eventually a surgeon in Honolulu convinced her to take the antidepressants, and he cut out some scar tissue where the hematoma had been. Jennie was fine afterward. But she and Warren were still bitter about their birth experience.

I didn't blame them, and I couldn't go back and change it, but I could and did resolve in future to fight the temptation to see things so simplistically. My experience with Jennie, and the teachings of the tipi ceremony about her, led to a dramatic change in the way I approached obstetrics. That change is still bearing fruit more than twenty years later. It led me to approach pregnancy and birth as an opportunity for healing. It led to my actually antagonizing some natural childbirth gurus, for I began to argue that normal birth is more than a simple combination of going to a midwife, staying away from the hospital, eating well, and thinking positively. It is the result of cultural beliefs, which sometimes must be challenged ferociously.

And I had learned something very important about what people say they want, and what they really want—and the difference between the two. True healing involves bringing these conflicting desires into harmony.

SEVERAL MONTHS AFTER Paul's ceremony for Doug, I witnessed a shamanic healing more powerful than anything I'd yet seen. Wesley was a Native American living in Duluth, about one hundred miles from the reservation where he and Paul had grown up. When I met him, Wesley's face was gaunt and he moved very slowly, wincing at the effort of rising from his chair. He looked like a man in his late sixties. I was shocked when Paul, who was in his forties, told me he and Wesley had been schoolmates.

Doctors at the University Medical Center in Duluth had diagnosed Wesley's illness as lymphoma, cancer of the lymph nodes. Wesley's had spread rapidly into his abdomen and chest, and his doctors told him he had no more than six months to live. They advised him to put his affairs in order. Wesley sought out an Ojibway medicine woman from northern Minnesota and asked her to conduct a ceremony for him. Carolyn, the woman, told him to come at the waxing of the moon. She told him to bring anyone who might help with his healing. (Professional jealousies and turf wars are rare among powerful shamans; the healers I respect welcome others to their ceremonies. I have seen the sort of ego-bashing battles physicians often wage, but only among amateurs.) Wesley asked Paul to come to Minnesota. Paul invited me.

At first Carolyn worked alone with Wesley, using what psychologists would call hypnosis to prepare him for the ceremony. The Arikara of North Dakota have a phrase for Carolyn's brand of hypnosis; literally it means "putting him to sleep so he thinks he sleeps when he's really awake."

After she had prepared Wesley, Carolyn took us all into the sweat lodge to pray for four straight nights. On the fifth day she took Wesley outside and walked with him. She told him that he might not think so yet, but he would still bend many bows before he died. She told him an eagle would be his sign of wellness.

When Wesley spotted an eagle later that day, he was ecstatic. Carolyn performed a ceremony on the spot, sanctifying the ground by sprinkling tobacco and cornmeal. Then she burned sage to chase away evil, singing sacred songs and smoking the sacred pipe and speaking to the spirits. Finally, she told Wesley that the White Buffalo Woman had told her he was well. When he returned to the city, Wesley's doctors could find no trace of his lymphoma—and they could offer no explanation of its disappearance, which was simply recorded on his chart as one of those rare, baffling spontaneous remissions. The doctors were not as quick as Carolyn had been to declare him well; because lymphomas sometimes go into remission and then reappear, judgment on a lymphoma cure is withheld for five years. When Wesley remained cancer-free for the required five-year interval, his physicians came around to the White Buffalo Woman's position and declared Wesley well.

I love science, and I understand the impulse to look for biochemical explanations for disease and everything else that happens in the body. I understand that our emotions are played out upon a molecular stage. But those levels of explanation fall far short in describing what made Wesley well. While healing can be described on a biochemical level, knowledge of the biochemical changes involved tells us nothing about how to start the process. How does a ceremony affect the lymph node's cancerous cells? How did prayers reverse the pattern of insufficient blood being supplied to Jimmie Left Hand's heart muscle? Miraculous cures apparently can change biochemistry, but how does that happen?

A neurophysiologist might dismiss lights flashing inside a dark tipi as hallucinations caused by exhaustion and excitement. Of course, physiological and psychological responses to heat, exhaustion, or hunger can trigger visual hallucinations and other phenomena. And so can substances like peyote. Even shared hallucinations or seemingly prescient powers can be rationally explained. The shaman who appears to have an uncanny knowledge of his patient could be working with everyday verbal and nonverbal clues—much like a good psychotherapist, or even an astrologer or fortune-teller.

I could, I suppose, find a similar explanation for the night in a tightly shut tipi when I felt something small and furry walk over my hand; why not also find a mundane source for the spirits of animals I saw walking in the dark? Others saw them too. I could offer any number of rational explanations, ranging from fraud perpetrated by the shaman's helpers, to the kind of mass hysteria that swept Salem village in the seventeenth century, when otherwise sane people claimed they had seen women consorting with demons.

I could, but I won't, because I believe rational explanations are destroying medicine today, as well as our society at large. To be healed, we need to believe in the possibility of healing, and in a greater world, and in higher powers than our own. We should not trivialize spiritual experiences, saying, "It's just *this,* it's only *that.*" It is a grave and sometimes fatal mistake to insist that every experience have an explanation that avoids the spirit. We cannot live without spirit. It is arrogant and in a sense dishonest—dishonest because scientific thinkers are not so much trying to explain as trying to explain *away* the miraculous.

Some people, for instance, postulate that Moses' parting of the Red Sea resulted from a combination of strong winds and hidden reefs that could have provided the fleeing Jews a land bridge across the waters. Does this make the story believable? Explanations like these ultimately backfire. A Native American shaman's ceremony, with the appearance of spirits and the healings that follow, is not incompatible with science. Science is one mode of explanation, and spirituality is another. Each addresses a different level or layer of reality. They are different, limited windows on a reality too expansive and complex for us to comprehend.

Anthropologists cannot do their work well without accepting that there are differing—sometimes wholly contradictory—valid ways to view the world. As a product of conflicting cultures and genes, I understand the balance of ideas anthropologists must maintain. They know that opposing world views can both be true—just as physicists know that light must be either a particle or a wave, though it can sometimes be both at once. Neuropsychologists such as the Nobel Prize–winning Gerald Edelman realize that life is multilayered, and that each layer holds its own sense and logic, often separate from and different from the logic that prevails at other layers. Levels can seemingly contradict one another, but only when we ignore the multidimensional nature of life.

In the end, I think you have to accept serious accounts of the miraculous on their own terms, or reject them altogether. You can't have it both ways. Scientific thinkers may feel that a rational exegesis of a miracle offers a back door into belief, but those who try to enter a spiritual life that way only find themselves in an empty room.

AFTER MY ROTATION in obstetrics, I moved to pediatrics, where I learned many valuable procedures that would help me care for children in a future family practice. I learned how to thread ventilating tubes past the vocal cords and down into the lungs of babies who are not breathing on their own, and how to suction out meconium from the trachea of babies who have aspirated it. I learned how to give dehydrated children IVs; how to distinguish between life-threatening illnesses and no-big-deal colds; and how to do spinal taps on very small spines.

I also learned that the idea of caring for the whole patient—the holistic philosophy that had attracted me to Lutheran—was as foreign to most pediatricians as it was to obstetricians and internists. Like other physicians, pediatricians tended to see themselves as mechanics repairing parts of a biological machine. The fact that their patients were children did not change anything. Children were simply machines with smaller parts accessible through littler apertures. The people who lived in those little machines were incidental, and getting to know them was unnecessary to the job of diagnosing and prescribing. Getting to know the little machine's family was an unthinkable waste of time.

I had to recognize that some of my patients and virtually all of my colleagues assumed that illness begins and ends in glands, tissues, and organs. I believed the less respectable view that illness also has its roots in the invisible world of the spirits, and in the stories people tell themselves. But I had signed on to become a doctor in a culture that separates the roles of physician and priest. I still dreamed of combining the roles as a healer. Perhaps psychiatry would offer an easier road to someone who believed patients were more than their brains and their bodies, who sought to honor the role spirits play in healing.

And after a year the double residency had gotten out of hand. The crisis intervention center wanted more than a half day of my time, and the family practice clinic was equally demanding. Residencies eat up between eighty and a hundred hours a week anyway, and by doing two at once, I was being asked to work even more. The family practice clinic wasn't turning out to be as holistic as I had hoped. Work at the hospital was discouraging, and the animosity aroused by my interest in home birth was getting tiresome. I decided to concentrate on the psychiatry residency in my second year in Madison. I'd be board-certified sooner, I'd be working bearable hours—and I'd have more time to spend learning from healers like Carolyn and Paul.

CHAPTER FIVE

Another Way

I F YOU ASK someone if he or she is a shaman, the closest you'll get to a positive response is, "People say I am." Native American culture discourages bragging about having spiritual power. True medicine men and women know that only the Creator and the spirits, or the patient, can really take credit for a healing. Besides, if we do not remain humble and respectful before the spirits, those who would otherwise help us in the work of healing are likely to desert us.

I have studied Native American healing for more than twenty years, and some people say I am a shaman. I'm reluctant, though, to claim the honorific for myself. One Apache shaman I revered told me, "I'm about as powerful as a dead chicken." At first I thought he was joking, or being modest; then I began to see why he was slow to take credit for a healing. "The patient must do 70 percent of the work of getting well," he said. "The Creator does 20 percent, and I do 10, which is barely worth mentioning." Most of what a patient can do to get well, he told me, is to make the firm decision to *be* well. This is where the medicine person steps in, by taking seriously a vision of the sick person as healthy, when no one else can or does. He or she creates with a patient a shared story of a mutual spiritual quest.

Medicine men and women live in almost every part of the Americas, from New York to San Francisco, Edmonton to Santiago, and not just on established reservations. They don't hang out shingles. They are not listed in the Yellow Pages, and for the reasons above will not always even admit to being healers when questioned by strangers. But they are out there nonetheless, quietly practicing their ancient ways of healing.

Some healers do live and work on reservations. Others live in the midst of—and invisible to—our modern culture. Obviously, no North American healers are untouched by modern civilization, as are the shamans still found in the South American rain forest. We can't know how closely we follow the traditions that dominated the continent before Columbus arrived. Some knowledge has been lost, but the tradition of healing is still very much alive and available to those who search for it.

Traditionally, shamans were trained through long apprenticeships. During these apprenticeships they usually maintained other tribal roles—taking their place among the hunters, for example—to sustain themselves and their families. Rarely did people learning to be shamans work as full-time apprentices, since then their teachers or families would have had to support them. Lengthy adolescent periods of schooling were not known in tribal society.

Today, in Western medicine, the pursuit of knowledge begins with schooling. The advantage is that knowledge accumulates more quickly through schooling than through apprenticeship. But there are still no formal schools for Native American healing. (This will change, I think, as reservations develop colleges and reclaim their heritage. Native healing will become formalized and taught as a legitimate profession, through departments of psychology or nursing or even colleges of medicine.)

What I know, I learned through years of apprenticeship and attending ceremonies and rituals, and also through my work with clients, which involved quite a bit of trial and error. Fortunately my errors were never grievous. As I learned, I made fewer mistakes. But all healing is an experimental process, of trying something that seems to work, then getting feedback about whether or not it did. Native American healing is no exception.

The first medicine men I sought out, after the sweat lodge in Wyoming that whetted my appetite, were a couple of Cherokee elders who had relocated to California. Both are dead now. Neither knew how to read or write. Neither had any national prominence. They were simple men who loved their religion and their culture.

One, Grampa Richards, was in his nineties, living outside Santa Rosa. I heard about him one day in the Stanford Coffeehouse. Like Coyote pestering Buzzard to take him to the Land Above, I kept bugging my acquaintance to bring me to see Grampa Richards until it became easier for him to say yes than no.

There was an etiquette involved in approaching Grampa Richards, and no way to learn it but by spending time with him. He had no phone, so you had to come to his spread and hope he was there. The first day I came I found a small group of followers gathered. Most were Anglos. Grampa Richards had two twenty-year-old blond girlfriends, both pregnant by him. There's nothing to stop a healer from being a rascal. And this was the 1970s in the Bay Area, when the ethics of the Haight-Ashbury culture still held sway.

After spending the day watching Grampa Richards tend to his business and speaking only when spoken to, I asked him if I could come visit again sometime. He said that would be fine.

Instruction was casual. People who knew his reputation would show up to be healed, or the group of us who made frequent visits would bring someone ill along. The repeated visits served as Grampa's screening method—because he could get to know you over time, but also because by the fourth or fifth visit he knew you weren't coming only out of curiosity: you wanted to learn something. If some of us acolytes were present, hoping to learn, he would let us tape the songs he sang while treating a patient. When the patient had gone he would explain to us what the songs meant in English. And we were welcome to take notes on the ceremonies he performed, and ask about them afterward. We helped him by fetching, as directed, the tools or sacred implements he desired.

Grampa had a briefcase. He'd hold it up when he was done talking or teaching for the day, and he'd say, "I'm afraid I've got some work to do." Sometimes he'd don an old businessman's raincoat to add to the comic effect—he had the right accessories, but the grizzled beard sticking out over the collar ensured that no one mistook him for a stockbroker. He'd wink at the group seated around him, step over our legs, and disappear into the forest. No one ever followed him. I don't know if he had serious work to do—prayer perhaps, or meditation, or herb collection—or if he just enjoyed his elaborate signal that it was time for us all to leave.

Much the same process held for Kosha, another transplanted Cherokee elder, who lived outside Ukiah. A follower of Rolling Thunder, a renowned healer at the time, told me about Kosha. This man did his healings in a lodge with a dirt floor covered with sandy earth his children had carted out to him from a sacred place back in Tennessee. The old man said that a person can go crazy simply by not being grounded, by not putting bare feet to bare earth at least once a day.

The strategy with Kosha, as with Grampa Richards, was to wait until recognized. For Native Americans, healing ceremonies are a group activity, as I've described. The healers' followers provide ready-made prayer helpers. The more serious the malady, of course, the more preparation a ceremony requires; the days I showed up when Grampa Richards or Kosha wasn't home often meant that he had gone to preside over a difficult healing somewhere else, with a patient perhaps too ill to travel. But many people came straight to them to be freed of relatively minor complaints, which responded quickly and well to treatment.

From these two men I learned primarily two things: how to approach ceremony, and how to improvise. Simply by watching these healers at work, I was learning how to sit down with a person who wanted to be healed. Holding a ceremony in an appropriate manner is as important to the patient as the medicine man; to be healed, a person must be convinced that he or she is well, after coming to you believing the opposite.

Improvisation keeps ceremonies vital. Students of any method tend to wish for a foolproof script they can memorize and practice. But there aren't any such scripts. Shamans frequently change what they do, based upon divine intervention and guidance. Through repetitive enactment, ceremonies can lose their power. Healers maintain a present connection with the spiritual realm, so they need not worry over whether or not a certain action is appropriate; they *know*. And healers respect the spirits of different illnesses by treating each one differently. The more I watched healers treat different patients, the more I knew there was to learn.

The Swedish anthropologist Ake Hultzkranz describes Native American medicine as "faith healing," akin to the "folk healing" of Euramerican societies.[1] I would call it spiritual healing, since it originates from the spirits. Faith helps the healing to occur—but the principal truth is that active disbelief defeats healing, more than faith promotes it. I have known animals and people to be healed who were unconscious or otherwise in coma, or unaware that ceremony and prayers were offered for them from some distance away. Studies have confirmed the power of prayer even when the patient being prayed for knows nothing about it.

The medicine person is both a medical and a religious practitioner—at once a doctor and a shaman. Hultzkranz calls Native American medicine a "religio-holistic" system when he compares it with the Western scientific system of medicine. This distinction is similar to one made by Dr. Andrew Stanway at the Institute of Complementary Medicine in London—between conventional medicine, which regards the body as a machine, and holistic or complementary medicine (the British use the latter term), which regards the human as an indivisible synthesis of mind, body, spirit, and environment.

The underlying ideas of complementary and Native American medicine are identical. Herbal medicine, manipulation, and massage

1. A. Hultzkranz, *Shamanic Healing and Ritual Drama.* New York: Crossroad Publishing Co., 1992.

therapies were among the methods available to the two Cherokee elders I first studied with. Some of their methods reflected what I was learning at medical school. But what drew me to them, because of what was most missing from my scholarly curriculum, was spiritual healing. This is not to say that my own approach is not eclectic. Today when I work I often use herbs, manipulation, and acupuncture in tandem with spiritual methods. After all, the path to the spirit runs through the body. Christianity asserts that the body is the temple of God. Likewise, Native Americans believe that the body is the earthly robe for the spirit; only through the body can the spirit interpret and understand earthly existence.

A medicine person uses spiritual energies to facilitate the healing of the body. This person may also have been trained to use herbs, manipulation, or other methods. But there is no degree. There is no certification. A medicine person is known by his or her works and by the testimonials of clients.

HEALERS, LIKE DOCTORS, do not always heal. Both callings have their share of incompetents and amateurs, even charlatans. Discrimination is required when it comes time to choose a healer. I chose stupidly shortly after Wesley's healing. Selfishly, I wanted to see in action two healers I knew primarily by reputation. Della, whom I had met at a workshop, lived in Utah. Scott, a man Della had spoken about at length during the workshop, lived in Nevada. I did not have time to fly to them. I gave up two frequent-flyer tickets (earned by flying around the country for residency interviews) so Scott and Della could come to Wisconsin and work with a couple I knew who were in serious trouble. I thought that while the healers worked, I could watch and learn.

Abdullah, another psychiatry resident at Lutheran, was a friend of Alex's and mine. He was a Sufi from Iran. His Protestant wife, Florence, from Nebraska, was extremely depressed and threatening to kill herself. None of us believed that the mental health system to which we belonged could do anything to help her. So I talked to Abdullah and Flo, and they agreed that we would call Scott and Della and bring them to Wisconsin for a few days. Flo was skeptical but willing. Abdullah was excited; this mode of treatment was not so far from his experiences back home.

When the healers arrived at Flo and Abdullah's, they met briefly with Flo, who was in a horrible mood. I sat with the three of them. She told the healers that Abdullah was largely to blame for her problems, because he didn't take her depression seriously. She wanted to be healed, but what about her husband? *He* was the one who needed to change. Couldn't the healers work some magic on him? Flo seemed acrid and sanctimonious. Scott was too stunned to speak. Then Flo turned and fled from the room, leaving behind her a bad energy as foul and palpable as the smell of skunk.

After a long silence, Scott turned to me. He talked with the characteristic accent of Northern Plains Indians; he had grown up on the Fort Peck Reservation in eastern Montana. Like many of his tribe, he was overweight, an almost inevitable result of the poor diet available to him on the rez. He said he wasn't about to walk on eggshells around anyone. Then he and Della retreated to the study, where Abdullah had made him a bed. For the next twenty-four hours—a time when we'd planned to finish building the sweat lodge and to sing songs in preparation for the ceremony—Scott and Della kept to themselves. I brought them flowers mid-morning, but they didn't seem to notice. They came out of Abdullah's study for dinner but hardly talked to me or even looked at Flo and Abdullah. The tension in the house was worse than before they had come.

The next morning Scott came outside to inspect the sweat lodge Abdullah and I were finishing. He told us the fire pit wasn't designed right, then asked how many people were going to sweat with us. I told him I'd invited some Chippewas Paul knew from northern Wisconsin and a few of Abdullah and Flo's friends from the university. He stared a minute at the fire pit and then shook his head. "You haven't invited enough people," he scolded. "And the Chippewas haven't showed up yet, which means they're not coming. Which probably doesn't matter anyway, because this couple isn't ready for a healing. Take me back to the airport."

I knew Scott only by Della's recommendation and didn't feel I could ask him to reconsider. I thought I had followed the few directions Della had given, but Scott was right to complain that we were poorly prepared. Between his work schedule and his depressed wife, Abdullah had too much on his hands to have been of much help. Neither Alex nor I had enough time, given our own work and family obligations, to have done much more than rush through building the lodge the day before. And one of the supplicants was clearly less than enthusiastic.

Della was more of a friend. I took her aside that morning and appealed to her, acknowledging that Flo's mood made things difficult and that I had not prepared for the ceremony very well. "I'm sorry the fire pit is wrong and there aren't enough participants. But Flo and Abdullah are in trouble. Can't you talk to them? Even if they aren't ready for healing, can't we do a sweat lodge and pray for them?"

Della was unmoved. She could do nothing, she said. Not without Scott. And he could do nothing in a situation where he had to walk on eggshells.

"Della," I said, stopping for a minute to catch my breath. "This isn't play-acting, or some game where 'They're not ready for healing' is a reasonable response. These people are desperate."

"How do you know Scott isn't right?" she asked.

"It doesn't feel right," I said. "If Scott had shown great wisdom and heard them out and *then* determined that he couldn't help them, that would be one thing. But it's like he's just put out by the whole situation and it seems to me he just wants to get the hell out of here. Maybe it's too dark and rainy and he's tired of being on the road. Or maybe his wife is screaming at him to come home and he'll take any excuse to do that. Or maybe he doesn't have the faintest idea how to help these people and he's afraid to say so."

"This is Scott's call," Della insisted.

"You know what I'd call this? Uncaring and abusive," I replied. "I've seen good and bad medicine, and this sure looks bad to me. And it's bad faith besides, maybe even a violation of a sacred trust. Please listen, give it some thought. And please make Scott think about it before he leaves."

But Della didn't think about it. In her eyes, Scott could do no wrong. So I drove them both to the airport. We rode in silence, mine an angry silence; I was cursing these two I had thought I could rely on. I knew I'd called them into a difficult situation. I knew we could have communicated better about the many details of organizing the ceremony, but I also knew that communication often broke down on reservations too, and most healers were more adaptable than these two. I regretted having given up two plane tickets for nothing, but much worse, I was certain this episode would leave Abdullah and Flo in despair about their future.

Grampa Richards or Kosha, Carolyn, Paul, my great-grandmother, even the snake-handling fundamentalists back in Kentucky—any of them would have done a better job than Scott and Della, because each of them went to great lengths to avoid judging people. First and foremost, true healers express and live out their heartfelt compassion. Healers are the kind of people who, having troubled to travel across town—let alone across the country—would offer whatever help they could. Even if the patient wasn't ready for their most intensive treatment or ceremony, they would offer something. I was amazed that Scott and Della couldn't be bothered. I felt they were acting like the unhelpful physicians I'd seen, peevish if the patient wasn't cooperative enough to have a problem that would respond to the treatments that were readily available. The only difference was that the healers were leaving town without collecting a fee, I thought as I paused at the last traffic light before the entrance to the Madison Regional Airport.

Miraculously, though, the two healers had no sooner been dropped off than a healer who was able to help showed up. Three Chippewa women arrived while I was driving back from the airport. They were plenty angry to hear that a ceremony had been canceled so capriciously. When I got to the house, a heavyset woman was already huddled in the study with Abdullah and Flo. The woman, whom we knew only as Turtle Woman, talked with them for several hours. Then she came out to ask me to start the fire for the sweat lodge stones. She promised to lead the lodge, since Scott had left.

Turtle Woman slipped quickly back into the study with Abdullah and Flo. For a brief moment I stood in the kitchen where she had just spoken to me. I worried what her qualifications were, but something about her was comforting to me. There was an oddly familiar scent in the air—the room smelled faintly sweet. Was it the herbs Turtle Woman had burned? She must have used some herb my great-grandmother had also used long ago. I went outside to prepare the fire. After a while, a short-haired younger Chippewa woman took over the tending of the stones. She had traveled many miles from Minnesota to be there that night, from the area near Mankato at the South Dakota border.

We had a beautiful sweat lodge. There was no moon to be seen, yet all around the lodge the landscape fairly glowed as the light from countless stars shone brilliantly in the clear night sky. The only light inside the lodge came from the glowing red stones, where they were first placed in the pit, and from the sticks used to light the tobacco in the sacred pipe. Turtle Woman was seated on towels just to the right of the door, in a place where the stars illuminated her large figure whenever the door was opened. Flo and Abdullah were seated in the west, in what she called the place of honor, directly opposite the door. Turtle Woman kept a weathered pouch beside her containing her sage and cedar and other mysterious things she needed.

This large woman, it turned out, was widely known across the Chippewa nation as a healer. The younger woman tending to the stones was her helper. It was the first ceremony led by women I had experienced. I was struck by the compassion they showed in all parts of the ritual.

Turtle Woman began the ceremony by draping a red-and-gray-striped towel around Flo's shoulders. Flo's long blond hair hung loose and straight over her shoulders and the towel. Soon Turtle Woman began to shake her large turtle rattle and sing. To my ear, the chant was unmelodic, at once haunting and monotonous. With the rattle going, I finally understood why people spoke of being "rattled." The noisy clacking began to reverberate in my eardrums, until the rattling seemed actually to be in my ears, not the healer's sacred instrument. At the end of each song the rattling sped up suddenly and stopped. I felt uplifted, as if carried on a cresting wave. I knew the unanticipated breaks in tempo would soon drop me into a trance. I could see Flo and Abdullah were entranced already.

Suddenly the lodge was silent, except for the hissing and crackling of the stones and the occasional sharp pop of the burning cedar—burned "to welcome the spirit of eternal life," said Turtle Woman. To ensure the success of this sweat, she had insisted that Flo and Abdullah sit beside each other. The couple's friends filled the lodge, along with one other Chippewa woman, the sister of the stone puller. I sat beside Turtle Woman, solidly ensconced in the north. All three of the Chippewa women wore towels wrapped closely over their heads and around their forms.

Turtle Woman told us Flo was sick because her spirit had left her body. She said Flo's spirit was lost, searching for its home. Abdullah later told me that in the hours Turtle Woman had spent behind closed doors with him and Flo, she had employed a wide array of techniques. She listened to them talk about how they felt but never let them focus on their complaints about each other. She asked them to talk about their cultural differences, which she said caused many misunderstandings. She burned sacred herbs and also did Native American body work on Flo, massaging her and rubbing pressure points. She asked them to speak words of love and praise for each other—as they had when they had courted and fallen in love—and then she held the sweat lodge to purify them both.

During the lodge, she again asked Flo and Abdullah to say loving things about each other, this time in front of all of us. She prayed for them and asked them to pray for each other. She fanned them with her feather fan—one that had silver, turquoise, and a light blue crystal embedded in the handle. Turtle Woman impressed us all with her power. During the ceremony she channeled a spirit. Goosebumps covered my body when the spirit spoke in a voice altogether different from Turtle Woman's own. The spirit told Abdullah and Flo to stay together and gave them instructions for renewing their love for one another. Afterward Turtle Woman chanted, shaking her turtle rattle and covering Flo with sacred smoke and drops of holy water.

Turtle Woman had beautiful long black hair. It shone in the moonlight as well as the sunlight, in contrast to Flo's paler locks. Flo was pretty and very tall—but still, her looks didn't hold a candle to chubby Turtle Woman's power. Abdullah sometimes looked funny next to Flo; incongruously short, he often wore thick-heeled cowboy boots in an effort to look taller. And yet the spirit said they were perfect for each other—soulmates, pushing their grocery carts up and down the aisle, oblivious to the picture they presented.

Over the next few months, Abdullah and Flo visited Turtle Woman several times at her house. Flo's depression lifted, and she and Abdullah began to repair their marriage. Turtle Woman also spent time teaching me how she worked. And from the two reluctant healers she had replaced, I learned the importance of preparing properly for a ceremony, and of being as discriminating in choosing a healer as you would be with a surgeon.

THE TIME I SPENT with Paul went very much the way time had with Grampa Richards and Kosha. The difference was that he had fewer followers, so I was able to learn more from him. (Alex stopped coming after a time or two; I think he had been mostly curious to try the peyote.) Paul also asked me along several times to more distant ceremonies.

Paul invited me to accompany him to one ceremony on the Devil's Lake Sioux Reservation in North Dakota. It had been "put up" by a family whose daughter's health was dwindling away. The doctors at a nearby hospital were unable to determine what was wrong. They knew she was severely anemic and not digesting her food. They knew she was vomiting frequently and had virtually constant diarrhea. But they could not determine a cause, and therefore had no therapy to recommend.

When we say a family "puts up" a ceremony, it means they are the ones who contact the medicine person and ask for his or her help. They offer gifts in return for that help, and build whatever structures are required. They invite others to the ceremony, plan how to feed all these people, and often are expected by tradition to give gifts to all who come. They must also pay the medicine person's fee.

When I first saw the girl, I thought she had gallbladder disease, but I didn't meet her doctors and would not have been in a position to make meaningful recommendations to them if I had. We don't often think of thirteen-year-old girls as having gallbladder disease, but this is becoming common among reservation women who are obese and eating a very high-fat diet. That is what is typically provided for them by the Bureau of Indian Affairs.

The girl's family was Christian, but their faith in Jesus had been shaken when their prayers and offerings had not changed the girl's condition. Paul's reputation for practicing the ancient ways had reached them, and they decided to call him. After they paid his initial "take the case" fee, he instructed them to build a tipi for the ceremony.

Building a tipi is no small feat. Twenty-foot trees of just the right thickness must be cut down and tied together at their ends with thick rope to support the canvas. Canvas must be bought, begged, or salvaged and then sewn. The sick girl's uncles pitched in to cut supports from a kind of fir tree common in their area. An aunt found some moldy canvas tarps in her basement. Everyone helped to repair them, stitch them together, then wrap them around the poles. By requiring the family to build the structure, Paul accomplished two things before he ever arrived in North Dakota: he established that the family was serious about the ceremony, and he focused their energies on the girl's healing. When the family was finished, they had a tipi that held about twenty people.

Most of those who would attend the evening ceremony also participated in an afternoon sweat led by Paul. Was it hot! He wanted to be sure that no evil would enter the tipi. One uncle who lived with the family said he was unable to miss work to participate in the lodge. And the girl was sweated for in effigy, since she was too sick to come inside. Her brother entered in her place and announced that he was sweating on her behalf. She lay outside the sweat lodge in a grove of cedars, close enough to hear the singing and the chanting. Close enough that the man tending the fire and the door could take her sacred water to drink, and the sacred pipe to smoke, at the appropriate times.

We entered the ceremonial tipi sunwise that night. Then Paul came inside dressed in his shorts with his towel wrapped around his waist. The girl followed shyly behind him. You could tell that this was not her idea—she was going along with it because her parents, aunts, and uncles were making her. She sat beside Paul. He had brought along a singer and a drummer who regularly helped him with his ceremonies. Another helper—Paul's son—lit a small fire in the center of the tipi and burned sage to dispel any evil that might have come inside with the people. Earlier in the day, Paul had blessed the ground, sprinkling cornmeal and tobacco around the outside of the tipi for the pleasure of the spirits who would come.

It was dark in the tipi. The fire was small, barely large enough to cast a shadow. In the darkness, the patient looked soiled and rumpled and stained. Paul's son used leather thongs to bind Paul's feet and hands, then extinguished the fire. The drummer began again, and the singer followed, his voice rising almost immediately to a frenzied pitch. Outside a host of other voices seemed to be joining his chant. The voices outside were stronger than the solitary singer inside, who grew more and more excited, singing feverishly loud, until there was an enormous crash. The tipi was shaking as Paul's main spirit helper arrived. A strange grinding noise came from somewhere underground. Blue lights flashed on and off everywhere.

It was at the height of this ceremony that I felt something furry walking over my hand. A long tail brushed against me. Moans and cries filled the air, some from the people and some from the spirits and spirit animals walking inside the tipi. An icy tentacle of uneasiness wrapped around me. These spirits were strong and powerful. Were they laughing at us? Trapped in the tipi and unable to move, I began to understand the fear that would drive a person toward a mental breakdown. I found myself reliving an unspeakable horror. Somehow I realized that the disintegrating mind I was receiving feverish impressions from was not my own.

That realization unlocked a door for me. I found myself walking unsteadily down a long, grand corridor. People stood grouped on either side, laughing and chattering. An ornate bronze clock guarded the top of a winding staircase. The clock's gilded hands struck midnight. A door opened underneath the staircase, and I wandered inside, disdainfully ignored by the people around me. In the small room under the stairs, I saw someone being raped. It was the girl who was sick. "Stop that . . . stop!" I cried thickly.

A man dressed like a butler appeared. "Please step outside, sir," he said cheerfully. "It's none of your business. The party's in the hall. Don't bother about this. Pay it no mind, none at all."

"Who is doing that to her?" I demanded. "Who is that man?"

The butler shook his head. "Never mind, sir. It's none of your business."

Hard as I tried, I could not see the rapist's face. I turned and saw Paul. While I was unable to move forward, he walked past me to the head of the bed. The butler seemed not to notice him. Paul stood silently, looking the rapist in the face; he did not seem to notice Paul either.

I turned around and walked out. I came to a precipice over the sea, which was as calm as a garden pond. No wind blew in any direction. The land around me was totally deserted. Clouds drifted lazily past the moon, its light shining upon the water.

A man sitting outside the tipi claimed to have seen paws and tails sticking out from underneath the canvas that night. Even the head of a fish. Other sightings were reported as well, by simple people who were not prone to exaggeration.

Paul spoke now, not in his old voice but in the crashing, thunderous voice of the spirits. We heard Paul's own voice at first near to the ground, which the spirit answered from impossibly high above. Then I heard the spirit's thunderous voice from deep within the earth, and Paul's from the heights of the tipi.

Suddenly Paul called to his son to stoke the fire. His son prodded the embers, sending up bright new flames, which showed Paul standing before us without his thongs. They were hanging twenty feet up from the poles near the top of the tipi. "I know what is wrong," he shouted, his voice ponderous and heavy. He pointed his finger at the patient's uncle, the one who had missed the sweat lodge. "The spirits have told me. Confess or you will die."

The girl's uncle was trembling. Even by the small light of the new fire, he looked pale and weak.

"Mikenak, the turtle, demands that you confess your crime," Paul shouted, while the patient broke into tears. She was stout and her extra pounds shook as she sobbed. Her uncle was wracked with sobbing as well.

"I touched my niece! My brother's daughter!" he sobbed. "I did wrong before Jesus. That's why he wouldn't help her, why our prayers were never answered." The uncle fell backward and was caught by the girl's father.

"Lay him on the ground," Paul commanded. I was sure the uncle had died, his body was so rigid. Meanwhile Paul was fanning the girl with his eagle feathers, waving cedar smoke over her. He reached down into his medicine bag and pulled out his eagle-bone whistle. He blew shrill notes through the air. He laid the girl down on the earth and put his mouth to her abdomen. Making a loud, sucking sound, he pulled something out and threw it into the fire, where it sizzled and burned.

"She is well," he proclaimed. "She is well." The singer and the drummer were going at their craft ferociously, cutting off his next words, drowning them with their furious sound.

He beckoned the father to bring the uncle before him. They laid the uncle down on the ground beside the daughter. Paul feathered him also, waving more cedar smoke over him. He sucked something out of the uncle, throwing it into the fire too. "Now he is well," Paul exclaimed. He lifted his hands in supplication toward the sky. "The spirits have forgiven him."

More chanting, praying, and singing ensued. Paul's head nodded to the rhythm. Eventually daylight appeared in the smoke hole of the tipi, the front flap was opened, and food was brought inside. The sky was quickly turning gray, and the rumble of distant thunder could be heard. A cool breeze, heavily laden with moisture, began blowing through the open front flap. Before we were allowed to eat, we were cautioned that whatever had happened inside the tipi must stay inside the tipi. We were warned that the spirits would punish anyone who gossiped about it. (I have omitted details of time and place and changed certain relationships and Paul's name, to honor this warning. But the gist of the story is as I've written.)

An electrical charge began to collect in the air. Lightning flashed overhead, illuminating the tipi walls, casting a ghostly light upon our faces. Another jagged fork of lightning split the clouded sky. It struck somewhere behind the nearby ridge, and in almost the same instant, a thunderclap sounded like a cannon barrage in our eardrums.

The girl miraculously improved. Paul's spirits had made clear to him that the incest taboo had been broken; that knowledge guided his work. The healing of the child and her uncle had begun with the ceremony in the tipi, but Paul stayed several days afterward to do counseling with the whole family, to prevent this taboo from ever being broken again, and to mend the broken pieces of the lives affected.

From reading I had done, I knew that the ceremony Paul used took elements from two historical ceremonies—the Lakota Yuwipi ceremony and the Ojibway Shaking Tent ceremony—and combined them into a new ritual. The Yuwipi ceremony is usually done in a house, after all the windows and doors are covered with blankets, to keep out any light. The medicine person is tied up, to be untied later by spirits who come in once the lights are extinguished. The Shaking Tent ceremony was originally done in a small structure only large enough for the medicine man. No one else came inside with him.

Many modern shamans, like Paul, pick and choose bits of different traditions, using a combination of things that work for them and their clients. In the ceremonies I do now, I find I improvise as much as Paul did. The shamans I sought out after him showed me practices closer to what I would call a pure tradition, and whenever I take a sick person to a shaman, I choose one who works in a traditional manner. But because I am not a white man or Lakota or Cherokee, and because I am all three, my way is to use a little of everything I have come across.

BACK IN WISCONSIN, I described my experience to Paul, of entering the uncle's deranged thoughts and coming across the girl being raped. I tried to find out whether Paul had shared in my vision, and what it might mean. His answer was a coy smile. I kicked at a rock.

"What do *you* think it means?" he taunted. I had heard this question from him often enough in the past; I should have anticipated it.

"If I knew, would I be asking you?" I said in frustration.

"Ah. Answering questions with questions. You're learning."

"It doesn't feel like it."

"Would it help if I was always around to interpret your visions for you? Maybe that would be good. Wherever you go, you can take me with you. It will get expensive for you, but it will be worth it. Your daughter can call me Grandpa. I can sleep between you and your wife, so if you have a dream, you can wake me right then and there . . . Look at him, he's smiling."

And then I started to laugh.

"Let me tell you a Zuni story, Lewis, about Coyote and the Burrowing Owl. Then, if you like, you can bring me home and I will explain it for you."

I suppose I deserved it. A dose of my own medicine.

Once upon a time there was an old, fat coyote who lived with his grandmother. The burrowing owls were having a dance. It was a very interesting dance they did, with a gourd full of foam balanced on their heads. And you know how owls are, sort of crooked and bowed. So they were pretty funny to watch.

But everybody knew to leave the burrowing owls alone, because they were having a sacred dance. Coyote should have known. But what does he do? He goes right up to the chief of the owls and says, "Whatcha up to?"

Burrowing Owl is pretty annoyed. "Well, Coyote, doesn't it look like a sacred dance to you?"

"Oh, can I dance? Can I dance too?"

Burrowing Owl looks at Coyote like he is the dumbest thing in the world, which maybe he is. So Burrowing Owl says, "Well, Coyote, you see what they're wearing on their heads? Everybody's wearing their grandmother's head, and it's full of foam. We have this special magic where we can cut off our grandmothers' heads and wear them, but our grandmothers are still alive and happy."

"Wow." Coyote is impressed. "But how do you get your legs to look all funny and crooked?"

"Well, I'll tell you what we do, Coyote. We take a very big stick. We put our legs across a stump. Then boom, we break our legs. And we have a special medicine to make them better, but they bend a little, so we can do this sacred dance in the proper manner."

"I want to do it too."

"Well, run right home and get your grandmother's head, and come right back. Then break your legs. We'll give you the special medicine, and you can join our dance."

So Coyote is so stupid he goes home, kills his grandmother, cuts off her head, ties it to his, and runs back to the owls. Then he smashes both his legs. "Okay, I'm ready for the medicine now."

All the owls can do is laugh. They laugh so hard they spill the foam, and that's why even today they have little specks of it all over them.

Paul laughed more than I did at his story, but I got the message.

There was no need to be quite so eager. There was no need to leave my brain behind when I visited him. I was as capable of interpreting my vision as he, and what did I expect him to do? Tell me it was true, reassure me it had really happened? I had a vision that gave me a partial diagnosis of what was wrong with his patient. It was a double message to me—that I was getting somewhere (to have the vision at all), but that I wasn't quite cooked yet (as I was unable to follow Paul to see who the rapist was). I had been encouraged and chastened by my first premonitory experience, and what more did I expect?

As I SPENT MORE time around shamans like Paul and Turtle Woman, I sometimes became frustrated with my psychiatric work at Wisconsin. But I told myself to stay on course. Completing the residency program, thus earning my board certification, was the key to finding a faculty position in which I could bring the shaman's perspective to a larger population. And toward the end of our second year in Wisconsin, Ellen and I had a son: a new reason to stick with the program and get the kind of job that could support our growing family. So I was plugging away at a trying but workable arrangement when everything suddenly unraveled.

My study of childbirth was the culprit. When I was finished matching home and hospital births, I ended up with 1,046 pairs of women and a few surprising statistics. All things considered, both groups of women should have had very similar outcomes. They didn't. The women giving birth in the hospital had many more forceps deliveries, more anesthesia, more Cesareans, more induced labor, and more babies that had to be admitted to intensive care nurseries. I described these dramatic results at conferences and was invited to appear on the "Today" show, "Good Morning America," and other network shows. I accepted the invitations, optimistically if naïvely thinking that it could only be good to get the word out.

I didn't realize that people at the hospital, and the university it was affiliated with, would be upset. I was twenty-two years old, idealistic, and a firm believer in helping consumers and doctors to make choices about medical care on the basis of the latest research. I also believed the American obstetrics industry needed a little shaking up, and I was excited to have the hard, scientific evidence to do the job. The dean at the university was likewise excited—sputtering with outrage, in fact—that I had presented my evidence on national television.

I was summoned, along with my lawyer, to a meeting with the director of the residency program, the dean of the medical school, and the university's attorney. The university's lawyer began by saying I must stop all research on home birth. My lawyer responded with an argument on behalf of academic freedom. No one could fault the research itself. And of course I had the right to pursue whatever research interested me, to publish my findings, and to make appearances talking about them, my lawyer said. The university attorney had to agree, in theory, but he wanted to put limits on where and how I could talk about my research—especially when the results might be embarrassing to the hospital or the university.

We had reached an impasse. The meeting lasted several hours, but I stopped listening to the details long before it ended. I had spent almost two years to that point trying to walk a fine line at Lutheran. This nominally holistic residency program was probably more tolerant of my views than most others would have been—and yet even here there was pressure not to disrupt the normal practice of medicine. Although the lawyers were speaking vaguely of compromise, I knew my only real alternatives were either to stop my involvement in home birth or to leave Wisconsin and continue my research elsewhere, outside the confines of a residency.

I was used to feeling sad and angry about what was expected of me as a doctor, but usually that happened when I was working for someone else, a doctor who ordered me to do something that went against my own inclinations. I was able to pull through by reminding myself of what I could accomplish under my own auspices. But now, even the work that was close to my heart was to be denied me. I firmly believed that my research could humanize the way women give birth in this country, could change an experience that had become brutal and abusive.

I was overwhelmed by the level of authority confronting me. I was beaten and depressed, on the one hand, while on the other I saw that the magnitude of the response I provoked proved how important and controversial my research was. As the meeting dragged on, I grew more and more disheartened with the idea of continuing in a hospital where I had to keep a lawyer on retainer. I was ready to move on. When the attorneys broke for the afternoon with the understanding that they would reconvene to work out the "parameters of acceptable research," I gave the dean my word I'd keep quiet about my work until the end of the academic year. At that point I would leave Wisconsin and say what I pleased. Then I drove home, and started looking for another way.

AT THE END OF my second year at Lutheran, Ellen and I returned to the West Coast. I helped start a community family health center in Berkeley that primarily served pregnant Medicaid patients, providing them with a wide variety of services, including home birth, birth at Mount Zion

Hospital's new alternative birth center, and, uniquely, the psychosocial support that many pregnant women need.

Over the course of four years there, I did hundreds of deliveries and continued to study childbirth practices and outcomes. Ellen, who had finished her master's in clinical social work in Madison, worked at the health center also. She used the clinic as an environment to earn her LCSW state license in clinical social work, which enabled her to set up a private practice as a psychotherapist. We collaborated on several books on the psychological aspects of childbirth in America. We also began leading workshops together around the country on related topics.

Berkeley being Berkeley, I was able to explore and employ unconventional treatments at the family health center, such as acupuncture, acupressure, homeopathy, hypnosis, visualization, nutrition, and anything else that seemed promising. But while the position allowed me to investigate holistic healing, I had no illusions that this work would allow me to make any essential changes in the way medicine was practiced. The childbirth research did have this potential, I thought, and I pursued it at every spare moment.

Unhappy about my lack of credentials, I decided to continue gathering them. Since I couldn't yet stomach the thought of returning to residency, I enrolled in a clinical psychology program in Palo Alto. I could do this while working, and the health center paid my tuition. Four years later, with Ph.D. in hand, I found a faculty job: Stanford, my old school, hired me to teach behavioral science research to med students and residents. The salary was modest, but I found weekend emergency room work at a local hospital to supplement my income.

I couldn't believe my luck. I had long dreamed of being on Stanford's faculty. Not having finished my residency made me feel grossly underqualified. (You must finish a residency to be board-certified for a specialty. Although you are officially a doctor upon graduating from med school, most jobs require certification, just as a professorship usually depends upon obtaining a Ph.D.)

Figuring that the best way for my students to learn about research was to do research, I designed a study around the patients who visited Stanford's Community Health Center in Sunnyvale. Most of the patients were Hispanic, Vietnamese, Laotian, Cambodian, and Korean, coming from the communities near the clinic. Some African-Americans came as well, but this part of Sunnyvale had fewer African-American residents than areas nearer Stanford (East Palo Alto, for example). Many of our patients came from cultures with living folk traditions. Mystical Mexican Catholics, for whom saints and spirits are synonymous, numbered among the Hispanics; the Asians had acupuncturists and herbalists and Buddhist shamans; we even heard of a few voodoo practitioners among the African-Americans. Given these backgrounds, I wondered how our patients responded to the medicine they encountered in our clinic. What did they remember from their visits to the clinic, and what treatments did they actually follow? These were to be our research questions.

The questions led a group of us one day to a ramshackle apartment in the barrio of Sunnyvale. We climbed the narrow, rickety stairs to a loft above a garage, to ask a Mrs. Machido why she had not returned to the clinic for her follow-up visit. The old woman wasn't being very helpful.

"It must be difficult for you to get down to the clinic," a blond medical student named Joe suggested sympathetically to the balding seventy-year-old Hispanic woman. Joe, in his second year at Stanford, was an intense young man who sat on the edge of his chair, his knees almost touching the old woman's. He scowled unconsciously as he struggled through the interview. Mrs. Machido sat on her sagging gray couch, flanked by two wide-eyed, preadolescent granddaughters.

"Not really," she answered politely, lowering her glass of ice tea. She had worked as a maid for a wealthy white family from Los Gatos most of her life, so her English was quite good. "I went out to the market this morning. These girls are my responsibility." She patted her grand-daughters' knees.

"The doctor at the clinic was worried when you didn't come back," Joe mumbled, sounding almost incoherent even to me.

"Don't lose no sleep over me," she said, getting up to turn off the gas burner. She'd been on her feet cooking when Joe and his two classmates and I knocked at her door. She closed her eyes briefly, shutting out the four visitors crowded into her little apartment. "I'm not coughing up blood no more. You tell them how I'm fine now."

"But you were very sick," Joe persisted, anxiety mounting in his voice as he scanned his long list of questions. "Your doctor wanted to see you again in two days."

I began to worry that we were badgering her. "Mrs. Machido," I broke in, then paused for a moment to show respect.

"Yes." Her eyes opened, and her attention returned to us.

"We're not really part of the clinic. We're not here to lecture you about keeping appointments. These are medical students from Palo Alto. We're trying to learn how to listen to people. When someone comes to the clinic and doesn't come back, we wonder why. If we can find out, maybe we can be better doctors."

"What can I tell *you* about being doctors?" Mrs. Machido said, but she smiled, and the shadow of fear in her eyes disappeared.

"Can you tell us how you got better?" I paused again before adding, "We won't tell the clinic doctors anything you say unless you want us to, and even then, only what you want us to tell them, and—if I may say so, I would be very grateful to you if you would help me teach these medical students here. They are *my* responsibility. I want them to learn from you, not just ride off in their cars, knowing nothing new."

"You want them to learn from an old person like me?" Her voice sounded suddenly loud and demanding, echoing off the cinder-block walls. She was clearly confident that there was plenty we could learn from her—and pleased to have, for once, been asked. "How can I help you?"

"Tell us how you got better. We know you were very sick, and now you are well, so this story would be of great value to us."

"Yes, I was very sick," she confirmed, returning to the couch. I offered my hand to help her sit down. It took her long moments to settle. She told us she had not wanted to go to the clinic, but her eldest granddaughter had made her. "I couldn't get a moment's peace from that girl until I went."

"How does your granddaughter know about the clinic?"

"She works in the same building. She goes there herself for the things she needs," Mrs. Machido said, "whatever they are."

"So you wouldn't have gone on your own?"

"Would you go somewhere only sick people go, where all they know is sickness, and not how to make people well? Where not all of them even believe in *God*," she said, whispering this last word to keep the blasphemy of the idea from tainting her.

"What did they do for you?"

"They gave me pills," she answered, frowning. "I don't know what kind of pills."

"So what did you do?"

"I went to Mama Barbosa. A *curandera*. You understand?"

I nodded. "And what did she do for you? How did she help you to get well? That is what I'd like you to teach my students." I hesitated and then added, "They may not learn this anywhere else; they may not have another opportunity to hear about a *curandera* again."

"Then I will tell them. But they could ask Mama Barbosa herself."

"We will talk to her, if that can be arranged. First I'd like to learn from you."

Mrs. Machido spoke quickly now, fixing each of us in turn with her gaze. She had gone to nearby St. Sebastian's, where her priest said a special mass for her. Then she visited the neighborhood *curandera*. This Hispanic Indian healer sat with her and prayed, then performed a ceremony for her. "She burned the sacred herbs. She used her fan to cover me with smoke while she sang the name of Jesus. She blessed me with the holy water, and then she took something from her altar and rubbed it onto me."

"I wonder what it was," one of the granddaughters said, giggling.

"She said I had been consumed by a sickness that I could not see or touch. She said that only the angels could heal me, that only the flying spirits could go high enough to look down and see what was wrong, because anyone living in the world would melt if they got that close to the sun."

"Did you see the angel, Grandma?" asked the younger girl, very excitedly.

"No, child, only the healer could see the angel," Mrs. Machido replied, touching the young girl on the cheek. "But the angels came like Mama Barbosa said and they lifted that sickness out of my body and I could breathe again. Mama Barbosa gave me herbs to drink so the angels could smell me and know where to come. She said they would be searching for a sign, a smell, a prayer to mark me, and they could not fail to find me if I drank the medicine after I burned some other herbs that she gave me."

"Did they come?" asked the younger child. "I want to see an angel."

"They came," Mrs. Machido said. "See how I am well?"

One of the more skeptical medical students smiled. "Is that the only way you knew they had come?" I glared at him and he backed down. He was welcome to be as skeptical as he wished later, but not in the presence of Mrs. Machido, not while we were trying to gain her trust to hear her story.

"There are always other signs of an angel's passing," I said. "Mrs. Machido may not want to tell us everything. She may need to keep some of the signs private, or save them for her granddaughters, as a special blessing to reveal. I don't think she should tell us unless she wants to." I paused a moment, and could tell from Mrs. Machido's broad smile that her trust had been restored.

"There was a sign," she said. "All the lights went off outside and inside and the cross on my wall began to glow. At first I thought I was dreaming, but I pinched myself and I was not asleep."

The students listened transfixed to the remainder of her tale. What she was saying was straight out of their books on shamanic healing; they could have heard it in a college anthro lecture. I had argued to the students that shamanism was thriving under their noses, and here was proof. I wanted them to understand the sacred trust involved in doctoring. I wanted them to learn that illness is a major life experience, and like any such experience, it must be handled gently. People are as open to being traumatized in these moments as they are to transcending illness and being healed.

Mrs. Machido finished her story, saying, "I prayed morning, noon, and night, just like Mama Barbosa told me."

"What happened at the clinic?"

"A nice young doctor examined me. He had them take my blood, and an X-ray, and then he gave me some pills, like I told you."

"What did he say was wrong?"

"He said there was some kind of bug in me."

In fact, the resident at the clinic had diagnosed bronchial pneumonia, probably caused by a bacterial "bug" named *Hemophilus influenzae*. Mrs. Machido was having so much trouble breathing that the resident wanted to hospitalize her and begin intravenous antibiotics. "What did you think of the treatment the doctor recommended?"

"He was very nice to offer me a bed in the hospital," Mrs. Machido said. "But I had to come home to fix dinner for my granddaughters. So he gave me pills I could take at home."

"Did the pills help?"

"I don't think so," the woman said reluctantly.

"Are you still taking them?" Joe asked.

The woman thought before shaking her head. "I'm not having trouble breathing no more," she explained with finality. "That bug is dead."

"How many did you take?" Joe persisted, almost shouting. He was frightening Mrs. Machido; I signaled to him privately. She faltered. We waited.

"Not so many."

"Mrs. Machido," I said, "whatever you did with the antibiotics is okay with us. You're obviously feeling well and we're really glad for that. We're just curious if we did anything to help. Or if we did something to keep you from coming back to the clinic."

The woman stared at me but spoke to all of us. "Children," she explained, "no one did nothing wrong. I just didn't have the heart to tell that nice young man I didn't take his pills. They seemed so important to him."

MY STUDENTS ENJOYED the project, intrigued by the cultural differences between these patients and themselves. Stanford Medical School had recently managed to restrict admissions to a conservative group of middle-to-upper-class science majors. Though different races were still represented, the values of the group as a whole were much more homogeneous than in my day. The admissions office had figured out how to select conservative students without breaking any laws—by excluding any candidates who had taken too many courses in the liberal arts, or who spoke too many languages.

Stanford prided itself on producing specialists and medical research scientists. Those who were likely to choose family practice or psychiatry as career specialties were not wanted. Too many students from my era had chosen these fields, the two most suspect career paths in the view of the Nobel laureates, molecular geneticists, and biologists who ran the medical school.

My students saw, when they made home visits to people like Mrs. Machido, a new world. They quickly discovered that clinic patients generally did not understand the instructions their doctors gave them. Sometimes language differences were at fault, but many of the patients spoke good English; cultural assumptions were just as often to blame. They also learned that many patients, like Mrs. Machido, took very little of the medicines prescribed to them. Others never even had their prescriptions filled.

If the students were surprised at how poorly patients complied with their doctor's instructions, they were amazed by what happened to the patients' illness. There were cases of deterioration from inadequate treatment, but many people just got better—too many to be due to chance, I suggested. My students set out to calculate how many recoveries to expect by chance. And they found my suggestion to be true: whether from prayers, the treatments of spiritual healers, or the natural restorative mechanisms of the body, many patients recovered completely without drugs, like Mrs. Machido.

When we saw how rarely patients followed through with the care their doctors had prescribed, we began asking why they had gone to the clinic in the first place. Most just shrugged and said they thought the doctors might help them. They didn't understand the language or tools of scientific doctors, but then they didn't understand the magic of saints and *curanderos* either. Modern medicine was one of a number of mysterious healing arts; the residents down at the clinic seemed nice enough, so why not give them a try? The doctors must be powerful, one man told us, to wear such expensive clothing and drive such nice cars. The striking thing was, most of the patients appreciated their doctors' efforts whether they followed their advice or not. Whatever was prescribed was a small part of the office visit, from the patients' point of view. Most thought the situation, the building, the small talk were all important to their recovery, even when they later ignored the doctor's instructions. In the end, patients felt that the time a doctor spent with them was more important than any medicine.

Our research findings were consistent with the shaman's belief that relationships are the key to healing. In Native American medicine, and in the holistic medicine I was exploring, healing grows out of a change in the patient's relationship to his or her self, or it grows through a relationship with the healer and the spirits the healer calls forth. A variety of tools—drugs and surgery among them—can be used to support a healing relationship, but the relationship is more critical than any tool.

I didn't discuss holism or shamanism with my students. I didn't have to. They were discovering for themselves that good doctoring has to include more than a diagnosis and a prescription. The drugs they were being trained to dispense and the surgeries they would learn to perform were not, in themselves, the most valuable things they could offer. I was convinced that this discovery was changing the way these students viewed themselves and would make them better doctors—even those who would eventually return to practice in middle-class communities where the cultural beliefs were not so diverse and exotic.

My faculty colleague Jonas Andrews was less enthusiastic. Jonas was a sociologist who had been hired to teach behavioral research techniques to Stanford's medical students, on the same grant that paid my salary. He believed in quantitative research and randomized, controlled trials, and was skeptical of our study.

"If it's not quantifiable, you don't know the importance of anything you find," he argued. "You don't even know if your findings are real. Your students listen to these people and hear what they want to hear. Worse, they hear what *you* want them to hear. And you've let them think they can call that research."

Jonas insisted that good research generates numbers and statistics, t-tests and chi-squares, distributions and product moments—objective results that can be disputed and defended. We, on other hand, were recording stories. Where were our rigorous controls?

I was overwhelmed by Jonas's fast-talking logic and didn't yet know the arguments I needed to refute him. I had no sharp answers to Jonas's criticism except a lame assertion that qualitative research had its own merits. But how, I wondered, when virtually no one at the clinic followed through with their care, could we find a control group? "How about we reverse it? Take the Palo Alto housewives who do everything their doctor tells them," I suggested, " send them to Mama Barbosa, and see what happens."

"Don't throw away your career," Jonas said dismissively, tossing my progress report down on the table. Today, I know how to answer his challenge. I know now that we were doing what are called "*N* of 1 trials." I know how to build computer models to test theories of healing, and how to talk about the deconstructionist view of reality, which has come to be mainstream thinking in the field of behavioral medicine. But in 1981, when we were asked to present our series of interviews at a teaching conference, all I had was an intuitive sense that our research project was useful.

Joe opened the conference by talking about how Mrs. Machido hadn't understood her diagnosis, how she hadn't filled her prescription and had sought out faith healers instead, and how she'd recovered without our antibiotics. I was next. I told the assembled doctors and students that Mrs. Machido was only one of many—that clinic patients often didn't understand our medicine and didn't follow our instructions. But I also delivered the good news: most of them got better anyway, and of those who didn't, few deteriorated.

Jonas proclaimed the work pseudo-science and the results meaningless. The director of the residency program came away from the conference worried that our study was undermining the clinic. Certainly the study threatened to undermine the prevailing view of doctoring. This presented the residency director with a problem, and Jonas had the solution: my contract should not be renewed. My departure would take time, but it was as inevitable as a witching. At first I wanted to fight it, planning to argue that the decision was racist. But after agonizing over what Jonas had done, I concluded that it was neither racist nor even your garden-variety backstabbing. Jonas was being true to his own beliefs of what could and could not be counted as science.

I hadn't viewed the research as challenging the validity of the clinic. I did think it might be worth reconsidering how medicine was *practiced* at the clinic, in light of what my students discovered. I never thought we should either give up the clinic or deny the lessons we were offered. If one approach wasn't working, why not try another? But the residency director preferred denial to change. He lacked courage. If there was any villain involved in my dismissal, it was he, not Jonas.

Some of the students wanted to fight the decision. Joe came to my office the next afternoon, perched on the edge of his chair, and asked what we were going to do.

I thought back to the pointless conference in Wisconsin, with the two lawyers yammering away. "You're going to continue on in medical school, and I'm going to clean out my office." I couldn't honestly see another way.

CHAPTER SIX

A Good Resident

A
T THE AGE of twenty-seven, I'd come to the end of yet another road. After having abandoned two residencies, I had been all but kicked out of my first academic appointment. My other options were rapidly diminishing. Still, though I'd left my psychiatry residency in Wisconsin, I had left it less from discouragement than from the unrelated controversy over my home birth study. Family practice clearly wasn't going to provide me an opportunity to deal with people as both emotional and spiritual beings, but I still held out hope for the field of psychiatry. By this time I was leery of any realm dominated by doctors, but there was nothing left to try, so I prayed for patience, summoned my courage, and filled out an application for the psychiatry residency program at Mount Sinai, a Jewish hospital in San Francisco. Fortunately I was accepted, and I enrolled the second day of January, in 1982.

My boss at Mount Sinai was a pleasant surprise. Luke was an iconoclast who came to work every day on a large motorcycle, wearing cowboy boots and leather gear over his dress clothes. A brash and successful man in his thirties, Luke had written a popular textbook on the psychiatric interview. Mount Sinai had recruited him to be chief of the hospital's locked adult ward. He advocated a "biopsychosocial" approach to psychiatry, arguing at every opportunity that we needed to do more than lock patients up and pump them full of drugs. Sounding almost like a Native American healer, Luke said we needed to keep track of the whole person in the context of his or her family and culture.

Luke was fierce in his beliefs about mental illness and had a combative style that brought him into immediate conflict with the older psychiatrists. As chief of the ward, he was able to win many of his arguments about what constituted appropriate treatment, but in the process he built up a large corps of enemies.

Luke's flashy dress and hard-charging temperament were consistent with his rural Colorado origins, but was it acceptable in San Francisco? This time out, I was trying to keep as low a profile as possible myself. I was definitely taken by him, though. Before long I had read all his books. Luke was as close to a thought leader as Mount Sinai Hospital, San Francisco, was ever likely to see. He was willing to bang away as long as it took to get a dispute resolved—and resolution according to Luke meant getting people to accept his gospel. It did seem to me he wasted time and energy on unnecessary fights, but I loved his biopsychosocial approach and considered him a kindred spirit. He felt the same way about me, I think. We started at Mount Sinai the same week; a week later, he'd made me his assistant ward chief.

Mount Sinai had a standing contract with the city to receive the steady stream of disturbed and broken people hauled in by the police—in one week, for example, a manic-depressive who had been walking naked through the streets; a schizophrenic who had chained himself to the doors of City Hall, an autographed photo of Allen Ginsberg pinned to his chest; and several suicidal people who were brought to us after being revived in area emergency rooms.

Most psychiatrists practicing at Mount Sinai believed that mental illness was either biological or, following Freud, the result of psychosexual traumas from early childhood. Certain types of mental illness could be treated through psychoanalysis—if the patient had the money and the motivation. Treatment for everyone else—and this was nearly everyone—consisted of a lot of drugs and a little group therapy.

I was glad I had witnessed how Turtle Woman treated Flo's depression back in Wisconsin. The Chippewa woman's deeply personal and humanistic treatment of Flo contrasted starkly with the way psychiatrists at Mount Sinai treated depressed people. Flo would not have been admitted until her depression got so bad she felt suicidal. Then her treatment would have consisted of antidepressant medications and of hours spent sitting by herself on a locked ward. She'd get a few quick interviews with a psychiatrist, who would assume her depression was biological.

Luke's biopsychosocial model was somewhere in between the prevailing psychiatric vision and Turtle Woman's view. According to Luke, the suicidal patients, the naked man wandering down Mission Street, the poet spewing prophecy on the steps of City Hall—these people were performing roles that had been shaped in give-and-take relationships with the other people in their lives. Luke did not doubt that their mental illnesses involved more or less of this or that chemical being released in their brains, but he argued that mental problems often *became* rather than *began* as biological problems. Luke's views and mine were not identical—he placed more emphasis on genetics than I did, for instance, and I thought his model should include a spiritual component—but we agreed on the key point that people's experiences interacted with their biology to produce mental illness. Today that doesn't sound like a radical idea, but as recently as fifteen years ago it was not the mainstream opinion—at least not at Mount Sinai. It was, however, compatible with what I was learning of the shaman's view of mental illness.

When I returned to California I had looked up Grampa Richards and Kosha again. Kosha passed away not long afterward. So while I was working with Luke at Mount Sinai, I was studying mainly with Grampa Richards, making trips to Santa Rosa as often as possible. He told me that people who are crazy have literally lost their way. The Creator made the seven directions so this would not happen. Anywhere you find yourself on earth, you have only to look to the west, the east, the north, and the south, the sky and the earth, and the center, which lies within your heart, and you will know where you are. Of course, being Native American, Grampa Richards placed great importance on the role families play in illness. He knew I was working at a psychiatric hospital, and when I'd tell him about a particularly difficult patient he would always begin by asking questions about the person's family.

I was often tempted to tell Luke about my Cherokee mentor. I hesitated, though, because I thought I'd finally found a place in medicine where I could work comfortably, and I didn't want to jeopardize it. Luke seemed open-minded enough to take shamanism seriously, but I didn't want to take even a small risk of losing his confidence. Eventually I'd share that side of my training with him, I thought—and I think I would have if things had continued to go smoothly for even a year or so.

LUKE'S COMBINATION OF intelligence and stubbornness made him a superb neuropsychiatric evaluator. He did unusually thorough evaluations of incoming patients. He often spent an hour or more in his first session with a patient, and he would have flown into a rage if a management expert tried to force him to see six patients in that time. Sometimes Luke found bits of information in people's biology, psychology, or social lives that would have gone unnoticed in the typical, more superficial admission evaluation. Because of the thoroughness he insisted on, Luke and I were sometimes able to provide a diagnosis that spared the patient from weeks or months, or even a lifetime, of inappropriate treatments.

Our first such success at Mount Sinai came when the neurological service sent us an acutely confused thirty-year-old woman with sudden and unexplainable delirium. In her anguished mental state, the woman was incoherent, but we gathered from her babbling that her complaints included headaches, dizziness, and lack of balance. Unable to identify anything else, the woman's neurologist had diagnosed schizophrenia. Luke and I were skeptical, and held off on the antipsychotic medications schizophrenics were routinely given. Schizophrenia does not usually appear out of the blue in a thirtyish woman who has worked as an engineer, made a happy marriage, and begun successfully raising two children. Luke figured the key to her predicament must be in the "bio"component of his biopsychosocial model. We hit the books and found a rare condition, the Arnold-Chiari malformation, that seemed to fit. Identified almost a century ago, the Arnold-Chiari malformation occurs when the bottom of the brain herniates, or protrudes, through the hole in the skull where the spinal cord descends. We obtained the necessary X-rays to show the condition and then treated the woman with calcium channel blockers to reduce swelling. The woman's coordination and balance improved almost immediately, and her confusion began to clear. Eventually she had surgery that completely cured all her symptoms of mental illness.

Another of our successes was a sixty-year-old woman who came to us with a diagnosis of manic-depressive disease (bipolar disorder). Roberta had become deranged quite suddenly and was found one night walking down a Nob Hill street clad only in a flimsy slip. She was an attorney who had spent her career with the public defender's office, representing the homeless and dispossessed—eccentric behavior for a lawyer, perhaps, but not crazy.

The morning we saw her, Roberta was flailing her arms and legs, inadvertently exposing herself, and talking incessantly and nonsensically. As she paced about the ward, chattering, her arms and legs flying and her hospital robe flapping open, Luke raised the question of how a very proper lawyer could suddenly burst forth as a raging manic-depressive. He called the psychiatrist who had admitted her the night before, and she said she didn't know what was wrong with Roberta, but she'd sure been *acting* like a manic-depressive, and the police didn't want the woman wandering the streets in her underwear. The psychiatrist had no choice but to agree to hold Roberta for seventy-two hours.

We reviewed Roberta's history and found she'd gone to her internist three days earlier because of spasms in her legs. She'd been given a prescription for a strong muscle relaxer. Working from the assumption that the woman was not crazy, we did not have much difficulty figuring out her problem. The *Physicians' Desk Reference* showed that the drug she was taking could in rare cases cause disorientation and other neuropsychiatric symptoms, especially with elderly people. The diagnosis was cinched when we learned that Roberta sometimes took extra doses of medications her doctor prescribed, and that she had a somewhat impaired kidney function—which meant that medications would stay in her body longer than in most other people's.

We stopped her medication, and by the following morning her speech had slowed and her modesty was returning. Roberta left the hospital five days later, deeply embarrassed about the episode, angry with her doctors for having signed her into a psychiatric ward, and greatly relieved that she had not lost her mind.

Six months at Mount Sinai passed quickly. I loved working with Luke to sort out the complexities of mental illness, sometimes pulling the rabbit from the hat and saving seemingly crazy people from standard psychiatric treatments that would have caused a whole new set of problems. Often, though, we could not find a problem as straightforward as a herniated brain or an adverse reaction to medication, and when the key wasn't biological or iatrogenic, we didn't do a whole lot better than anybody else. We tried to make sense of the psychosocial part of people's lives, but we were groping. For many of our patients we couldn't improve much on Mount Sinai time-tested, one-treatment-fits-all strategy: hold them; medicate them; wait until their bizarre behavior abates; send them to an unlocked ward for a period of stabilization; discharge them back to the families and communities in whose bosoms they had gone mad in the first place.

Luke freely acknowledged that we were not helping most of the people who came to us. More than acknowledge it, he insisted on it. He almost rubbed our noses in it. At staff meetings he would interrupt a routine presentation to challenge an attending psychiatrist's quick and easy diagnosis of schizophrenia or manic-depressive illness. Or he would ask a resident if she thought her treatment plan (which inevitably centered around one of our powerful neuropsychiatric drugs) was going to make any significant change in the patient's life.

"We prescribe Thorazine or Haldol or lithium for bizarre behavior as casually as we prescribe antibiotics for bacterial infection," Luke would say. "Isn't chaining yourself to City Hall and reciting passages of *Howl* a more complicated problem than strep throat?"

Some of the other psychiatrists thought Luke was stubbornly playing devil's advocate, whereas in truth he was simply stating the obvious: we didn't know enough about most of our patients to even begin to understand why they were behaving bizarrely, and we had no idea if the therapies we offered them—or more often forced on them—addressed their problems at all.

To his credit, Luke was equally critical of his own ability to help patients. Some of the psychiatrists who bristled at Luke's challenging manner were quite happy to agree with his self-criticism. A few of his residents, ignoring Luke's successes with patients like Roberta, began to grumble that they were being led by a man who bragged about his inability to help his patients.

At the same time that he was irritating the psychiatric staff, Luke was making political enemies in his various battles with the hospital administration. I didn't pay much attention to these battles. As his close assistant, I was guilty by association, but I trusted Luke to take care of the politics while I tried to learn how best to provide care.

ONE FOGGY NIGHT I was called to the seclusion room on the locked ward to see an orange-haired woman named Sylvia Bowers. She was tied spread-eagle to the bed, cursing and writhing and trying to bite any-one who came within range. Eight burly orderlies were jammed into the room, looming over her bed. One was holding a long tube that the night nurse wanted me to insert through Mrs. Bowers's nose and down to her stomach so we could pour some medication into her. On the wall, too high for any patient to reach, was the requisite figure of Jesus on the cross—suffering very much like Sylvia Bowers, who had a parodic halo of her own just then, from the light of the ceiling's single naked bulb.

"You're not gonna put any fuckin' tube down me!" she shouted, arching her back and struggling valiantly against the leather wrist and ankle restraints. "I'll bite your fingers off."

"She will, too," said an orderly who was rubbing his forearm. "She's a biter and a scratcher." He showed me where she'd gouged his arm.

The room stank. The floor was puddled with urine and the bed was smeared with feces. Feces were also splattered on the wall near the door, where Mrs. Bowers had hurled her waste at the orderlies back at the beginning of the battle, before she'd been tied down.

"You know I don't have a choice about giving you medication," I told the woman. It was true—as a resident I had to do as directed. Sylvia was smart enough to have figured that out. She bared her crooked teeth in a snarl and redoubled her efforts to break the restraints.

As she arched and twisted, she swore savagely at me. "You asshole lackey! You come near me with that tube and I swear to God I'll bite your fuckin' fingers off!"

I was feeling pretty sorry for myself just then. I felt like more of a victim than I imagined the patient did. Jesus, I said to myself, realizing what an incredibly absurd thought that was. The idea that I could feel like more of a victim than did a shit-covered mental patient suddenly made me want to laugh. Not at her, for she was a piteous sight—but at myself for having such thoughts. I remembered a psychiatrist and teacher back in Wisconsin who used to say, "The only solution to an absurd situation is to make it funny." I searched for the dumbest, funniest thing I could think of to say.

And that was, "If you bite me, I'll break your leg." Sylvia immediately stopped thrashing and looked at me in astonishment. The orderlies were also struck dumb, and the room was suddenly still.

"You can't break my leg," the woman said with quiet disbelief. She lifted her head off the bed and peered at me quizzically. The orderlies hadn't moved a muscle. The one with the nasogastric tube was still holding it out toward me.

"Anyway, you really don't want me sticking that thing up your nose," I said. "I'm pretty bad at it. Who knows, I might miss and gouge your eye out by mistake." She stared at me, more puzzled than anything else. The truth was, I was about equally afraid of being bitten and of injuring her throat if I had to put the tube in while she struggled. Medically it's a terrible idea to attempt any procedure on a struggling patient.

As the woman stared at me, her outrage grew. "You can't break my leg," she decided, "and I don't even think you're allowed to say something like that."

"Well, are you allowed to say you'll bite my finger off?" I asked, feigning outrage in response.

"I can say any fuckin' thing I want to," she said. "And I can bite off all the goddamn motherfuckin' asshole fingers I want to. I'm a mental patient, for chrissakes, or hadn't you heard? I'm not responsible for my actions. I'm crazy! *Fuuuck-in' craaa-zy!*"

"I'm crazy, too," I told her when the echoes of her curse died away. "I'd have to be crazy to work here. Right? So I'm not responsible for my actions, either. And if you don't take the medication, whatever it is, I'm gonna break both your legs. And if you don't do it soon, maybe I'll break an arm, too, just for good measure. Maybe I'll put a voodoo curse on you and make you vomit for twenty-four hours, maybe I'll make you watch 'Captain Kangaroo' every morning in the day lounge, or worst of all, maybe I really will stuff this stupid tube up your nose."

"You can't do anything to me," Mrs. Bowers proudly announced, "because you're the doctor and I'm the patient, so it would be malpractice."

"Really?"

"I have rights. All patients have rights. And I'm going to exercise those rights."

"Okay," I said with an air of regret, "but it's still Okay for me to break your nose with this tube by accident, as long as I don't break your legs or arms. Thing is, I haven't put one of these into someone in years. I hardly even remember how to do it."

"You're shitting me, aren't you?" She was smiling now, no longer acting crazy.

"Never," I replied, smiling also. I kneeled on the floor beside her, careful to avoid the puddles. "Like George Washington or Sitting Bull, I never tell a lie."

"Like hell."

"Would you believe almost never."

"You lie."

"Okay. A little white one every now and then. Do I still get to break your leg?"

"You do and I'll sue you, for every last dime you've got."

"Done," I said, and put a dime on her cot.

"I really will bite your finger off if you try to put that tube up my nose," Mrs. Bowers said, a little more plaintively now.

"I don't want to put the tube up your nose. But you've got to take the medicine; neither of us has a choice about that."

"Okay," she said, "I'll take it, but not because I need to, only because I have to, Okay?" I sensed her searching for a way to give in with dignity.

"You are only taking it," I told her, "because you have no other choice. Pills or liquid?"

She chose pills. "In case I decide to spit one out at the last minute."

"Don't start. We'll end up having to think up new threats for each other." I sent one orderly to the nursing station for pills, and another for a mop and bucket, and linens, and a fresh nightgown for Mrs. Bowers. Then I reached down to untie her right hand restraint. George, the orderly nearest her, tensed up, ready to spring.

"I'll bite your fingers off!" the woman growled.

"I'll bite off his fingers for you. You're busy. Take your pills. Now. Quick. Before I lose patience and have 'em tie you down so's I can break your legs."

"Fuck you," the orange-haired woman said good-naturedly. Then she threw the pills in her mouth, washed them down with water, and opened her mouth wide to show me she wasn't hiding anything. "Now you can get me a beer, George," she said, smiling, "or maybe some wine." The orderly looked embarrassed for a moment.

"How about a little drink of whiskey?" he croaked.

"I really would have bitten your fingers off if you tried to put that tube up my nose," she said to me.

"I know you would. You seem to be a person who keeps her word."

"Yes, I am," she said proudly. "I need some more water, George. Maybe a Pepsi. I got to get my fat and sassy fighting weight back. You sure are a goddamn crazy doctor, but I like you."

"I'm relieved," I told her. "Maybe you can go back to your room now—if you give me your word you'll behave." Sylvia stood up abruptly on her wobbly legs and walked toward the door. "Now that you know I'll break your legs if you don't behave, I'm sure you'll do what you're told and follow all the rules, and we can get things cleaned up in here in case someone else needs this room." I left the seclusion room with her and escorted her down the hall. She told me I was her favorite doctor and that from then on she would make the nurse call me every night to give her the medicine.

"If I ever come back here again, I'm bringing my nasogastric tube," I told her.

She said she'd be sure to bite my fuckin' fingers off if I did. Then we discussed the San Francisco Giants' prospects that season, after which she disappeared into the women's bathroom to clean herself up.

So WE DOCTORS stumbled along as best we could, given our vast ignorance. I began to think I'd finally found my spot in medicine. I actually enjoyed spending time on the chaotic locked ward, and then on the weekends I wasn't on call I loved visiting Grampa Richards, talking about the broken people of Mount Sinai. Back in the city on Monday mornings, I'd ride to work on the public buses or the BART train over the bay. Every day on Market Street I'd see wretched and confused souls wandering around lost in their own private worlds. Sometimes I'd see people we'd discharged from Mount Sinai, walking around like zombies in medication-induced stupors. We had a long way to go in learning to help these people, but at least we admitted it and were looking for new ideas.

Then one morning in late June I arrived at Mount Sinai to find that Luke had surrendered to pressure to leave. "Ah, hell," I moaned. "How did this happen? What are you gonna do, and what's gonna happen to me?"

"They've already recruited someone to replace me," Luke said.

"Why is this happening?"

"I can't say much," he answered. "We've struck a deal that includes my keeping quiet."

"So basically you can't tell me anything."

"Basically. Politics, Lewis. It's all about politics . . . who you piss off and who you don't. I didn't play the game. You don't play the game either, but maybe it's time to learn. Some of the people who were after me have it in for you too."

"Why?" I whined over the noise of the funky air conditioner he had brought in from home. "Seems to me like those guys'd have something better to do than care about me." Knowing myself, I was going to obsess about this the rest of the day, and all that evening, too. I've had a lifelong terror of authority, probably stemming from my stepfather's beatings. Luke stood, pushed open his office door, and held the heavy gray door for me. I wondered if I had been sitting there in shocked silence so long he had to throw me out—gently, really, but I felt like a dog he was pushing away with his boot.

"I don't know how to be political," I said as I stepped slowly into the doorway.

"Then you'll have to learn, same as me. If you want to be employed in ten years." He smiled—but I didn't see anything to smile about. "You'll find out more at the supervisory meeting. You're a good resident," he said. "You work really hard. But it's time to learn how to fit in."

With that he shut the door. I was numb. Later I would feel the anger of abandonment. And later still I would realize how much heat Luke had been taking for me, protecting me from. When we eventually did have our supervisory meeting, I learned that Luke wasn't really being fired, at least not on paper. An arrangement was being made that included severance pay and relocation expenses.

I wanted Luke to fight his severance, but he'd already lined up a position he preferred anyway, on the faculty at a major medical school back East. He didn't have any incentive to get wrapped up in a nasty legal battle. "Maybe if it was about treatment or diagnosis, or some real psychiatric issue . . ." he said. "But, Lewis, this is about money, and as far as I'm concerned, to hell with it. If they want to call people suicidal or homicidal to fill beds, that's their business. But I won't make it mine. I've already said too much. Forget what I'm telling you."

It seemed to me it *was* about treatment and diagnosis. Luke had refused to follow Mount Sinai's long-standing practice of declaring people dangerous, either to themselves or others. When we established that patients were dangerous, we were accomplishing two important goals: the court would allow us to hold them, and their insurance company, or the federal government, would pay for their treatment. Of course, by calling them dangerous when they really weren't, we began our relationship with a lie. And since I believed that a relationship is integral to the healing process, this struck me as the worst possible way to begin one. The coherent patients knew we'd labeled them dangerous, and they resented it bitterly.

Luke and I agreed that what most of the faculty did—calling people suicidal or homicidal so that Medicaid would pay for their admission—was unethical and probably illegal. I certainly didn't want to be around if Medicaid ever investigated us. But our bosses were confident that such an investigation would never take place, and that they were doing the right thing by buying patients more time and treatment at Mount Sinai.

Luke had come and gone quickly, barely long enough to get his face in the 1982 faculty photo. The reality of how quickly he had gone from welcomed expert to persona non grata was daunting. Luke could have grabbed Mount Sinai's administrators by their necks and pinned them against the wall. I was disappointed that Luke, for all his combativeness, was walking away from such a righteous fight. And if he could get axed so quickly, what was going to happen to me?

LUKE WAS GONE by the end of the week. The following Monday morning the director of the residency program called me into his office to ask about my threat to break Mrs. Bowers's leg. Luke had heard about the incident the morning after it happened, and he had laughed and congratulated me for getting medication in the woman without the nasogastric tube. He criticized the night nurse and the orderlies for letting the situation get so ugly, and that was the end of it. Or so I thought.

Now that Luke was gone, one of the reprimanded orderlies had filed a formal complaint accusing me of brutal and inhumane treatment. The situation was brutal and inhumane when I arrived, I argued, describing the eight orderlies hovering over a woman lying in her own waste. I had a fleeting notion of calling Mrs. Bowers in to defend me, but that was of course impossible. Instead, I told the residency director that I'd seen the woman a number of times since that night, and that we were on friendly terms. Whenever we saw each other we talked about the headlines of the morning *Chronicle* and how the Giants were doing. I told him she said I was her favorite doctor. I should have known better than to say such a thing to a Freudian psychoanalyst.

"Only because you stimulated her masochistic fantasies of self-abuse," he promptly replied. " 'Take your medicine or I'll break your leg'—that's quite a choice."

"That was just to get her attention."

"Oh, it got her attention, Dr. Mehl. Her attending says you awakened her unconscious fantasies of dismemberment and annihilation.

She's now struggling to suppress a fear of doctors, for which you are directly responsible."

If so, she was struggling successfully. When I passed her in the day lounge after the meeting, Mrs. Bowers interrupted a monologue she'd been directing at a catatonic woman and rushed over to me waving the *Chronicle*. "We beat Nolan Ryan last night," she said. "What do you think of that, crazy doctor?"

Whatever she told her attending, I was sure she had been pulling his leg. Sylvia would say anything to get a rise out of someone. She was whip-smart, and could figure out just what buttons to push. Her attending had used her verbal bantering as the evidence he needed to say that I was a bad doctor. I realized the meeting I had just left had very little to do with Sylvia Bowers, or the deeper question I needed to answer—was it right for us to keep her against her will and stuff her with medicine nobody was really sure she needed? That question would never be addressed in this hospital, not in the climate that prevailed with Luke gone.

Things got steadily worse for me at Mount Sinai. No longer the assistant ward chief, I was now assigned to the locked adolescent ward, where I was introduced to the theory that it was a patient's fault if we weren't able to help. It was Dr. Mann, the director *of adolescent services* and a newly graduated resident, who proposed it. Jackie was his twenty-three-year-old patient, a diabetic whose illness had been poorly controlled since it was diagnosed when she was twelve years old. Over the years she had been hospitalized repeatedly for a host of problems, including gastroparesis (protracted and uncontrollable vomiting caused by diabetic-related disorders of the stomach and esophagus) and diabetic ketoacidosis (blood sugar elevations so severe they sent her into a coma). She'd also been treated off and on for bulimia. Jackie came to us in a state of profound regression, urinating on herself and defecating in her bed. Dr. Mann diagnosed depression.

I met Jackie on her first afternoon on the adolescent ward, a Friday. Her psychiatric treatment would not begin in earnest until the following Monday. Over the weekend we planned to monitor her eating and adjust her insulin in order to stabilize her blood sugar. Dr. Mann was scheduled to see Jackie Monday morning, after I presented her case to him.

This Friday afternoon was quiet on the adolescent ward, and I was able to sit with Jackie for an hour in the day lounge, listening to her litany of complaints. These included uncontrollable vomiting, perpetual nausea, headache, back pain, and intermittent fever. Jackie admitted to feeling lousy and demoralized. She described constant anxiety, irritability, and fatigue. But she adamantly denied being depressed. I can remember how deep and dark and how terribly sad her eyes looked. I am still haunted by her sadness.

That afternoon I did imagery work with her. Imagery is close kin to visualization and hypnotic storytelling. The therapist uses mental images (suggested sometimes by the patient, sometimes by the therapist) to reduce anxiety, bypass resistance, or prevent obsessive defenses from thwarting therapy. Imagery can be used both in general psychotherapy and with psychotic clients. It has also been shown to be useful in treating physical illnesses.

I didn't tell her I was using imagery; I just chatted with her about her symptoms at first. I asked how she felt about being committed again.

"Are you kidding? It's a *joyful* experience, really. Puh-leaze. I can't believe they put me on the adolescent ward. Do I look like an adolescent to you?"

"It says here you're twenty-three."

"You can *read* that chart. *Good* for you. Every doctor I've ever met is an idiot. Present company included. Not that I mean to offend you," she said.

"You didn't," I assured her. "You remind me of a Hopi friend I had at Stanford. He grew up in Shongopovi Village on Second Mesa on the Hopi reservation in northern Arizona."

"Good for him."

"He was about twenty-one then, younger than you are now. He stayed with me one Thanksgiving—he didn't have the money to go home and didn't want to stay in an empty dorm. Too depressing."

"I'm not depressed."

"Yeah, but I think my friend was, a little. So each night he entertained me and my kids with Hopi stories. It's like Indian television, you know, what else is there to do at night but sit around the fire and tell stories? So one of his stories was about the first Hopi leader and his battle with the Spirit of War and Death, whom they called Matsu'ua."

Jackie didn't look at me, but for the first time she didn't answer my words with sarcasm, so I knew I had earned the right to continue.

The people had been forced to migrate for lack of food and water. They had been starving. I guess you know what that's like better than I do, Jackie. The Leader went ahead to scout out new land; his people were supposed to follow him. When they did not appear at the appointed time and place, he had to backtrack to look for them. He found them trapped on a mesa, surrounded by the Spirit of War and Death. They were cowering on top and would not come down. They were terrified and unwilling to descend, because of the terrible spirit, Matsu'ua, who ran circles around the mesa each night. He had devoured the few people who tried to escape starvation in their mesa prison. When the Leader found them, he discovered a way to sneak past Matsu'ua up onto the mesa to his people. Their food was gone and they were near death. So the Leader offered to go down and confront the oppressor on their behalf.

I was offering myself as the leader, the one who could venture out with Jackie to defeat the evil that had been encircling her. At least, this was my intention; I wanted her to take away an unconscious sense of optimism about working with me.

The Leader went to meet Matsu'ua. That awful spirit came when the Leader challenged him to do so. And, Jackie, he was something terrible to look at. He had a face, but no skin—only clotted blood and raw bloody muscle, held together by ligaments. But the Leader was fearless. He said, "My people live in peace. We have no wish to live in your service. We want you to go back where you come from. If you fight me I will defeat you."

With a roar Matsu'ua rushed the Leader. And they wrestled a long time. But because the Leader was so strong, and so young—just about your age, Jackie—the Leader overcame Matsu'ua. And you know what that spirit did next? He pulled off his bloody head, which was only a mask, to reveal a young and noble face.

This young man said to the Leader, "You have done well. You have demonstrated your courage. I would have killed your whole tribe if none had the courage to face me. I was angry with your people because they have been denying my existence."

The Leader promised Matsu'ua that henceforward his people would honor the Spirit of War and Death properly. A covenant was made with the people, that Matsu'ua would no longer stalk them and entrap them, as long as they would honor death with a shrine and make prayers at Matsu'ua's altar.

The metaphor of the story fit Jackie's situation well. She was starving from the combination of bulimia and gastroparesis. The spirit of death was clearly stalking her. She was trapped in the prison of her own fear of living. I wanted to communicate to Jackie (indirectly, via metaphor, for now) that I could work with her to save her from Matsu'ua's jaws, and that we could do that by respecting and acknowledging her diabetes, instead of pretending it didn't exist.

Jackie talked freely after the story. After we talked for about an hour I told her I was on call for the weekend and asked if she'd like to talk again. She said she would, and we met again on Saturday afternoon and Sunday morning.

Jackie's treatment began first thing Monday morning. Dr. Mann went to her room and pulled a chair next to the bed, where she lay grimacing and holding her stomach. He asked how she was feeling, and Jackie said, "Horrible. Same as every morning."

"Horrible in what way?" Dr. Mann asked.

"Don't you guys talk to each other?" she asked. "I feel shitty this morning in exactly the same way I felt shitty yesterday morning and the morning before that. He was on duty this weekend." She pointed to me. "Ask him."

Dr. Mann raised his eyebrows, a little surprised that I'd bothered talking to Jackie over the weekend, after the first interview. He told Jackie I'd given him a report on her physical discomfort, but he was really there to find out how she was feeling in a larger sense.

"I don't have a larger sense," Jackie said. "All I have is an overpowering urge to throw up. So unless you can help me with that, why don't you just go away."

"Well, Jackie," Dr. Mann told her, "we're not here to help you with your nausea, but we can help you with your feelings of depression."

"You can't help me with feelings of depression if I don't have them," Jackie said. "Just give me a plastic bag to vomit into."

They went around in circles for a while. Then Dr. Mann switched tacks and asked what she did with her feelings of anger.

"What difference does it make to you what I do with my anger?" Jackie shouted. "What business is it of yours? Why don't you just move me back to the west wing, where someone knows something about diabetes? That's the only thing wrong with me."

Dr. Mann explained the importance of dealing appropriately with anger. "The real source of anger has to be identified, not suppressed or misdirected. I don't think you're really angry at me. And I don't want you to turn your anger against yourself. Anger turned inward is depression."

"I'm not depressed!" Jackie snapped. "I just feel goddamn terrible. It's not in my head; it's diabetes. Any real doctor would know that. You are such an asshole to come in here talking to me like this when I'm sick. Wanna know what my real feeling is? My feeling is I'm going to throw up. So leave me alone."

"Jackie—" Dr. Mann spread his hands, appealing to her to be reasonable. Jackie rolled over and vomited on his shoes.

"Fuck you and get out of my room," Jackie said, rolling back toward the wall.

Dr. Mann saw Jackie every morning that week and the next. Their conversations consisted of shorter and shorter arguments over whether or not she was depressed, until she stopped talking to him altogether. And because I had to accompany him, I was "as useless as he is," Jackie said. We never talked again as freely as we had the first three days she was in the hospital.

Dr. Mann was unfazed by Jackie's sullen silence. It was important, he explained to the residents, that he continue to confront her. Jackie's acknowledging that she was depressed would be her first step toward dealing with the emotional problems that actually preceded her diabetes. I agreed with Dr. Mann that she was depressed, but I could see no hope of getting her to acknowledge it, and no hope of helping her until we let it go. I wondered what would happen if we looked instead for an approach so nonthreatening, so indirect, that Jackie could not see anything to fight. Why not set aside the question of depression and just begin wherever Jackie was comfortable beginning? I suggested this to Dr. Mann, but he insisted that if we didn't confront Jackie we were wasting her time and ours. I didn't argue with him, but I did note the irony: having been reprimanded for confronting Mrs. Bowers, I was now scolded for wanting to avoid confrontation with Jackie.

Dr. Mann continued to go to Jackie's room every morning, usually with me or one of the other residents in tow, but soon Jackie would not even acknowledge our presence. The battle of wills lasted a few weeks before Jackie decided to break the stalemate and prove that her problem was deteriorating diabetes and not depression. One Sunday night, Jackie figured out how to put herself into an insulin coma. I still don't know precisely how she did it, but she was comatose by Monday morning. Her blood glucose was twenty—very low. I had to inject a 50 percent glucose solution directly into her internal jugular vein, which brought her back, barely.

So we lost the power struggle and Jackie "won." She succeeded in getting herself transferred off the adolescent ward and out of Dr. Mann's care. Her victory had almost cost her her life. But she was willing to pay the price; being right was more important to her than being alive. Dr. Mann was satisfied he had done everything in his power to help his patient. Her treatment failed, he told an assembly of residents during rounds, because she refused to participate in it. Listening to Dr. Mann's discussion of Jackie made me miss Luke. He might not have known how to help this angry young woman, but he would never have blamed her for being the one to fail. He would have acknowledged that confronting her didn't work, and at least considered a different approach.

@ @ @

NOT ONLY DID WE fail with patients who resisted treatment, we were often unable to help people who had sought us out. At the same time as our futile struggle with Jackie was going on, I admitted a San Francisco State student named Kristin. She was suicidal and had been cutting her arms. This was Kristin's third stay with us, and her twenty-second psychiatric hospitalization in ten years. Already, at the age of twenty-four, Kristin was a textbook of failed treatments. The psychiatrist's tool kit includes four major categories of drugs—antianxiety drugs called benzodiazepines, antidepressants, antipsychotics, and mood stabilizers—and Kristin had tried them all. She'd been treated with various combinations of Klonopin, Valium, Xanax, Librium, Ativan, Loxapine, Haldol, Mellaril, Pamelor, Lithium, valproic acid, Tegretol, Elavil, Zoloft, Parnate, and Nardil. She'd also slogged through sporadic sessions of group and individual psychotherapy.

Nothing helped, and Kristin kept cutting herself. She told me she wasn't really trying to kill herself—"not yet, anyway." What she told me next was chilling: she cut herself to get readmitted when she got too lonely. She thought our therapies and drugs and diagnoses were a waste of time, but she was comforted by the other patients she found on psychiatric wards. Even more than college students, psychiatric patients were willing to stay up all night with her, talking over the deepest existential issues: the meaning of life, its value, the various ways it could be ended, and the reasons for deciding to end it or continue on. Kristin was asking the right questions, the ones Grampa Richards had told me were important: Who are you? Where did you come from? Why are you here? Anyone who can answer those three key questions will be well, he promised. But Kristin was making no progress because she didn't know how to look beyond the questions for answers.

And we weren't prepared to help her. As psychiatrists, we didn't believe that confusion about the meaning of life had anything to do with mental illness. We saw Kristin's philosophizing as a type of defense we called intellectualization. We assumed she engaged in metaphysical musing to distract herself from some real problem, which if not biological was undoubtedly some long-repressed emotional or psychic injury. But since we couldn't find anything biologically wrong with her, and we couldn't identify any repressed trauma, we had no idea how to help her. By her third admission her treatment plan was being written by reflex. We scanned our list of drugs and therapy groups, assigned her something in a different dosage than she'd tried before, and moved on to more interesting patients, knowing perfectly well that nothing we had to offer would make any difference to Kristin's life.

Before delving into psychiatry, I had expected its theories to be grounded in the mysteries of the mind and spirit. But modern psychiatry can just as well be called psychopharmacology. It's no surprise that drugs are the only reasonable choice to psychiatric professionals, when most are incredibly pessimistic about the capacity of human beings to change. Also, not coincidentally, their fatalism leads many psychiatric professionals to overuse drugs themselves.

We live in a world without fixed points of view. It is Einstein's legacy; there is no longer any absolute reference point from which to view anything. Like the postmodern literature critic, who does not believe that any story has a set message, or structure, or even author, we are postmoderns who can see no intrinsic point to life. Like the academic who believes that stories by themselves don't mean anything, that they are written only by being read, we postmoderns look at life and see something essentially meaningless, something that we pretend has meaning in order to be comfortable.

This is of course a discouraging and depressing way to go about life.

The postmodern view has much in common with the shamanic view. For most people, these views inspire nihilistic despair; for a few, if we agree with Nietzsche, they inspire artistic brilliance and creativity beyond bounds. Few are happy living according to the postmodern stance of a world without absolute references. This position works for a shaman, however, because he is a rarity in the context of a traditional society. The majority of Native people live with a structured set of ideas, within which life is simple and meaning is rather fixed and concrete. The shaman lives in a different world from his people—this is what gives him a clear vision of what to do for those who are stuck somewhere in their lives.

The shaman specializes in finding meaning by venturing outside its borders into chaos and meaninglessnes. Paradoxically, the venture is possible only because of the strong faith the shaman has in what is true, because of the traditions, teachings, and tools that aid in his spiritual journey. In his personal life, the shaman reverts to the premodern stance, finding comfort in the old ways, being surrounded by rituals he finds to be meaning-*full*.

The depressed person, or the person suffering from psychotic disorders of the self, is suffering from a lack of absolute reference points. Without limits or boundaries, emotion becomes unbearable—it is out of control. Few are strong enough to survive without reference points. Those of us who try suffer from a loss of meaning, or loss of world, or loss of self. We look at the world and see nothing there. Even among the few artists who can make something out of chaos, there are many who destroy themselves. We need to either return to the premodern beliefs or adopt the way of the shaman and create meaning out of nothing. When a shaman finds a psychiatric patient who has no world, who sees no meaning, she says, "Well, Okay then, let's make up a new world for you. Let's create a world that you can enjoy."

If I were to work with Kristin today, I would no longer be afraid to meet the challenge she was presenting. I was too shy then, worried that the attending would see it as inappropriate if I tried to help Kristin to a world view she could live with, and learn to contain her emotion. Today when I am able to help people heal themselves, it is often because I have been able to do one thing: coax them back to a view of life where their soul exists. Where there are forces with agency and will overseeing and guiding life on earth. Where the absolute reference point is that our lives are purposeful.

Finding the soul and connecting with other souls, even spirits, with whom we can enter into a respectful relationship can have a powerful comforting effect on those who suffer deeply. Such external agencies— "guardian angels," as many seem inclined to call them these days—can assuage our pain. Finding direction means recognizing that life actually has a purpose. Once we believe that it does, then we have it in our power to heal ourselves. To me that is proof enough that our lives are meaningful.

I HAD LEARNED to keep my doubts to myself until about three months after Luke's departure, when Dr. Mann sent me to court. I was to testify in a commitment proceeding for a fourteen-year-old boy who was repeatedly running away from home, getting in trouble at school, taking drugs, and stealing. Dr. Mann and the boy's parents wanted him committed for a long stay on the locked adolescent ward. The family had good insurance that would pay for a six-month stay, and the boy clearly needed help. But Xavier didn't want our help, and we couldn't hold him against his will unless he was dangerous to himself or others.

From the moment I learned I was expected at the court hearing, I felt despondent. In some respects, like the traditional Indians on an isolated reservation, I was overwhelmed by the inexplicable, irresolvable demands of modern society. If I displeased Dr. Mann, I was in danger of being terminated from the residency. If I lied in court while under oath, I ran the risk of losing what little self-esteem I had—the self-esteem that came from always trying to "do right," as Archie had taught me.

Preparing for the hearing was like preparing for a funeral: mine. I was losing my bearings, having been cast adrift by Luke in a sea of conflicting theoretical models and frameworks. I felt powerless, lacking any significant impact on any situation I encountered. Furthermore, I had come to doubt that our treatments were always superior to no treatment at all. Should I tell the truth to the judge, even if it did get me fired, even if Xavier lost his opportunity to be locked away from his demons?

When I heard my name called in the courtroom, I knew what I must do. I prayed continuously to the ancestors as I made my way to the witness chair, wanting desperately to be receptive to their universal wisdom as a means of transcending my dread. The judge asked me if Xavier was suicidal or homicidal. I told him that Xavier had poor judgment and was in continual conflict with his peers, parents, teachers, and the law.

"But is he suicidal?" the judge asked. I said no. The judge ordered Xavier released. Mount Sinai lost the admission, and Dr. Mann lost confidence in me.

"That boy needed hospitalization, Lewis," Dr. Mann said that evening in his office.

"He wasn't suicidal," I said, "even if he did need treatment."

"He takes whopping doses of street drugs," Dr. Mann said. "That's at least a serious disregard for his personal safety, if not evidence of inner turmoil. Don't you think a disturbance as severe as that could lead him to kill himself?"

"I told the judge that he had lousy judgment," I said, "and that he was abusing drugs. But I couldn't tell him Xavier is suicidal when he's not."

"He needs treatment, doesn't he?" Dr. Mann snapped. With effort, he adopted a gentler tone. "Look, Lewis, we're trying to help this kid. We didn't snatch him off the street. His parents brought him to us because they can't handle him. The boy needs help, don't you think?"

"He absolutely needs help," I agreed.

"Well, the only way to help him," Dr. Mann offered pedantically, "is to hold on to him for a while. Sometimes you have to lie to do right by someone."

"I just couldn't lie under oath."

"You know," Dr. Mann said, his patience draining away and his voice rising, "we're fighting to do the right thing for people. To do the right thing, we have to go to battle now and then. And when we do, I can't send you because you're a loose cannon and I don't know which direction you're going to shoot. How can I deal with parents and judges and crazy kids when I don't know from one case to the next whose side you're on?"

Sweat was glistening on his forehead when he finished his tirade. He wasn't really looking for answers from me, so we ended the meeting without resolving anything. As I passed through the adolescent ward, I saw that Jackie was back, sitting in the same chair she'd sat in on her first weekend, when she was still talking. Her pale cheeks were flushed and her eyes red, as if she'd been crying. She had recovered from the esophageal bleeding caused by her incessant vomiting and had been transferred back to us against her will. I said hello and she rasped, "Fuck you and go to hell."

When I left the hospital that evening I imagine I was no happier than Jackie. The evening was hot for San Francisco. No breeze, no fog. I got in my compact car thinking about Dr. Mann's argument. In the long run, maybe it would be justifiable to hospitalize people against their wishes or bill insurance companies for nonexistent suicidal tendencies—if those deceptions allowed us to help people. But we weren't helping people very much, so we had no Machiavellian justification for massaging the system. Of course nobody admitted that. Why be honest with ourselves, when we weren't with judges or insurance companies or patients?

I passed children from the Western Addition spraying themselves with garden hoses in front of ramshackle tenements. The buzz of city traffic sounded in my ears. The successful residents were the ones who played the game, smiled, and did what they were told—making up progress notes each morning, detailing how the patients were still suicidal, homicidal, or gravely disabled. Why should they consider new methods of treatment when they were so busy denying that the old ones were failing? There was no reward for risking saying something off the wall to a violent patient, or trying imagery on an angry one, when everyone else assured themselves that our methods were sound—whether they worked or not. I just didn't think I had it in me to be a good resident any longer, at least not a well-behaved one.

Children in diapers were running along the sidewalk. I feared for their safety. One false move and they would be in the street in front of cars speeding toward the 101 Freeway. I was starting to agree with my wife's opinion of late, that I was a failure. The places where I had succeeded were invisible to the modern world. I had been developing healing skills, studying Native American spirituality, witnessing miracles. I felt proud to be a part of changing people's lives. But my awkward combination of idealism and stubbornness seemed to prevent me from finishing a residency.

I came up fast behind a flatbed truck, not noticing that it had stopped for a red light. I stamped on the brake and in the few sickening seconds it took to skid into the truck I thought my life was over. I braced for the impact, and a moment later the windshield burst and something shiny flashed past my head. I don't remember the crash that followed, but I remember shortly afterward sitting behind the wheel looking at the crushed hood, the billows of steam rising from the engine, and the shattered windshield. I ran my hand over the shiny metal beam that had punched through the windshield, past my head to the backseat, where it was embedded in the rear seat cushion.

According to the Native American belief system, there are no accidents. Everything has a cause, and everything happens for a reason—usually a very personal one. Later that night, as I lay in a hot tub soaking my bruises—miraculously my only injuries—I thought again about the story Archie told about the ship captain. The beam that narrowly missed killing me was a warning. I was fortunate to be alive, and doubly fortunate to be unhurt, but I wasn't out of danger. The stress of being where I was not meant to be was draining my spirit and making me accident-prone. My determination to finish a residency and find a faculty position had passed from selfless dedication through stubbornness and into pig-headed resolve. I was only one year away from finishing my residency, but I had already learned that I did not belong at Mount Sinai.

I'd been telling myself that I was sticking it out for the sake of a larger good, but maybe I was only collecting credentials so I could feel legitimate. Legitimate—even as I thought the word, I recognized what I had been trying to do: give myself a legitimacy my mother had been unable to provide. My job was to learn to be a healer, and that would have to be enough. If, in the process, I changed anyone else's view of medicine, good. If not, okay. In the morning I took the BART train in to Mount Sinai and resigned. I had walked to the end of the family medicine and psychiatry paths. I had stubbornly continued on a quest for legitimacy so against my nature that it had almost killed me. Now I had been given another chance. Now it was time now to walk the good red road.

CHAPTER SEVEN

The Sacred Fire

I N 1984 I was invited to a conference on Native American medicine in Tucson, Arizona. Ed, the conference organizer, was an Apache medicine man working at Tucson's Catholic hospital. He scheduled me to talk about how Native American philosophy can be integrated into conventional medical practice. I would be on a panel with two others; each panelist was to speak for forty minutes.

In January of 1983, not long after I left Mount Sinai, Grampa Richards died. I had intended to spend more time with him. After his death, unsure of how to find another healer to study with, I concentrated for a while on other things. I spent my workday hours in a postdoctoral fellowship at Berkeley, earning my psychologist's license; I also worked some weekends in the emergency rooms of Sacramento, Woodland, and Davis hospitals. That left me with little time to spend on the new path I had chosen. The conference would be, I hoped, a turning point.

Having taken clients to medicine people for years, I wanted to learn how to lead ceremonies myself. I had to choose a teacher carefully. Many New Agers were leading "Indian" ceremonies they had invented themselves, but this approach was not what I was interested in. The customs I hoped to master had remained essentially unchanged for hundreds of years. When I told Ed that all the teachers I had known had passed on to the spirit world, he assured me I would find a teacher at the conference. He believed the spirits worked in that manner. If I put out a sincere request for help and kept my ears open for the spirits' advice, a teacher would be waiting for me.

I was apprehensive about speaking at the conference. I still felt inferior about being a half-breed, and my skin seemed conspicuously light in

Tucson, among darker-skinned Arizona Indians. I was so nervous I was shaking when I got up to give my talk. Later, Ed told me I had been very inspiring, but I don't remember a word I said. I do remember the relief I felt afterward, to look up and see people clapping and know I was done.

After the applause, I turned to leave the podium. I tripped on a microphone cord and landed in the lap of Marilyn Youngbird, one of the other speakers, an Arikara-Hidatsa medicine woman. Ed made a joke I didn't hear; everyone laughed. My face flushed red. Marilyn told our audience the accident meant we would be seeing more of each other. She invited me to give her a call when I got back to Berkeley (she lived in Santa Cruz). Then she got up to give her talk, about the sacredness of women, givers of life.

When I returned from Tucson, I did call Marilyn. I had gone to Tucson looking for a teacher and I literally fell in one's lap. The spirits couldn't get much more direct than that (however embarrassing their sense of humor was for me). Marilyn bade me to come see her in Santa Cruz.

Marilyn, born in 1939, was raised in a traditional Arikara village in North Dakota. The fact that she lived through childhood at all was something of a miracle: she had a heart condition that left her paralyzed and hospitalized by the age of nine. Her doctors told her parents that she was unlikely to live very long. That's when Marilyn's grandmother, a medicine woman, stepped in. Her prayers, and the loving care of an Arikara nurse (one of the first of her tribe to earn a degree in nursing), made the difference. Marilyn walked out of the hospital on her own within a few months.

By the time she turned thirteen, she was completely well. Her father sent her to a boarding school so she might learn the ways of the Anglos. He wanted her to be comfortable living in both worlds. Marilyn's father was a strong believer in maintaining open lines of communication between the Native American and Anglo cultures. He passed those values on to his daughter. By the early 1970s Marilyn was the commissioner of Indian affairs for the state of Colorado. She established a forum for her people, and the people of other tribes, to air their particular concerns with the state and federal governments.

Marilyn views her own cure as proof of how well Western and traditional medicines can work together. Since she believes her cure was due to a combination of scientific medicine and the power of traditional prayer, she has made it her life's work to promote communication between the two disciplines.

Like Marilyn's beloved nurse, I knew something of both kinds of medicine. At any rate, we got along well. After several months of getting to know Marilyn, I brought her a patient. She resolved to teach me how to lead a sweat lodge ceremony in the traditional Lakota style. She had learned the ceremony from Wallace Black Elk, a relative of the man whose biography is the subject of the book *Black Elk Speaks*. The first lesson for me was in tending the sacred fire used to heat the stones for a lodge; when Marilyn decided to hold one for my patient, she named me firekeeper.

The patient's name was Homer, and he was a retired engineer. He had prostate cancer, and it had metastasized (spread). He was trying everything he knew to treat his illness, including alternative healing. We had been working together using hypnosis in the office, and I had gradually introduced the Native American world view. Homer was intrigued. Marilyn met with him several times, practicing her own brand of hypnosis. I attended those sessions as an observer. Like any medicine woman, she was making her own assessment, her own diagnosis of what was going on with Homer. When she was satisfied, we planned his ceremony.

The night of the sweat was cold, clear, and dark. Oak trees leaned over the path to the lodge, their shadows commingling, their leaves blocking the light from the house. The wind whispered through the dark night of the new moon, rustling branches outside the circle of light cast by the fire. I was far enough along in learning to be firekeeper that Marilyn left me alone with the task. Trees shivered in the cold, rubbing their dry leaves together for warmth. The night was full of the sounds not only of foraging animals but also of deeper, more primordial grunts and gurgles. Each sound heightened my awareness of the powers the night held. Terror welled up as my childhood fear of darkness returned. An oak tree's dark, tangled leaves were dancing in the updrafts from the fire.

The fire prescribed my orbit. Within its circle of light I felt safe; outside it I felt terribly exposed. I tried to calm myself, releasing my fears with a sigh, reminding myself that many more spirits would come that night, and they would come for the good of us all. I remembered Grampa Richards saying, "Good is always more powerful than evil. Just remember, when you are scared, call upon the Creator. Ask for his help and you'll be fine no matter what's out there."

I called upon the Creator as I built the fire. I remembered what Marilyn told me, that every thought is a prayer. I prayed for the spirits' help as the fire grew higher and hotter.

I prayed, too, for Homer. He had attended his first sweat lodge one month earlier. That had been a group lodge, held during the day, and not dedicated to Homer. It was after that first lodge, as Marilyn listened and wove a horsehair blanket, that Homer asked her for a personal healing ceremony. He told her the spirits of loved ones who were no longer alive had come to him in the afternoon's lodge. This was at once thrilling and frightening; he wasn't sure what it meant. Continuing to weave, Marilyn told him she would do the lodge, but with only four people, one for each of the directions. After Marilyn, myself, and Homer, that left one other person—he chose his daughter to make the circle complete.

I was startled by the call of a hoot owl. I took a deep breath and returned to the fire, which I had to keep burning strong in the four directions. Each direction's spirit has its own color and meaning. North means strength, and its color is red; south, compassion, is white; east, vision, is yellow; and west is black, because it means fear. If I let the fire take its own course, the experience of the lodge would be offset according to the fire's imbalance: too much fire in the compassionate south would make for too mild a lodge; a western fire boded an almost unbearably hot, fearful lodge.

Right now the wind was blowing steadily from the east, so the eastern side of the fire burned most intensely. The wood was starting to glow bright red. The Spotted Eagle Nation brings us vision and alertness from the east tonight, I thought to myself. But the western side needs bolstering, to burn away the fears we'll carry into the lodge. I waved a blanket to move the wind through the fire and encourage the western flames.

I smiled as I thought of the typical Lakota logic, whereby the Four Directions song we would be singing later that night actually includes three directions beyond north, south, east, and west. There is also sky (up), which is blue and means protection; earth (down), which is green and healing; and center, the direction from which all relationship proceeds. Because all colors are related to center, no one color can signify it.

The eyes of the night were upon me, the eyes that come when the sun goes down and humans retire indoors. Science hides in the light of the library. When the doors close and light is extinguished, science is gone. Magic and nature enter through the cracks in the door, seeping into the rational volumes, flowing over the factual tomes that try to explain away their existence. There are eyes in the night which are denied existence by the modern scientific world. These eyes watch, assess, guide, cajole, and encourage. The spirits behind them lead us through the darkness back to the dawn.

The silence between noises is night's most profound offering. Between the rustling of the branches and the creak of tree limbs, between silence and sound, is the tension of flesh and spirit. Portals to other worlds lie within that tension, portals that science is terrified to imagine but that native peoples have known for centuries.

A tremendous crack sounded behind me. I jumped up, wanting to look. I could feel the fear welling up inside. Did I doubt the power of the fire to protect me? Scenes from old werewolf movies replayed themselves in my mind. Always there was a desire to call out and warn the character of what was in store. Voices in my own head were warning, *Look around! Quick! See what's threatening you before it's too late!* I calmed myself. I did not look around. I prayed again for help in calming my nerves and trusting in the power of Nature, within me and outside me.

I thought of the Dinehs I had met in Chinle, Arizona, after Ed's conference, and of the Coyote-Way ceremony I had the honor to participate in. (Their tribe has historically been known as the Navajo, but Dineh—"the people"—is what they call themselves.) They sang the same song over and over while a fire was lit, until it was burning pure and sacred, suitable for the purification of all who took part in the ceremony. I began singing a Dineh tune, the First Morning, Fire-Making Song, hoping no ancient Lakota or Dineh spirits would be offended that I was mixing the practices of two cultures. I'm sure I misused the Dineh language, but the song sounded pretty to me and I was comforted.

I knelt by the crackling fire, holding Homer's image in mind. "Remember," Marilyn liked to remind me, "the greatest gift you have been given is freedom, and your greatest freedom is in choosing your own thoughts, words, and actions." With my thoughts I dedicated the lodge to Homer's healing. Silently I prayed for his wellness, for his sake and the sake of his children. His only brother had died in the past year, shortly after his twin sisters. The recent deaths frightened Homer, and demoralized him. But their spirits had come to him in last month's group lodge, I was sure, to encourage him to fight his cancer. I asked the night for help. I called upon the spirits of the beautiful Santa Cruz woods, so tame by daylight and so powerful by night. Gazing at the stars, I asked them too to lend us their energy. "Under the two rising stars I bring these to you." These were the words of a prayer Marilyn had taught me to say as I made an offering to the evening stars. "Beautiful tobacco I bring to you," I said as I threw on the fire some dried flowers that my new Dineh friends had brought me.

I also prayed for myself. Homer wasn't alone tonight in needing help. I needed the strength, courage, and endurance of the spirit of the north. It was a time of great uncertainty for me. I wanted my own healing. I pocketed my folded glasses and stared intently at the fire.

Not long after Grampa Richards died, Ellen and I had separated. I continued to take care of the children at home, cooking them dinner and helping them with their homework (Ellen saw her clients mostly in the evening). I was relieved to be free of the tensions with Ellen but concerned about maintaining my relationship with my children.

That night, by the fire, I prayed for help in releasing whatever bitterness I still felt toward Ellen. And for help in releasing my fear of not making enough money because of my lack of credentials. I swallowed hard. I tossed some more of the white-blossomed Dineh tobacco onto the fire. I prayed that any pain our separation had caused my children be transformed into health and happiness. I gave thanks for my teachers, for the beautiful spirits of my children, and for the abundance that I still had. I did my best to be altruistic and pray for Ellen's happiness. And I prayed to the north for the strength I would need in the upcoming months of transition in my life.

Before the Dineh's Coyote-Way ceremony, we had made reed prayer sticks as offerings to different spirits. These were for the spirits to smoke. We cut four-inch sections of common reeds. We placed pollen inside these reed sticks, then tobacco, then plugged the ends with a paste made of water and corn pollen. We painted the sticks according to whichever direction they were intended to signify. Finally, each stick was "lighted" by touching a quartz crystal to its tip.

Inside the house, Marilyn, Homer, and his daughter were making prayer ties, the Lakota version of the Dineh prayer sticks. Prayer ties are made from one-inch-square pieces of cloth, tied onto a cotton string. Six colors may be used for the ties: red, white, yellow, black, blue, and green, the colors of every direction except center. Earlier, Marilyn had chosen the colors to be used, and now she and her charges placed tobacco on each piece of cloth, folded it up, and tied it on a string. A finished string of prayer ties can hold as many as 405 of these "dancing robes" for spirits to come and sit inside, the better to hear our prayers.

I watched the shadows of flickering tongues of fire on the ground beneath me. A tall redwood creaked. Some of its branches hung close to the rising sparks. I watched carefully to make sure the fire did not endanger the overhanging tree branches. Water was nearby if I needed it.

More and more birds congregated around the fire. I thanked one for coming. I found myself speaking out loud to the redwood the birds rested in. "Thank you, tree," I said. "Thank you for your life, thank you for the life of your brothers who burn to heat our stones. Thank you, stone people, for taking the heat into your bodies to help us heal. And thank all of you spirits for coming."

As my inner awareness was opening, I was overwhelmed by the consciousness of the spirits around the fire. I stared off into the trees, where more consciousness waited in the darkness the flames could not reach. I lit a cigar and blew smoke toward the fire, excitedly anticipating the night's events.

The fire was hot enough. It seared my face as I bent close to prod the logs with the pitchfork and rearrange them side by side. This was to provide a platform for the stone people. Wood sparks worried me as they lifted skyward, until they extinguished themselves like so many shooting stars. I laid the platform east to west. I was careful that the directions were properly acknowledged. By the time I had finished, I was sweating profusely. I stepped away from the intense heat to rest before laying down the stones. When the heat had passed, I chose the largest, roundest stone and placed it on the west side of the log platform.

"Help us with our fears," I said to the stone. "Help Homer to be well."

I picked a second stone and stepped back from the heat again for a moment. I carefully placed this stone on the platform to the north.

"Help us to have strength, courage, and endurance. Help Homer to use his strength to withstand this lodge. Help him to find the healing that he seeks."

I placed the third stone to the east, asking for help with alertness and vision. The fourth stone went to the south, honoring love and compassion. The fifth stone was for the sky; the sixth, for the earth; and the seventh, for all our relations. For all beings are related, sharing one mother, the earth.

When these stones had been placed upon the platform, I stepped back to rest. Marilyn had received guidance that twenty-eight stones were to be used. I stacked the rest of the stones upon the first seven in as compact a formation as possible. Then I built a tipi of logs around the rocks to fully cover them and concentrate the heat. When this was done, I sat down near the fire.

I sat at the border between the cool of the night and the fire's heat, close enough to be a part of the fire's energy, but far enough away for comfort. I watched the fire; I would need to add more wood if any rocks became uncovered. The rocks had to be protected, respected, and kept as hot as possible until it was time to place them in the pit at the center of the lodge.

I heard a sound like gravel being thrown against a window pane. I prayed. "Today we smoke tobacco together." The fire hissed and sputtered. "Today you will remake my feet." The wind started blowing again, and other sounds started. "Today you will remake my legs." As I sweated from the fire and accepted the reality of the presences around me, my troubles began to melt away. "Today you will remake my whole body." I was remembering the First Morning Prayer. I could feel the presences answering my prayer, reminding me, "These things you think are so important are inconsequential. What is around you is what is real! Look at your hands. Look at your body! You are alive! You are well! This is what matters. Let go of your fears. Let go of your worries!"

A spark struck my T-shirt, burning a hole before I could brush it away. The fire had reminded me some wood needed rearranging. When I was finished doing that, I used the blanket to again create a draft and keep the fire burning brightly in every direction. I continued to tend the fire, all the while requesting help for Homer, until the other three joined me, ready to enter the lodge.

The low, round structure was made of willow saplings lashed together and allowed to dry. Sheets, canvas, blankets, tarps, and plastic were stretched over the saplings to hold the heat inside. What power must there have been when actual skins and furs, the robes of animals, were used to hold in the heat. Today we make do with modern coverings.

Marilyn, Homer, and his daughter came by the fire with their towels, Marilyn's suitcase of ceremonial supplies, and the prayer ties they had made. The ties were ready to be hung inside the lodge. Marilyn had called for Homer to make black prayer ties, since he was full of fear. His daughter made white ties, the color of love and forgiveness, to balance his fears. And Marilyn made green ties, for healing.

The lodge had a small oval door through which we entered. We all followed Marilyn, who crawled sunwise around the central pit to sit near the door. After Marilyn was Homer's daughter, followed by Homer, who sat directly opposite the door. This is the hottest place in the lodge and also the place of honor. Finally, since I was the firekeeper and stone-puller, I came last and knelt just inside the door. When Marilyn finished hanging the prayer ties in their proper positions, she was ready for a shovelful of hot coals.

When I left to fetch the coals, I was overwhelmed by the power and energy assembled around the lodge. A part of me was afraid, but I was too much in awe to be fearful for long. A hot wind blew at me from the north. At first I thought it was coming through the fire. Then I realized that the fire was in another direction. I acknowledged the spirit wind's presence silently as I retrieved coals from the fire. I brought the coals into the sweat lodge, kneeling just inside the door.

Marilyn placed New Mexican sage on the coals, which burst into flames. Its pungent smoke filled the space. She asked each of us to bless ourselves with the smoke, by using our hands to direct the smoke around our bodies. Then she placed cedar from the Big Mountain area on the coals. When this had burned, she laid down a braid of Manitoba sweetgrass to smolder, and began to fill her sacred pipe with Dineh tobacco. She took a pinch of tobacco and held it over the smoke from the sweetgrass to bless it. Then the tobacco was held toward the west while she prayed to the spirits of that direction, placing the tobacco into the bowl of the pipe when the prayer was finished. She wove intricate prayers to each of the seven directions. After she made a prayer to each direction, another pinch of tobacco was placed into the bowl.

The pipe is the most sacred object of the Lakota. Its use parallels Christian communion. When the pipe is smoked during the ceremony, prayers placed into the tobacco are carried to the spirit world. Marilyn reminded us that all our thoughts were prayers and were going into the pipe. "Be alert. Know what you're praying for. There is craziness and sickness loose in the world," she said. "Ask for protection from that. Creator, keep us on our feet and watch out for us. Thank you for looking down on us and picking us up when we fall."

Our attention was focused upon Homer, since he had requested the healing. We all directed our prayers and attention to Homer, helping to increase the strength of his request for wellness. The prayer ties began to move and sway above us. Robes in all the colors of the directions (pieces of fabric a square yard in dimension, with tobacco ties at one end) hung majestically from the wood frame of the lodge. The red, northern robe began to dance as if the wind were tossing it. No breeze blew through the lodge; every possible opening had been covered but for the door. I could feel the presence inside the lodge of the same strong energy that had been blowing outside in the hot northern wind. The black robe began stirring, too, with our mounting fears.

When the pipe was filled, I took the hot coals out. The energy outside had continued to build. I knew a miracle could happen that night. More energy than I had ever felt before had assembled in one place. I moved the logs with a pitchfork, preparing to carry the stones beneath them into the lodge. The first seven stones are blessed by the sacred pipe. They represent the directions, and are laid in the pit accordingly. I took the first stone from the fire and dusted it off with a cedar branch. I made sure no coals remained on the pitchfork before I carried the stone into the lodge.

As I returned from the lodge to get the second rock, out of the corner of my eye I saw a short, golden man. He was about one foot tall, wearing clothing, but with the most amazing skin, as if he were made from gold itself. I turned my head sharply to see him and he was gone. I turned my head back to the pitchfork and glanced from the corner of my eye again. There he was. Who was he? Later Marilyn told me he was one of the little people, well known to Native Americans. I marveled to have been granted such a vision, and was grateful to this being for letting me see him.

I carried in the second stone and placed it in the pit, then brought in the third, fourth, fifth, and sixth stones. After I placed the seventh stone in the lodge, I put the pitchfork aside and took the sacred pipe from Marilyn. I placed it on the mound of earth serving as an altar, directly outside the door. In awe of the energy surrounding me, I continued to carry the remaining stones into the lodge. When all twenty-eight were in, I took the pitchfork outside and stripped to my underwear.

After coming inside, I closed the door, which was made of blankets hung on a large stick, supported by rope stretched across the top and secured in back of the lodge. It was completely dark inside except for the red glow of the stones. The sweat began to pour off my body. I remained alert to what was happening with Homer. In the dark, Marilyn poured seven dippers of water onto the stones, and the steam rose upward. We sang one of the sacred songs together and then sat quietly in the darkness. I could feel the toxins pouring off my body. I could feel myself releasing aspects of the spirit of Homer's illness that I had absorbed while working with him.

The compassion and sympathy a healer works to develop have their perils. According to the traditions Marilyn was passing on to me, the medicine person takes on the illnesses of a ceremony's participants, releasing them later through a purification and cleaning process. Medicine people sometimes pass out during or after an especially intense sweat lodge. Wallace Black Elk actually had a heart attack following one.

I try not to subscribe to this belief, but I find that I occasionally absorb some manifestation of a patient's illness, especially when the treatment is going well and a patient is able to release a lot of energy. Now I do periodic purifications with a simple ceremony, or, if there isn't time for that, exercise—anything to work up a sweat. If I neglect to do this, I can develop an uncomfortable headache, a throbbing knee, or the symptoms of a low-grade flu.

In the lodge, I breathed in the presence of the spirits. I felt them releasing the toxins even more with each breath. I felt a presence, one that was becoming familiar: my spirit grandfather. He is usually the first to come in response to my prayers for guidance and help. I had been having visionary experiences sporadically since working with Paul in Wisconsin in the mid-1970s. With Marilyn's help, I was becoming more adept at welcoming these experiences. Besides my spirit grandfather, I was (and still am) frequently aware of the spirits of Archie, Wolf, Coyote, and Christ.

A spirit can appear and speak in a physical form. To a Native American, a spirit is likely to adopt the form of an animal, such as a wolf or a coyote; to a Christian it might take the form of an angel. The spirit chooses a form that is culturally acceptable to the person who has the vision. When I say I am aware of Christ during a ceremony, I mean there is a spirit present who means to me what my background has taught me Christ means. To another, the same spirit may appear in another form. Marilyn's spirit helpers come in the form of seven different and powerful women, not all of them traditional—besides the White Buffalo Calf Woman and the Mother of Corn, for example, Marilyn is aided by the Lady of Guadalupe and Pele, the Volcano Goddess. Some of her helpers were unknown two hundred years ago; other counterparts would have taken their place.

Around Homer a white glow appeared, resembling the white-hot glow of the hot stones. Marilyn announced that the White Buffalo Calf Woman had come. I could see the outlines of her presence in white. She was covering Homer with her light. Through that light I could see him stretched out upon the eucalyptus-covered earth. Grandfather stood behind me on my left.

I felt the White Buffalo Calf Woman reach out and begin to explore Homer with acceptance and compassion. This was important for him because he was self-critical and judgmental. I traveled with that spirit toward him, maintaining an awareness of how Homer was doing. I watched as she entered his skull and began to rearrange the electrical patterns of his brain. She allowed me to see how she perceived his brain waves—to her they were colorful patterns of electromagnetic energy. She straightened and adjusted the waves as a weaver might untangle strands of yarn on a loom. His fear dissipated; it had been removed and realigned. "I'm teaching him to love himself," White Buffalo Calf Woman told me. Grandfather grunted an affirmative. In a state of heightened awareness, I was given to understand how electromagnetic patterns create all the forms of the body.

I didn't know how long we'd sat there when Marilyn said to open the door. I moved through the darkness clumsily at first, unsure where to find it. Dirt mixed with the sweat on my legs and arms. I found and pushed open the flap. Some of the heat inside rushed out into the cool night air. The fire still burned brightly. I went outside to adjust the door and bring in more water. The night remained pregnant with activity. Sounds, tapping, rustling, whistling—everything was alive.

I could hear Marilyn praying inside. "Hau Tunkasila, Wakantankan, this man has made a promise which he is here to fulfill. He has promised to do what he can to help others and not just himself. So he comes here to pray for his health and that of his family. Therefore, Wakantankan, grant him and his family good health and happiness. If there is any more sickness in his family, I pray for you to help them, and in this way they may walk again in happiness. This is why we pray to you."

Everyone responded, "Hau," in a common, deep, musical tone.

"Tunkasila, hear his prayers. And if you hear them, he will continue to offer thanks to you in this way for many years to come. This is why we pray to you in this way with this pipe."

Again everyone responded, "Hau."

"And look favorably upon us, smile on us, those of us who are hurting or are sick. Bless us, Tunkasila. Give us health and happiness and a good life. Help us to walk the good red road from north to south, from wisdom to compassion. These are the things we ask, especially now as the leaves turn and we prepare for the winter, especially now for Homer and his family. This is why we offer you this pipe."

I had reentered the lodge by now, and joined in responding, "Hau."

Marilyn continued. "Tunkasila, Wakantankan, help all our relatives with their daily needs. Look after their land, their home, their livestock, their crops, what they do to feed their families. Help those of our people who are not as fortunate as we are here. Help us, for we know that our prayers will be answered when we pray in this sacred manner with this pipe. The White Buffalo Calf Woman has told us that this is so, and that is why we offer this pipe to you in this manner."

"Hau."

There was some silence and then Marilyn repeated, "Hau . . . hau . . . hau . . ." to the spirits who were talking to her. Then she spoke again, now in a deep, authoritative voice. Another entity seemed to be speaking through her. "If you pray with all your heart, all of you, Homer will be well." The spirit continued, telling Homer that he was a beautiful person and that he would come to love the parts of himself of which he was ashamed. The spirit wanted to be certain Homer knew he was well.

Homer acknowledged the spirit, whispering, "I am well," then more strongly affirming, "I am well."

"Hau," we all chorused again. We sat quietly with the door open, letting out some of the steam. Then the time came for prayer and I closed the door. Marilyn asked me to start. She would finish.

The door is closed four times during the ceremony. Four is a sacred number. Each of the four rounds (also called doors—the first door, the second door, and so on) is dedicated to one of the directions, always beginning with the west. After the second closing of the door, each person prays silently or aloud. The route of prayer travels sunwise around the pit of stones. I prayed mostly for Homer, feeling and thanking the presence of the spirits I had seen during the first door. I prayed too for other clients with whom I was working, asking for help and health for them. When I was done, it was Homer's turn to pray.

During sweat lodges, people are incredibly honest. I've experienced few other places where lies are so rarely spoken. Homer told the truth about his fear. He was afraid of living and afraid of dying. He asked for help. Marilyn helped him formulate his prayer, reminding him to clearly state his desire for health and help. After Homer prayed, his daughter took her turn. During her prayer, I was again aware of the White Buffalo Calf Woman massaging Homer's spirit and helping it return to his body. Further brain-wave adjustments were needed.

During her own prayers, suddenly, Marilyn cried out in pain. She had just felt the metastasis in her back, in the same place that Homer had developed it. She prayed that this area be healed.

Marilyn directed that the door be opened. The night world around us was engulfing the lodge. Again I felt the ecstatic pleasure and fear of the spirits and beings outside. The fire's light cast a red-orange glow into the lodge, throwing eerie shadows. We talked more, but with a quiet awareness of the deep, powerful processes at work.

I closed the door for the third time. Marilyn tossed water onto the stones with her eagle-carved ladle. The steam rose into the darkness and we sang, our voices filling the night. The song, translated, goes like this:

> *I send a voice above.*
> *With the pipe I send a voice above.*
> *I do this because I want to live with my relations.*
> *Saying this over and over, I pray to Tunkasila.*

Glowing lights appeared in the lodge as we sang in Lakota. They were bright blue and green. These were lesser spirits showing themselves. I felt something releasing from my liver and breathed it out onto the stones. I rubbed myself with the eucalyptus leaves, covering my chest with their scent. Some of them were gritty from the earth beneath me. My sweat mixed with the dirt and poured off my body. Again Marilyn said to open the door, ending the third round.

Then we cleaned ourselves with our towels and smoked the sacred pipe, representing the one the White Buffalo Calf Woman brought to us so we could pray to the Creator and be heard. The bowl represents the earth, and feminine energies; the stem, the masculine energies of the sky. When the two are joined, the pipe is activated and ready to work. The tobacco smoke carries the prayers skyward. The pipe was lit and smoked around the circle. Marilyn finished, making sure all the tobacco was gone.

I set the pipe on the altar outside, and closed the door for the fourth and final round. We began with a silent prayer for anyone we had forgotten earlier. We sang another song. Marilyn used her eagle-bone whistle and eagle feathers to usher in a spirit. I had a vision of Homer walking on a beach in a tropical land that resembled Hawaii. He looked well. I enjoyed the palm trees swaying in the wind. The balmy ocean breeze was in turn enjoying the yielding natures of the trees. In that moment, I knew that Homer was well. I sensed that there were many choices remaining to him, and that his path had turned toward wellness. I saw an eagle spirit flying around the roof of the lodge.

Sometimes, on a new path, the way becomes frightening and a person chooses to return to being ill, just as an abused wife returns to the husband who is the only source of love she knows. Nevertheless, those moments when a healing journey has begun are truly magical. This was one of those moments. Just now, neither the shaman nor the patient was important. Even what choices would next be made, the moment after returning to mundane life, did not matter. The process transcended all the individuals present, and in transcending, was a blessing to us all.

With the door closed, a lodge is dark and hot, and it is never easy to determine how much time has passed. Even the level of heat cannot be assessed. When we are hot, it is not just temperature. An energy is being held in. The stone people know this and increase the heat to facilitate that release. When the heat becomes uncomfortable, it is time to look within for the fear, for the toxins that need to be let go.

That night, when I started feeling hot and restless, I tried to find what energies were struggling for release inside me. I took a slow, deep breath and allowed the spirits in the lodge to fill my body with love and acceptance. That day I sensed, waiting for release, the little boy who craved his stepfather's approval, only to feel his criticism and the sting of his belt. The White Buffalo Calf Woman helped me to cradle that little boy. Grandfather put his hand on my shoulder.

I let go of the image of Homer I had been holding and honoring. I knew he would be fine. I let myself return my thoughts to a vision of my own, one that I had had several months before.

As PART OF MY training to learn the sweat lodge ceremony, Marilyn had encouraged me to do a vision quest. She wanted me to consider why I was traveling down the healer's path. The quest, she believed, would help me to clarify who I was, where I was coming from, and why I was here.

After a purifying sweat lodge, Marilyn guided me to the hilltop spot she had chosen for me, where I would sit and meditate for the next four days and nights. Flags and prayer ties had been posted in a square around the spot, and inside it was where I sat—with my pipe and a star quilt, waiting for a vision.

For a long time nothing happened, as I was filled with fear. I didn't know what I would do with myself to fill such a long time. It seemed as if four days would take forever to pass. And what if a bear or some other terrifying animal came to dislodge me from my spot? Would I be disqualified from having any kind of experience?

I finally started to pray just to quiet my thoughts. Before long, I drifted into a trance state and lost track of time. The vision that came to me in bits and pieces, as I went in and out of the trance, was of my spirit grandfather. He was my father's ancestor. I saw his life as it would have been in the early 1800s in South Dakota. For a long time I watched him from a perch in the branches of an oak tree.

When Grandfather was asleep, we went on fabulous journeys. When he was awake, I watched him instruct a young man I was led to understand was my spirit brother—not a blood relation, but a soulmate in another place and time. I found I could let my consciousness enter my brother's. For those moments he felt himself to be larger than life, expanded, more whole. I was never far behind when my brother made his way to the corral, for he was an excellent rider and the pace of the horse thrilled me. I loved the sensation of riding bareback across the prairie at a gallop. We rode together toward the setting sun on a horse that could anticipate the prairie dog holes faster than we could spot them.

Eventually I woke from these strange but stirring visions of my genetic heritage. I had no idea how much time had passed. I looked around at the hilltop and the prayer ties as they flapped in the early evening breeze. I stretched, smoked my pipe, and returned to my vision. Soon I was back in my perch on the branch in the tree. I saw my spirit brother approach Grandfather's house. I quickly merged my consciousness with his—I started seeing things as him. He was being taught a lesson in patience by our grandfather. These were his thoughts:

I watched Grandfather closely. He stretched on tiptoes to brush his horse's mane. His eyes were the window of his soul. He could wither you with a glance or beckon you into a cradling embrace.

The prairie sloped gently upward to the black mountains beyond. It was Corn Mother's time and the grass was brown. The Thunder spirits had not brought rain for some time. The land was hot and dry. A lone eagle lazily carved circles overhead. In the distance lay hot rows of canyon ridges.

Grandfather was a healer, a man to whom people came in times of sickness or trouble. He was teaching me the ways of the medicine man. The training was slow, for Grandfather taught that life was long and should be enjoyed slowly. Sometimes I would sit for hours watching him tend his horse, make prayer ties, or create a sacred object. "You are learning patience," he would say. "This is a virtue few young men know."

I found the soothing voice he used while brushing his mare's hide transporting. I closed my eyes and leaned back against the wall of his stone house. I opened up my inner vision to the eagle flying through the clouds, riding the updrafts and gliding on the breeze. Grandfather's voice stayed with me, following the eagle through the clouds. Suddenly we were perched on the eagle's back, flying through the clouds of the Sky Country, to the hole in the sky. Through that hole we would be able to walk out onto the Milky Road, to the Creator's lodge at the end of the Sky Rainbow.

The land dropped rapidly away as we climbed higher. The Sun Chief had just begun his journey above the horizon. The day was young, the air invigorating. Eagle's wings lifted and folded, lifted and folded, beat-beat-beating against the air. Slowly but surely he carried us upward. I held Eagle tightly, but Grandfather rode erect, hanging on with his legs as he would a horse, galloping across the prairie. He wore his deerskin leggings and his fringe shirt — "since," he explained, "it will be cold up in the Sky Country. We'll go so high we'll be looking down on the Sun Chief, scattering his rays like seeds upon the land." Grandfather's medicine bag hung around his neck, a small, worn skin pouch filled with the few things he thought he might need.

I saw the hole in the sky, opening on to a cave. Eagle flew inside and we landed.

"Thank you, Brother Eagle," Grandfather said ceremonially, "for the wonderful ride."

"I am happy to serve you," replied Eagle. "Call sharply on your bone whistle when you are ready to return. For now I leave you with my brother, Spider, who came with us. He will ride behind your ear and keep alert for danger. For spiders can warn you if anyone is planning treachery or speaking from a dishonest heart."

"Always I am grateful to you, Brother Eagle. We gladly accept the help of Spider." Spider crawled off Eagle and onto Grandfather's proffered arm. "Welcome, brother. We appreciate your help. Ride on my grandson, please. He is learning the ways of the eagle and the spider."

The spider crawled across Grandfather's arm and onto mine; he crept up behind my ear, where he whispered a promise to warn and advise me.

We walked through the cavern for quite a way. The walls were smooth. There were small stones scattered on either side of our path. At the end of the path, the cavern opened into another world. The greenery was lush, the bushes thick and small-leaved. The trees stood tall with thin, peeling bark. "You will experience three challenges," Grandfather said, "and once you've met them, you'll receive a medicine gift. Pay attention and be alert. You don't know when the gift will come."

"Be alert," said Spider into my ear. "I sense your first challenge."

"Grandfather," I said, "Spider senses something up ahead."

"Then go first and alone," Grandfather said. "I will be there with you in spirit and will come quickly if you need help. This challenge is yours to approach."

I took a deep breath and went ahead. I trusted the power of good. Whatever challenge awaited me, I would call upon the Creator, Grandfather, and my other helpers, as I needed them.

As I rounded the corner, a giant appeared. He walked among the tree-tops and was taller than they were. He was made from stone. I had heard stories about stone giants and their powers. I was afraid. He growled like a wolverine, fierce and menacing. He beat stones together with his hands. The rocks crumbled with the force of these powerful blows and the earth shook beneath his feet.

"Speak first," said Spider. "That will offset his power."

"Giant!" I said. "I call upon you to tell me your message."

"I have come to destroy you," he replied. His misshapen stone face was impassive. He raised a stone above his head, preparing to hurl it at me.

"Only your fear can destroy you," said Spider. "Have courage."

My heart was pounding with fear. I called upon the Creator for help, to give me the strength and courage to withstand this challenge. A hole opened in the earth and I jumped inside. The giant's stone sealed the opening with a powerful crash. I slid down a slight incline and stopped with a lurch. There was a tunnel, and crouching in it was a strange man, dressed very oddly in an embroidered shirt. Could he be one of the Sky People?

With a shock I realized that the strange man my spirit brother was looking at was me. It was oddly dissociating to be conscious both of myself and of the first impression I made on another person. My embroidered shirt—the one I was wearing on my vision quest—was nothing unusual for 1984, but I could see that it might look extraordinary to someone from another time.

From behind the oddly dressed man stepped a coyote.

"Oh no," I said. "How did you get here?"

As a response, he belched, and a foul smell spread through the tunnel.

"He ate the gopher who made this tunnel," the stranger stated with some distaste.

"I enlightened the gopher. I delivered his spirit to the Great Beyond." Coyote giggled.

"You can trust Coyote, for now," Spider whispered. "But you don't have to make friends."

We traveled a long way through the gopher's tunnels. Coyote led haphazardly; it was dark, but I could tell where the tunnel's walls were because Coyote kept running into them. The stranger followed me. He was also clumsy, sometimes running into me, always apologizing.

Finally, traces of light dappled the tunnel walls. We arrived at an opening, curving upward and to the right. Coyote wriggled out of the almost-too-tight-to-exit hole. On his way out, he farted in my face. Grandfather was waiting, laughing, as I struggled out myself.

"Sorry about that, friend," Coyote said. "The hole pretty much squeezed it out of me."

"Thank you, Brother Coyote," I answered, as ceremonially as I could. "For leading me away from danger. Not for farting."

"No problem." He gave a toothy grin and trotted away. The stranger was stuck in the hole.

"Welcome," Grandfather said, "my other grandson." He grabbed the stranger's hand and pulled him out of the hole.

"Who is he, Grandfather?"

"He is your spirit brother. He will be living in another time, another place. He has been coming here for my teachings, for soon he will be born into his time. Welcome him into your vision, for today you have entered his as well. This is his journey as much as it is yours. The giant had meaning to him, as it did to you. He is learning your lessons as you learn."

I looked at my spirit brother. He smiled. "My name is Lewis. Truly we are brothers," he said in the ancient tongue.

"That is a strange name. How do you know to speak in the ancient manner?"

"In the dreamtime we all speak the same language."

"Come, my grandsons," called Grandfather. "Our journey must continue." We stood on a small plateau. Below us were the clouds Eagle had flown us through to get to this land. Jagged peaks towered high above us; our path led toward them. Our feet crunched upon the scree. Occasionally the decaying remains of a fallen tree softened our footsteps. Each step required testing to be sure the footing would hold. Sometimes the path disappeared among large boulders. We climbed up them on all fours until we could walk again.

When we reached the pinnacles, the view was breathtaking. We could see in all the directions. Only the way we had come was enshrouded in clouds. Above the pinnacles a gentle landscape marked the top of the Sky Country. Other peaks loomed in the distance.

Sitting on a rock in the near distance was a white-haired, bearded old man, staring at us intently. I looked away. When I looked back, he was gone.

"That is the spirit of the mountain," Grandfather said. "Your task is to go to him and ask his help."

"Come," said Lewis, "let us seek him."

We walked to the highest peak. A beautiful alpine lake stretched before us, deep blue, reflecting the peak upon its surface. To the north, the trees disappeared as the mountain rose above the timberline. To the west, snow still clung to the summits. We sat to await Grandfather Mountain. Closing our eyes, we opened our inner vision to an awareness of his presence.

"Spirit of the mountain," I called out, "thank you for showing yourself to us. We come to honor you and to ask your blessing. We come to ask for your help in the sacred work of healing. We come for assistance with our strength and our courage. You have the power to rise majestically above the clouds, to provide nests for eagles and a home for the bighorns. At your top even the trees cannot grow. We are here to seek your wisdom."

"I have come," came a deep, thunderous voice, both comforting and rumbling. "You have done well to mount my slope. I offer each of you the gift of myself. Take a piece of the stone beneath your feet. Place it in your medicine bag. When an illness requires my medicine, take out the stone and place it on the affliction. Call upon me and I will come."

"I will do so," I answered, dropping my forehead to touch it upon the rock. I kissed the rock, giving thanks for this blessing.

Lewis did the same. "Thank you for this gift of yourself," he said.

"Your task is the greater," the old man of the mountain thundered in answer. "For in your world and time, they do not believe in spirits. They will not believe where you have been and what you have seen. They are possessed by the spirit of nothingness, of that which has never existed and never shall. Your task is more difficult, for they will not know to honor you when you return from your vision. You are lucky they do not throw the very stones of my body upon you."

"I know this, Grandfather Mountain," he replied. "I will do my best to bring you to my people."

"As you must," the old man insisted, "for they are on the brink of destroying their world with their belief in nothing. Nothing is something to them. Doubt is their stock in trade. You will speak of this and only some will listen. Now rise and depart."

Both of us rose from the stone floor, then retraced our steps down the mountain. A lightness had come over us, a joy, from being honored by the mountain spirit's presence. I thought about the trivial matters which led so many people to squabble. Here in the bosom of the mountain these matters were grains of sand in the path. I thought of the careful words of my grandfather, that we each choose our paths and our moccasins. Grandfather said, "Always walk behind the sacred pipe that the White Buffalo Calf Woman brought to the people. On one side of the pipe is hatred; on the other, jealousy. Only behind the pipe lies the path of truth." Coming down that mountainside, I vowed to follow the path behind the pipe of truth.

Suddenly Lewis almost ran into a solitary dead cedar reaching out of the rocks. He jumped backward, into me. "Careful," I admonished him. "Stay alert."

"I saw this tree before, on the way up the mountain," he said. "But then it was shaped like a snake. Look at it now. It's shaped like a great feathered serpent. See the beak, and the plume? It almost has wings, stretched out behind it."

"I see. He looks almost ready to fly."

I ran my hand over the gray wood. The tree was weathered smooth, and stooped, evidence of the terrible winds that blew there. Having asked permission of the cedar spirit, we broke off small twigs of the tree for our medicine use, then carefully picked our way back to Grandfather. The dusk breeze whispered the sly mysteries of the mountains.

When we reached him, Grandfather held out his hands.

"The old man of the mountain has told me both are worthy. Both have purity of heart and of purpose. Both will serve the Creator and are blessed because of that. You have done well. You make an old man proud." He pointed to Lewis. "Soon, Grandson, you must face the giant that Coyote helped you escape from. Alone."

"No!" he cried, fearfully.

"The giant will one day be your stepfather. You must make friends with him. Then the ghosts who haunt you will depart."

"He speaks the truth," said Spider. "Ghosts of the giant follow you both. They seek to pull you down onto the rocks below. You must learn the language of the giant and befriend him. Through that friendship the ghosts will be released."

Grandfather beckoned toward the southwest. "Before you face him, Grandson, one things remains. You must both meet the Feathered Serpent. He has already examined you, disguising himself as an old cedar. Walk toward him; his home is in the southwest. He awaits you."

"Let me down here," Spider asked. "For you do not need my help to meet this final challenge."

I gave Spider back to Grandfather. Lewis and I walked together down that faint path. Darkness settled as silently as a blanket upon us. We looked upward and trembled in the shadow of a great, winged serpent. A column of animals trudged in his wake. A wolf led the way, then Coyote, who winked at us. He was followed by a brown bear, a bighorn, the mountain chipmunk, and all the birds of the sky. We knelt on the ground.

"We honor you, Feathered Serpent," I said. "We come to ask your blessing and learn your medicine."

The bird landed, becoming a man as its feet touched the earth. "The earth draws me toward you," he answered. "I appear as one of you. I felt your heart when you stroked me on the mountain. What I felt was good. You respected me even in the pose of death. This is necessary for a healer. I have come to offer you my medicine to drink. The taste is bitter, but its powers are great. You will learn to see what a man cannot see within himself."

When the feathered serpent became a man, his rainbow plumage transformed into gold and silver garments, which shone brightly in the sun. He offered a wooden bowl to us. Lewis took the bowl and held it up to the serpent spirit.

"I thank you for this medicine," he said, "and for the gift of sight. I pray to use this gift always in the service of the Creator." He raised the bowl to his lips and drank. Quickly he handed the bowl to me. I did the same.

It was bitter, like rancid meat. I almost vomited the liquid as it trickled down my throat. It burned my stomach; soon Lewis and I were brought to our knees by the power of the Feathered Serpent's medicine. I called upon the wolf who led the procession for the strength to withstand this medicine. The wolf came and stroked my forehead.

"Rise," he said. "The medicine is bitter, but it will protect you from the bitterness and anger that others hold in their hearts. It is bitter like the sounds of mothers paining in birth, a weeping that brings joy." Remembering the lessons of the sweat lodge about endurance, I rose to my knees and began to sing with the medicine. The words were strange, but the sound returned my awareness. Suddenly the world was crystal clear. I was a stone who could see in all directions. The world moved swiftly about me while I slowly followed my life cycle. I marveled at how swift were the lives of men and animals. Hundreds came and went as I blinked my eyes. Only the giant sequoias seemed to stay long enough to mark the time. Occasionally a man would hold me and I would speak to him and aid him, but quickly enough he would be gone. Another might come in years or centuries. With this awareness I saw our lives against the backdrop of Creation.

"Now you are ready to meet the Great Spirit of the Land Above," said the Feathered Serpent. "Rise and follow." We followed without knowing how our feet rose and fell. We flowed with the animal procession, among the many pilgrims come to pay homage to the Great Spirit. As we reached the top of the summit, the Milky Road lowered itself to meet us and we stepped onto that bridge. Darkness and starlight fell around us. The Feathered Serpent had given us a potent enough medicine to assuage our doubts of stepping onto a bridge of stars, for we did this and the bridge held, and we were carried skyward.

A thunderous greeting rattled the very bones of my body. The words were unintelligible, but the sense of peace was so vast I began to dance. Words could not contain the joy of that communication. For minutes or centuries we were all transfixed in a song of joy. And then, too soon, we found ourselves descending the Milky Road, back toward the summit. The echoes of the Creator's song moved in on both sides of us as we walked down the star-lined path. In the blink of an eye we were sitting upon the scree, our ordinary vision restored. The Feathered Serpent was preparing to depart.

"What is the medicine?" I asked.

"It is the essence of the unspoken tears," he said. "When they are never spoken, they become bitter. You are given them to drink because 'like cures like,' and you must know this bitterness to work with it. You are ready now to go forth and do healing. You have seen the Sky God and you have passed the tests. Now go."

As we returned to my grandfather, Lewis nodded to us both. "I am ready now to face the giant. He grew with my fear. Now that my fear is gone, he should be a midget." He embraced me and Grandfather, and then continued on to the last place we had seen the giant. Grandfather and I prepared to call Eagle to return us to the Land Below.

"Will he survive the giant?" I asked.

"He walks with courage," Grandfather replied. "The giant will have shrunk so much that he may have trouble finding him."

Grandfather pulled out his eagle-bone whistle, and soon we were back leaning against the walls of his stone house. It was hot again and the horse needed combing. I was certain we had been gone for days, until we got back to the house and the sun was in the same place in the sky, with the same eagle making lazy circles around its rays. Maybe only seconds had passed. The warm wind played with us, blowing fast one moment and slow another, turning in swirls when it wished. I caught a glimpse of a blue spark in the oak tree by the corral. It sat steadily on a branch in the tree.

"Grandfather," I said. "That blue spark. Is that a spirit in the tree?"

"That," he said, in a voice more like memory than sound, "is the spirit brother you met on our journey. He comes here often to visit me. Now you are honored to see him."

"Why does he come?"

"He is sad in his world. His mother is ashamed to carry him because she is not married. He wears her shame like an old buffalo robe. He cannot see that she loves him anyway. He feels unhappy, so he comes to this place to visit us. In his dreams we talk. He lives here through you. You are his spirit brother and he yours. It would be harder for you to go into his world, but you can try. His world is more complicated than ours. The Creator has given them the means to destroy the earth and is waiting to see what they will do."

"What will they do, Grandfather? How can we live today if our earth is in danger of destruction?"

A fly settled on Grandfather's head. Grandfather did not bother to brush him off. He waited patiently for the fly to be done. "Our earth is in no danger, as only one image is of theirs. Lewis will choose that image of the world in which the earth will live. Others there will cross over onto the earth that is destroyed. It is their way and they will learn from this, and will start again. Next time will be easier for them."

I left my spirit brother's consciousness and returned to my perch in the tree. Before long I knew I would be delivered to 1953, to my mother's womb. For now I flowed with the South Dakota wind, dreaming of the father who had roamed those hills. Once I visited him in spirit, but he had no sense of me. Then I floated toward the Badlands, dancing upon the strange formations that settled there. When I returned to my uterine cradle, I cried fetal tears for my mother, for her pain, for my sadness at causing her shame. I heard my thoughts from the future, calling out to me to stop. "It's not your fault," he says. "I am you. There is pain to come, as there is pain now. But it will be better if you also feel your mother's love, and let go of the blame."

Morning came. Marilyn approached to lead me down the hill. I was amazed to see her—I was certain there were still three days to go. My vision quest turned up plenty of material for consideration. I experienced my father and grandfather, whom I had never personally met; I faced down my archetypal stone giant of a stepfather; I reexperienced my mother's womb.

How much of this was "real"? I had enough Anglo blood in my veins to worry about this a moment on my way down the hill. But I quickly decided, what difference would it make if the vision were "real"? Would its power be diminished if it were not? And by what measure could I quantify its reality? I was giddy with the insights I had been offered, and I found myself giggling. Marilyn joined in my laughter. I was in love with the world again, as much as I had been after Jimmie Left Hand's healing back in 1973.

WITH THE MEMORY of the vision quest flowing through me, I opened my eyes to find myself in the lodge. Marilyn had asked me to open the door. We were done with the ceremony for Homer.

We walked carefully through the darkness back to Marilyn's house. Homer was so weak that at first he could not stand. I supported him, holding him up, letting him lean on me as he walked. Homer was reluctant to accept the help, but I encouraged him to let go of his pride. He had been through a lot; he could allow himself to lean on me now. I picked my way carefully in the darkness. None of us had thought to bring a flashlight. In time, the footing became surer, and lights shone through Marilyn's windows to illuminate the ground before us. We came to her gravel driveway and crossed to a concrete walk. The wind followed us, as did the rustling of the trees.

Inside, Homer showered. Soon we would sit down to a traditional meal of buffalo, blueberries, corn, fried bread, and a soup of tripe and hominy. But first it was my duty to return to the fire and the lodge and make sure that all was in order. I took a flashlight but challenged myself to walk without it. At first I walked so quietly that I could have eased through a covey of quail without their stirring a wing.

Soon I realized that however quiet I was, the spirits would see me anyway. So I addressed the assembled energies out loud. "Forgive me my fears, for truly I am pitiful. Thank you for coming tonight, healing Homer, and helping me to understand my vision. Protect me on my way to tend to the fire and on my way back." I walked on. The night cries pierced me. I picked up one foot and set it down slowly, letting my weight settle onto the uneven ground before moving the other. By starlight I could see the outlines of branches soon enough to avoid them. Finally I came to the fire. It was smooth and raw; most of the logs had burned down to red-hot coals. Again I spoke out loud.

"Thank you," I said. Tears fell from my eyes. "Thank you for this honor, for protecting me, for healing me, and for healing Homer." I raked the coals and the unburned logs together and covered them with dirt, allowing them to smolder safely and die. The light from the fire faded from a brilliant red to the shady brick color of the almost sunken sun in the Kentucky hollows of my childhood.

The feel of the old rake was new to me. In that instant of putting out the fire, everything had changed and nothing could return to its familiar state of being. I had been transformed. I was at the threshold of many potential pathways. I felt sad when I left the fireside; life cannot be conducted inside a sweat lodge. Problems would return. I had much more to learn before I could lead ceremonies on my own. But in that moment I felt a state of grace, and it was a feeling to which I could always return.

People need ceremony. It's not enough just to think about life or healing. Ceremony creates the magic that allows healing to happen. It doesn't much matter which ceremony, as long as both the healer and the supplicants believe in it.

I retraced my steps to Marilyn's house. By the end of the path, I was following the smells of the wonderful food more than any visual cues. Miracles had happened in the darkness of that spirit-filled night. Now was a time for feasting.

CHAPTER EIGHT

The Gift of the Sun

WITHIN SEVERAL months of Homer's healing Marilyn took me with her to an isolated California spring. The surrounding land was vast and open. An unexpected valley hid the spring behind a screen of trees. Upon arriving, we drank eagerly from the pure water. Above us, tree branches formed a rim around the sky, a sky already turning pink in the distance.

We prepared a fire. The night sky was filled with the campfires of the star people. The stars floated and bobbed in the nearby spring, playing at holding still in the clear, fast waters. The moon broke over the hills, only a quarter of it left after Sky Badger's nibbling.

"Every story has a spirit," Marilyn said, her hair braids falling forward across her chest, reaching to her waist. The flames danced, taking pleasure in Marilyn's voice. "Stories have preferences about where they should be told. I want to tell you one about how the medicine lodge came to the people—the same lodge I have taught you to lead. This is an important story which you will tell for years to come. The story must be told for the first time in a sacred setting, so I have brought you to this medicine spring. The animals here will also want to hear it. The stars will listen in, too. It is proper to tell the story here."

We leaned back against the gnarled tree roots that traveled out and down across the damp earth banking the spring. Green leaves shook above us in a wind that rose and fell like waves on a stormy lake. "We begin with a prayer." She spoke in the ancient language, turning her face toward the west, where the sun had disappeared. She took a pinch of tobacco and held it out in that direction. The trees shook above her, ready for her to begin.

"Creator," she said, "as you sit in the west, hear our prayers tonight. We have fears of the night and of darkness. Take these fears from our hearts and minds. Transform them into health and help, for we are pitiful and ask for your guidance. Hear our prayers as we share the story of your medicine lodge." Finishing, Marilyn placed the tobacco in the blood-colored pipestone bowl of her pipe. She took another pinch of tobacco from her fringed and beaded leather bag.

"Creator, Grandfather, Grandmother, as you sit in the north, hear our prayers." Marilyn held out the tobacco to the north. "Give us the strength to carry this story to the people who need to hear it. Give us the wisdom to honor this story. Help us to use it wisely." Cradling the pipe against her body, she placed the tobacco in its bowl. Her hands were strong yet gentle. They were scored with the lines of one who had witnessed much and endured more.

She offered a third pinch of tobacco to the east, praying, "Creator, Grandfather, as you sit in the east with the Spotted Eagle Nation, the Wambligleska, hear our prayers. Give us the vision to see where to use this story, how to travel with this story, to see its spirit, and to honor it through telling it." She placed the tobacco in the pipe; taking another pinch, she turned toward the south.

"Creator," she said, "Grandfather, Grandmother, as you sit in the south with Corn Mother and the Deer Spirit, hear our prayers. Give us the compassion to understand this story. Give us the love to feel the pain of people and to bring healing to them through this story. Hear our prayers, for our prayers are for the good of all." She placed the tobacco into the pipe's bowl. She raised another pinch toward the Milky Road, pathway to the Creator's Lodge.

"Sky Spirit, Wakantankan, as you sit in the sky and look down upon us, hear our prayers. Show us how to walk with sacred footsteps. Show us the proper path to walk, behind the sacred pipe. Neither to the right where jealousy abounds, nor to the left with hatred. Show us the path behind the pipe where we may walk as two-leggeds, in balance and harmony with all your ways. Let your blessed rain wash away our pain, wash away the impurities from the earth and our bodies, and cleanse our hearts and minds." After putting that tobacco in the pipe, she touched the earth with another pinch.

"Mother, Maka Ina, as you sit below us, hear our prayers. Sustain and nurture us, for we are your children. Give us the fruits of your womb, the foods of your flesh. Give us our daily corn and our meat. Give us the nuts and the roots of your children, the plants. Bless all of us who walk upon your beautiful skin."

Then she held some tobacco toward the center of the fire. "Creator,"

196 • LEWIS MEHL-MADRONA

she said, "and all my relations. As you sit in the center of Creation, as you sit in the center with all our relatives, hear our prayers, for we are one. Our prayers are their prayers, and their prayers are our prayers."

Marilyn sat up on her knees and held her pipe toward the stars. A tear streaked her check as she cried out, "Creator, Tatuskanskan, we have filled the pipe in the sacred manner, the manner taught to us by Wohpe, the White Buffalo Calf Woman. Hear our prayers, for we offer them in this sacred manner, in this way that she taught us." Marilyn's voice trembled as she said, "I thank you, for I know you will hear our prayers and they *will* be answered."

She touched the earth with the bowl of her pipe, letting it rest upon the ground. "Maka Ina," she prayed, "thank you for the herbs you grow. Thank you for the tobacco and all the sacred things we use that come from you. Bless us, for you have made it possible for the Creator to hear us."

She took her pipe and, holding the bowl stationary, made four great arcs with the stem. She called out, "To all the Sacred Beings who have gathered here. Thank you for hearing our prayers. Thank you for helping us, for carrying our prayers across the Milky Road to the Lodge of the Creator." Marilyn lifted the pipe once more toward the heavens and then brought it to her lips. I fished a stick from the fire and held it up to light the pipe.

Marilyn took several puffs and passed the pipe to me. I savored the flavor of the tobacco. My soul was touched by the prayers it carried. I was ready to memorize the story Marilyn would tell. I was confident the story would come to me when its message was needed. I took several more puffs and passed the pipe back to her.

She, too, was deep in reverie as she blew the smoke skyward and into the fire. The flames threw her face into sharp relief. A coyote howled, returning a message from the spirit world that our prayers had been received. A crash just behind us startled me. A dead branch of the tree had fallen to earth. I slowed my breathing and concentrated on returning to the reverie of the moment before.

"Don't ignore what happened, for it is good," Marilyn said. "The dead weight is being discarded so the tree can live. It is a sign that the unwanted burdens you carry are being released. The spirits have heard our prayers. They are pruning your spirit. Nature rejects all that is useless. Your body rejects and eliminates the poisons that form inside it. Your body, like the tree, rejects what it no longer needs to maintain good health. Only now are you ready for the story."

Marilyn thoughtfully smoked the rest of the tobacco, blowing smoke to the four directions. Rays of firelight passed through the clouds of smoke, refracted amber by them. The moon set and the earth was as lightless as the womb. Marilyn rested her pipe upon the makeshift altar she had built and began her tale.

A long time ago there lived a young man named Scarface. This partic-ular young man had no relatives on the earth. All had left for the Sand Hills and the Spirit World beyond. He had no possessions save those he wore on his body. He had no food save those scraps others left for him or gave him to eat. He was strong and he worked hard, but he lacked weapons with which to hunt. He had to borrow them, and so had to share much of his kill with their owners. He frequently sat with old Tunapai, who doc-tored the sick and saw visions. He performed errands for the old man and assisted him when needed. But Tunapai did not think Scarface was in line to receive the sacred knowledge of healing, and so Scarface took away only scraps of knowledge, much as he did his food.

In the same village, there was a beautiful young woman, whom all the young men adored. Each young man of the village, and indeed of many neighboring villages, wanted her for his wife. Each set out to impress this woman with his finery, or his skills at hunting and providing, or his exquis-ite dancing at the ceremonies that brought the villages together. But none of these young men found fancy in the young woman's eyes.

Her parents had begun to worry about her. The Raven Dance was soon to be held in the village, drawing many young men from the neigh-boring villages. Her mother hoped to marry her to an ideal suitor at this upcoming event. When her mother approached the young woman about her marriage prospects, she only shook her head and declined. "I have all I could want here in my parents' lodge," she said. "Why should I leave prematurely?"

Her mother began to suspect her daughter of hiding something. By the time the father returned from hunting, the mother was certain, and quite upset. "Our daughter is having a secret union," she cried. "She will become pregnant and disgrace our family! You must speak to her."

The father approached the daughter with the mother's concerns. "No," said the young woman. "I am not having a secret relationship. But I can-not marry, and I will tell you why. One day as I was gathering berries three summers ago, the Sun Chief approached me. He acknowledged me. I stood unable to move, basking in the golden light and heat of his face. 'You are a good woman,' he said. 'You have found favor in my eyes. You must not marry. You must save yourself for me.' What could I do, Father, but agree with him?"

Her father nodded thoughtfully. "That is so. When the Sun Chief speaks, we must listen. Therefore, no further words will be said about the subject of your marrying. The matter is closed." He so instructed his wife and there the matter ended. Or at least, if his wife complained, she knew better than to complain to him.

The Raven Dance came and all the dancers approached this young woman with their finest dancing clothes. The best dancers begged for her hand, but to all she gave a firm "No."

Soon after the dance, many of the young men were sitting together telling tales of their prowess and skill. They boasted in the way young men do, before they have been tested and have tasted the bitterness of their limitations. They agreed that none could win the eye of the beautiful woman. Scarface sat listening at the edge of the group, hoping not to be noticed, for he had neither handsome finery nor status. But one young man did notice him and began taunting him. "Surely the great Scarface is not afraid to ask for the hand of the beautiful maiden. We have all failed, but Scarface has not even tried. Surely she could not refuse him and his magnificent scar. With such a beauty mark, she will swoon on sight and be his in an instant. Isn't that so, Scarface?"

Scarface smiled and rubbed his toe in the dust. He knew this game, but he decided to play along. His pride was greater than his wealth. Secretly he longed for the young woman, but he had never dreamed of asking for her, given his lowly position in society and the scar that disfigured his face. Scarface stood tall. "I will ask her then," he said, smiling. "Why not." Everyone laughed. "As you say, who could refuse anyone as handsome as I?" This was so funny that some of the young men were soon rolling on the ground, laughing uncontrollably.

Scarface left the group before they could mock him further and went down by the river where the women gathered water. He hid in the rushes. He vowed to himself and to his spirit guides that he would propose to the young woman the very next time he saw her. He had his honor to uphold.

Scarface did not have to wait long. Before Sun completed his journey across the roof of the sky, the young woman came with her basket to gather water. Scarface sprang out from the rushes, startling her. She jumped back.

"Do not be alarmed," he said. "My intentions are honorable. I wish to ask you here in the open, under the eyes of Sun, who notices and hears everything, to be my wife. I have loved you from afar for years and have watched all the others ask you. I have never had the courage to ask you myself, but I do so now."

The young woman covered her face with her robe, as is the custom when such a request is made. She peeked out at Scarface. Truly, she had never noticed what a fine man he was. The scar had drawn her attention away from his many good qualities. She was impressed by his courage. She had an idea.

She lowered her robe and smiled. "I accept your proposal," she said. It was Scarface's turn for shock. "It is true that you have no possessions, but my parents have many and can provide us with what we need to begin our lives together." Scarface could barely restrain himself from jumping up and down. "But there is one problem."

"What is that?" asked Scarface nervously. He feared that what he had received so easily might just as easily disappear.

"I have promised the Sun Chief that I would save myself for him. You must travel to the home of Sun and ask his permission. I will know he has agreed when he has taken the scar from your cheek. When you return we will marry."

"B-b-but," Scarface stammered, "I don't know where Sun lives. No one has ever visited his lodge. How will I find him? Where will I look? How long will it take me?"

"That is your problem," answered the young woman. "But you are resourceful and wise. If anyone can accomplish this task, you can. Surely I am worth such a journey," she said, smiling. "Besides, it is necessary, for I cannot break my vow to Sun." She leaned over to Scarface and gave him a kiss to seal her commitment. Then she ran away before Scarface could muster his wits to ask more questions. Her empty water basket lay where she had dropped it; Scarface summoned a child to return it to her lodge.

Scarface vowed to leave the next morning. He could not remain in the village another day without being mocked. He would have to find the Sun Chief and obtain his permission to marry the young woman, or never again return to his village. Those were his choices.

Marilyn stopped a moment to take a sip of water. "You know that life is this way," she said to me. "We want our dreams to be granted to us, but they require sacrifice and effort. There are conditions we must meet before we can attain our desires. Scarface had to choose to follow his dream, or not. But those who do not follow their dreams are broken men. Their spirits are never fully with them.

"Many times we ask for something. We are told how we may attain it, and what we are told seems totally ridiculous and impossible, but if we've had the courage to ask for something, we must have the courage to hear the response. Like Scarface, we must not belittle the response but take it seriously. What we have been told is no joke." Marilyn resumed her story.

Scarface went to a woman who frequently fed him. She was a widow and had taken pity on Scarface; in return he helped her with chores\and other tasks. "I am going on a long journey," he told her. "I cannot tell you the purpose of my journey, only that I may be gone a long time. Please, if you can spare me moccasins, do so. And if you can spare me food, do so. I must leave early in the morning."

The woman worked all night, for she valued Scarface and wanted to help him. She made him seven pairs of moccasins. She collected all the dried food she could spare and put it in a pouch for Scarface to carry. When she was done, she awoke Scarface, who had slept outside her lodge, and gave him the gifts. She restrained her curiosity about where he was going, only begging him to come see her when he returned and explain his mysterious journey. He quickly agreed.

Scarface left the village and headed west. He knew the Sun Chief disappeared in the west at night, so that must be the direction of his lodge. He would ask for directions when he reached the Great Mountains, the Backbone of the World.

Scarface walked for longer than he could remember. Time blurred. A great fog seemed to creep into his vision. He could not remember eating, but he must have done so, since the dried food the widow gave him was slowly disappearing. He could only vaguely remember sleeping. By the time he reached the Backbone of the World his first pair of moccasins had worn away. He put on the second pair and resolved to ask Wolf for directions. Some said Wolf knew every inch of the mountains; therefore, Wolf should know where Sun slept at night. Scarface could see frost high upon the mountains and knew that it would creep down to cover the valleys long before he returned. The thought made him shiver.

Scarface walked along a riverbank calling Wolf by his true name, the name Tunapai had taught him. Finally Wolf emerged from a nearby thicket. "Please!" Wolf said. "Not so loud! I don't want every last mouse and rabbit in the mountains to know where I am. Now, Two-legged. You have called my true name, so I must help you. What is your wish?"

"I wish to know where the Sun Chief's lodge is," said Scarface. "I must go to where Sun sleeps at night and ask him a question. You are wise, so I ask you, where does Sun sleep at night?"

"Actually, I am wise," answered Wolf, after a long pause. "But I do not know." He stroked his chin whiskers lightly. "If you had asked me about the Backbone of the World, about the calls of the animals who live here, about the spirits that prowl the canyons and the heights—those things I could tell you. But I do not know where Sun sleeps at night. I'll tell you one thing, he doesn't sleep here, because I've been to the heights and watched him cross over and go far beyond where I can see. But listen. I'll

take you over these mountains, and you can ask Bear on the other side. Bear is wise and meditates the longest of any of the animals. If anyone can tell you what you ask, it'll be Bear."

Scarface thanked Wolf and carefully followed the magnificent animal as he wound his way up a narrow trail covered with pine needles and wood chips from fallen trees. They passed the burnt stumps and other signs of the Thunder spirit's work. New growth was already appearing in the areas that had burned.

"Life is just this way," Marilyn remarked. "What dies is replaced. And the first helper you ask may only point you on the path to the next. When you have just begun, the path looks too difficult. This is when most people give up and settle down beside the path. It took courage for Scarface to walk up the mountain behind Wolf. A lesser man would have given up when Wolf didn't know the answer, and would have looked for a lesser task to accomplish. Some of us do not live up to our potential, to the tasks the Creator has given us to do."

Scarface followed Wolf all the way over the mountain. Snow covered the top; they had to pick their way carefully over the glacial ice they found there. The western side of the mountain was less steep. The narrow cliff trails they faced, going up one side, were replaced by broad paths they ran down on the other. At the end of the trail, in a lush mountain meadow, was a cave tucked away in a sheer rock wall. "That is Bear's lair," Wolf said. "It is close to time for Bear to awaken. Call to him that Wolf sends his spring awakening. But stay away from the center of the cave; when Bear emerges after such a long sleep, he tends to eat the first thing in sight. Sing this song to wake Bear and you will be safe." Wolf taught Scarface a song, and when he was satisfied Scarface could sing it, before two pecks of a woodpecker's bill, Wolf had vanished into the tall trees.

Scarface carefully approached the cave, hugging the left side of the sheer rock wall. When he reached the edge of the granite opening, he began to sing the song Wolf had taught him.

> *Bear wake up, Bear awake,*
> *The sky is blue, the snow is gone.*
> *Bear wake up, Bear awake,*
> *The meadow's green, and spring is come.*
> *Bear wake up, Bear awake,*
> *The animals await you here.*
> *Bear wake up, Bear awake,*
> *Or you will sleep through summer!*

Scarface heard stirring and growling inside. Bear was awake! He watched as Bear charged out into the sunlight, looking for something to eat. There was nothing there but a sapling, which Bear tore up from its roots, chewed twice, and spat out again. Then he called out for Wolf. "Wolf is not here," Scarface answered timidly. "He sent me instead to awaken you and ask your counsel."

Bear stopped short and growled. "He sent a two-legged?" Bear's eyes narrowed into little slits. His ears flattened backward upon his head and he showed his teeth. "Make it quick, Two-legged," he said menacingly, "for I am hungry."

Scarface told his story briefly and asked for directions to the lodge of the Sun Chief. Bear became calmer and friendlier as he listened to Scarface. "Truly you have undertaken a great quest, my young friend," he answered thoughtfully. "I do not know where Sun lives, but I have heard that he lives across the Great Desert. He certainly travels that way every afternoon. In that direction," Bear said, pointing out a path for Scarface to follow. Then he made Scarface memorize an elaborate and flattering speech for his friend, a badger. "Take this greeting to Badger, who lives on the other side of the Great Desert. Ask Badger which way leads to the lodge of the Sun Chief. If anyone can tell you, it will be Badger. Now, go in peace."

Scarface thanked Bear and made prayers to the Bear spirit. He discarded his second pair of worn-through moccasins and entered the Great Desert on the third pair. Time blurred again. Nights turned into days. Days blended with nights. Sleep came and went, perhaps while he was on his feet. Scarface did not know how long he had slept or walked. His mind soared with the winged spirits as his body crossed the desert. Always he was led to water. Always there was just enough food. By the time he came to the mountains on the other side, he had worn through his fifth pair of moccasins.

How will I find Badger? he wondered. Then he remembered that the widow had told him once how Badger could not resist being told what a beautiful face he had. So Scarface sat down beside a spring, where the many deer tracks told him animals came to drink. Soaking his calloused feet in the water, Scarface began to sing the Badger song the widow taught him:

> *Badger who rules the forest,*
> *Badger who stalks by day and night,*
> *Badger who rules the forest,*
> *Who has the prettiest face in sight?*

Scarface waited a moment. When he heard no answer, he resumed his song.

> *Badger who rules the forest,*
> *Badger who stalks by day and night—*

Before Scarface could finish, Badger appeared. "You are wise, Two-legged, to sing of my great beauty. I will tolerate you in my forest. Tell me why you have come."

Scarface again told his tale, this time adding Bear's greeting and telling Badger what Bear had said about him. Badger brightened at Bear's praise. "Bear speaks the truth. If anyone knew where Sun sleeps at night, I would. But I don't. So nobody knows. Good-bye."

"Wait! Have you ever noticed where the Sun Chief is headed?"

"Every afternoon, he crosses the top of these mountains. He must live on the other side. Wolverine lives over there. You could ask him. Good-bye."

"Wait! Over where?"

"I'm very busy. Very, very. You could follow me, I suppose. I'm headed over there on an errand. Follow me over the top."

Scarface heaved a heavy sigh and began to follow Badger. It reminded him of his journey behind Wolf over the Backbone of the World. He had never heard of these mountains before, but they were just as soaring—and just as steep. Beautiful lakes awaited at the summit. Badger wanted to linger and fish, but Scarface begged him make haste, for his true love awaited. Badger hissed and complained about women but complied with Scarface's request.

When they had come down from the rocky path over the steepest part of the mountains on the other side, Badger motioned him to stop. "We're here, in Wolverine territory. I'm gonna leave you here. Wolverine makes me nervous. Anyway, I have my errands to return to. Don't worry about finding Wolverine—he'll find you!" Badger giggled nervously, then vanished.

Soon Scarface heard Wolverine's low growl. "Why do you come to my forest?" demanded Wolverine. "I saw that silly Badger bring you. Why did he do that? Does he not respect me? Who are you? Why are you here!" Wolverine's fur was puffed out and he wore his fiercest face.

Scarface respectfully told his story and begged Wolverine for his help. When Scarface had finished, Wolverine sat for a long time without a sound. Then he answered, "I will help you. Sun sleeps on the other side of the Great Water. I will take you to its edge. There you can see Sun enter his lodge at night. I don't know how you'll get to his lodge, but at least you can see it."

Scarface was overjoyed. He put on his sixth pair of moccasins and gratefully followed Wolverine down the foothills, into the great valley, and on toward the Great Water.

The Sun Chief was entering his lodge when they reached the edge of the Great Water. Scarface watched in awe as Sun descended. "Does he live beneath the waters?"

"No," answered Wolverine. "Did you hear the hiss of something red-hot dipped in water? Did you see any steam? The entrance to his lodge must be above the water. But we cannot see it because it is so far."

"Then how will I get there?" asked Scarface.

"Is that my problem?" And in a moment the fierce animal was gone. He had left Scarface at the edge of the Great Water, as he had promised. His other duties needed attention.

Scarface was desperate. He had never imagined such a body of water. He could not swim so far. His face grew long and tears formed in the corners of his eyes. They began to roll straight down one cheek and crooked along the scar of the other, leaving clean trails on his dusty face. Without the sun, the air grew cold. He was ready to give up. He imagined lying there until his spirit left his body. He was at his wit's end.

Scarface had never felt so cold, alone, and afraid. He began to pray. He prayed to the Creator. He prayed to his guardian spirits. He prayed to his helper spirits. He prayed to everyone. Before he knew what had happened, two beautiful swans materialized on the water. "Where did you come from?" he cried.

"We are your helper spirits. We would have come long before if you had asked. But since you didn't, we assumed you wanted to make the journey on your own. Now you have asked and we have come. Climb on our backs and we will carry you across the Great Water to the lodge of the Sun Chief."

Scarface was overjoyed. The swans were so white, they shone even in the darkness. If only he had remembered to ask the spirits for help sooner! It was a lesson he would not soon forget.

"You remember that, if nothing else," Marilyn said. "When you need help you must ask for it. Remember how it took you almost two years to ask for help finding a teacher? And here I was living in California the whole time. Next time I hope you will not wait so long."

She looked carefully through the darkness at me. "Everyone comes to such a place in their journeys," she said. "No person escapes this moment of despair. We can only pray for the strength to walk through it, to know how to handle it, to know how to solve this crisis of faith that always comes."

The shadows were listening, flickering with the firelight. Tongues of flame leapt out, and flashes of heat, so we would not forget the fire's presence. All beings in the vicinity were entranced by the power of the story. I could feel the depth of their combined consciousness welcoming us like the fresh, cool air of a deep cave in summer. Marilyn resumed, her voice returning to the storyteller's cadence.

Scarface climbed onto the backs of the swans, who carried him across the Great Water. They flew a long way, farther than he could imagine, and finally landed on a beautiful garden island. "This is where the Sun Chief lives," said one swan. "There is a path here on the cliff. Follow this path as far as it goes and you will come to the home of the Sun Chief. When you are ready to return, call upon us and we will come."

Scarface thanked the swans and watched them disappear in graceful flight. Soon they blended with the sky and the water. Great turtles surfaced, traveling in the direction of the swans.

Scarface turned to face the cliffs upon which the Sun Chief lived. Unhappiness could never exist here on this island. He remembered the faraway snow drifts of winter, the hours spent inside a tiny dwelling waiting for a storm to pass. The warmth of the sun was too great to allow that here.

The mountains were dizzyingly high. Waterfalls covered their dark green surfaces. Patches of black volcanic rock poked through the greenery in high places. Scarface walked with awe upon this land. Each footstep fell in a sacred manner as he prayed for guidance. When he had walked only a short distance, Scarface came upon the most beautiful suit of clothes he had ever seen. They shone, generating their own light from glowing white cloth and gold weaving. An exquisite bow, quiver, and arrows lay beside the clothes. The inlaid design was exotic and unique. Scarface longed to touch the bow, to feel the arrows and stroke the feathers. But he did not. These belonged to another, and no one would leave such finery without planning to return for it. Scarface reluctantly walked on toward the center of the island.

When he had gone another few stones' throws, he turned a corner around a large boulder to see the most handsome youth he had ever gazed upon. The man was radiant. His muscles were well developed, rippling as he walked. His skin was the color of bronze. Scarface dropped to one knee, for he was sure this was a god.

"Welcome," the young man said. "We do not see many mortals here. I am happy you have come. By the way, did you see my clothes and my bow and arrows, back there on the path?"

Rising, Scarface answered, "I certainly did. They were the most beautiful I have ever seen. They are fitting clothes for such a god as you."

"Why did you not pick them up?"

"They were not mine. And such beauty could not have been abandoned."

"Then you have passed the test!" exclaimed the youth. "You are welcome here. Whenever mortals come, we leave something to test their honesty. If they are honest, they are welcome. Few come and fewer pass the test. My name is Morning Star, and Sun is my father. My mother is Moon. My father is away each and every day, but I will take you to meet my mother. She will be glad to see you, for she loves mortals and is happy to meet the few who manage to come our way."

Scarface followed Morning Star down the path toward the lodge of the Sun Chief. He was surprised when he saw the lodge. It was half red and half black. Stars shimmered on the black side; the Milky Road was there to see. The lodge was immense. When they entered, Morning Star greeted his mother and introduced Scarface. Moon invited him to feel at home, and the three spent the day in conversation about matters upon earth and Scarface's village.

When the time came for Sun's return, Moon told Scarface to hide quickly under some fur robes. She pushed him down and threw the robes on top of him. "My husband is quick to anger," she said. "He will accept you when he hears about you, but a sudden flash of his temper might burn you to ash. Stay under here until he calms down."

Scarface waited beneath the robe, fearful of melting in the searing heat before he could accomplish his quest. He prayed to his guardian spirits for protection. Sun roared in; Scarface cringed at the sudden blast of heat and began sweating profusely beneath the robes.

"I smell a two-legged from the earth! What is this about? Why is he here in my lodge?"

Quickly Moon and Morning Star placated Sun and explained to him that Scarface had passed the test of honesty and had been welcomed into their home. Sun's anger passed and the heat diminished, and when it was safe, Moon bade Scarface come out from under the robes. Scarface did so and knelt before Sun, asking his blessing. Sun rose majestically before him, giving his blessing and asking Scarface to remain and hunt and be a companion to Morning Star. Scarface graciously accepted and left Sun's company, quivering and happy to be alive.

Each day Scarface and Morning Star hunted. The animals of the island were many and various, and each brought its own unique challenge. They hunted throughout the summer; fall did not come. Soon Scarface realized that it never would—not to this island. Moon cooked their kill and served a joyous feast each night. Moon told Scarface with a mother's appreciation that Morning Star hadn't been this happy since before his brothers were killed. Scarface wondered how that had happened, but he knew better than to ask. He also wondered when he would have the opportunity to ask his favor of Sun. He longed to see a fall and a winter again, though he had complained about those seasons often enough in the past. For the time being, he dreamt of his love at home, and passed the time pleasantly with Morning Star.

One day before hunting, Moon told Scarface the story of how her other children had died. There were ferocious birds who lived in the waters. Her sons had gotten too close and had been eaten. She feared for the life of Morning Star, for he had reached the age at which the other youths had grown curious, sought out the birds, and died. She begged Scarface not to allow Morning Star to go down by the water's edge, for the birds were quick and would devour him before he could let an arrow fly. Scarface promised to look after Morning Star and keep him from harm.

Later that very morning Morning Star dared Scarface to race him down to the water's edge and see what strange creatures could be hunted there. Scarface called out to Morning Star to stop, but the youth had already begun running toward the water, pretending not to hear. Scarface had no choice but to race after Morning Star. Sure enough, Morning Star won the race. As he turned to taunt Scarface, three great birds rose from the water. They were the largest birds Scarface had ever seen, looking like lizards with wings. They aimed their fearsome beaks at Morning Star.

Scarface grabbed an arrow and prayed to the Creator to send Wind to carry it swiftly toward its target. He prayed with all his heart as he fit the arrow, drew back the sinew, and let go. Not even waiting to see the path of the arrow, he drew another and released, another and released. Three arrows traveled almost simultaneously toward the creatures. Three arrows struck their necks and killed them. The sound of Wind was enormous.

Grateful and exhausted, Scarface fell upon the ground. He thanked Wind and the Creator with all his heart. Morning Star was too stunned at first to know what had happened. When he finally understood, he ran toward Scarface, apologizing for his foolishness and thanking him for saving his life. Together they prayed to the Creator and to Wind, thanking them for their lives. Then they went to work, sawing off the heads of the creatures to take home to show Moon. She would never need to worry again.

Dragging the heads back took time, for they were as large as bears. Even before Scarface and Morning Star reached the door of the lodge, Moon heard them coming. She ran out to see what was causing such a commotion. Humbly Scarface recounted the story. Morning Star embellished it, praising Scarface's courage and piety. Moon hugged Scarface in gratitude. "Now my son is truly safe. When his father returns home tonight, I will tell him the story and he will grant you whatever you wish."

The next few hours were long ones for Scarface. He was raising the courage to ask for what he truly wanted. When Sun returned, Moon told him the story. Sun questioned Scarface to his satisfaction and examined the heads of the great birds. When he turned to Scarface, he said, "Truly, we are in your debt. As my wife has said, ask for what you seek and it will be granted."

Scarface told the story of the young woman whom he wished to marry. He told the story of his journey to Sun's lodge. He recounted what his bride-to-be had told him about the scar on his cheek. He asked Sun to remove the scar to indicate that he had blessed the marriage and had released the young woman from her vow so she could marry Scarface.

Sun listened carefully and nodded. "I know that young woman. She is a fine woman and full of virtue. She will make you a good wife. I give my blessing." Sun took an ocher medicine and rubbed it along the scar on Scarface's cheek. "When this medicine wears off, the scar will be gone. This is a sign of my blessing."

Sun gave Scarface many more gifts. He taught him Sun medicine and gave him the gift of the sweat lodge to take to the people. "When the rocks are hot and are brought into the lodge, you will feel my presence, for I am the source of all fire and warmth. My heat will cure your people. It will enable their illnesses and the bad spirits they carry in their bodies to be sweated out, and will restore them to health. My wedding gift to you is the healing power of Sun."

Sun taught him about other medicines, plants, and ceremonies, all of which would make his people healthy. When Scarface learned all he could absorb, Sun pronounced him ready to return to his people. He was given the greatest finery ever seen upon the earth and a simple brown robe with which to cover it. Scarface called for his helpers and, after waving good-bye to Sun, Moon, and Morning Star, was carried back to a hill above his village by the swans. He sat there in the darkness, waiting to feel the warmth of Sun above him as the great spirit began his daily journey across the sky.

When the light of day came, the people noticed the thickly clad stranger sitting on the hill above their village. He sat there the entire morning, cloaked in brown, despite the heat, which was so great that the lodge coverings had been rolled up to let drafts of air blow through. When midday passed, the chief could sustain his curiosity no longer. He asked some of the young men to go to the stranger and invite him to share drink and food. When the young men reached the stranger and asked him to remove his robe, they were dazzled by his clothing. Then they recognized Scarface and noticed that his scar was gone. "What has happened?" several exclaimed at once.

"I will tell my story to the chief," answered Scarface, "and all will hear." A procession followed him down the hill toward the lodge of the chief. Scarface asked that Tunapai, the widow, the beautiful woman, and her parents all be given places of honor in the chief's lodge. Once this was taken care of, everyone settled down and listened spellbound to Scarface's story. The marriage was arranged, and the village celebrated for an entire week. Slowly Scarface instructed the people in the medicine ways he had learned from Sun. Sweat lodges were built and the people learned how to sweat away their sicknesses.

Scarface and his wife lived a long and good life and had many grand-children. When they had lived over ninety summers, they departed together one night in their sleep for the Sand Hills and the Spirit World beyond. All were happy for them, and a great celebration was held for these two who had lived so well and so long. And that is how the sweat lodge came to the people.

The fire was burning down. The eyes of the coals glowed dully. Marilyn placed tobacco on the fire in appreciation of the spirits who had gathered to hear the story, and of Scarface himself, who Marilyn said was in our midst whenever the story was told.

"Learn well from this story. Remember the gift of the sweat lodge, and why it was given us. Remember, too, that any journey is always hardest in the middle. You must ask for help from those around you when you need it. When that has not solved your problem, look to the spirits for help and guidance. Look to the sky, look to the earth, and take help from the Creator. In this way you will prove your honesty and reveal your intent, and the spirits will reward you. You will receive great gifts, which you must then share with everyone."

I thanked Marilyn as the final flames flickered out. I thought of Scarface often as I watched the stars that night until I entered the land of sleep. There I visited the land of Sun, saw the heads of the great birds, and asked for guidance from Morning Star, who woke me once he was satisfied that his advice had been absorbed.

MARILYN ENCOURAGED my plan to move, early in 1985, to Santa Fe. Ellen and I had been separated for over two years but hadn't yet taken the time to be legally divorced. For a while we had been on relatively good terms. We even led a few birth-psychology workshops together. Tension between us increased over time as we each became romantically involved with other people.

Not only was it time to legally sever the ties between Ellen and myself, it was a good time to move, as I was between projects. I had finished my postdoctoral training program and was now a licensed clinical psychologist, as well as an emergency room physician. Friends had explained to me that it was often better for children to have some distance between their parents; the children could spend summers and holidays with one parent, school time with the other.

New Mexico appealed to me for other reasons. I had been doing regular trainings for a group of psychologists and midwives in Albuquerque since 1981; I felt I had many contacts to base a practice on. And I was already flying out there once a month to consult, see clients, and supervise the psychologists I was teaching. I also wanted to spend time with some Dineh elders I had heard were living within a day's drive of Santa Fe. The transition to a full-time lifestyle seemed desirable, and I felt the need to put my California past behind me. Sometimes a move is as much symbolic and psychic as it is physical.

An acquaintance who attended a lecture I gave brought me to see a Dineh elder named Hosteen Begay. Hosteen lived in a hogan on the Dineh reservation in northeastern Arizona, just south of the Utah border. The road to his place was nothing more than a set of well-worn tire tracks running over the dry, sandy earth. To drive a car onto his property you had to know the combination to a padlock on the gate across the road that led from the highway. It wasn't hard to remember—it was the year of the Pueblo Rebellion, when the Hopi rose up in arms against their Spanish conquerors.

Hosteen's hogan had sat there for at least nine generations; rooms were sometimes added to it, sometimes taken away. The last time I was there, a small second hogan had been built for a ceremony, about one hundred feet from the main structure. Both stood at the edge of a wash—called Hanging Woman Wash, after some unfortunate, forgotten soul—which was sometimes overflowing with water roaring down the hillside. The main hogan was padlocked in front but open in back and badly in need of repair. Next to it was a summer shelter made of aspen logs. It was roofed over with green aspen boughs and had an east-facing entrance.

At the south end of the shelter was Hosteen's bed; its mattress frame rested on pine logs. A square piece of old shower curtain, starting to mold, was attached to the beams overhead to keep rain from dripping onto the bed. Two thick sticks were suspended by rope from the roof. Sheepskins and neatly folded blankets hung over them. On the northeast side of the shelter was a fireplace built of sandstone and mud. Sometimes Hosteen Begay would burn a fire all day to stay warm. Between the bed and the fireplace stood a shaky table. Thick pine stumps served as chairs. Wooden crates nailed securely to the west side of the shelter held household items like pots and pans, canned food, utensils, spatulas, and a fly swatter. Nearby Hosteen had an ancient wood-burning stove he used to heat his coffee. His bolt-action Mauser rifle stood next to it, always within reach but never looking as if it had been used.

Hosteen was remarkable—in the same way as Nelson and Archie—for the warmth of his personality. Hosteen was also a bit like Coyote. He liked to be outrageous. He made it easy for people to laugh at their own foibles, because even when he teased you, it was easy to tell you were cared for by him. Once, having asked about my family, he was treated to a longer history of my separation than he expected. He looked askance at me a moment and then commented, "If you'd just go get your balls cut off like a sheep, you'd be a much happier man."

Besides being a shaman, Hosteen was a shepherd. He regularly rode the fence along the blacktop highway to repair any holes that his sheep might be tempted to wander through. He also kept a few chickens. One of the funniest things I ever saw involved one of them. Hosteen and I were sitting outside his hogan drinking the thick, black, sweet coffee he loved to simmer all day long. His gun was loaded as always, and leaning against a wall. He usually put his chickens in a coop to keep them away from the coyotes, but on days when people were around, he let them wander free in the yard.

Soon we saw a coyote stagger into the yard. We laughed at her, and Hosteen wondered aloud whether the predator had stumbled across the town of Gallup, where they drank all day long—because that coyote was zigzagging, falling down, hardly able to stand on all four feet. Neither of us noticed how close she was getting to a particular chicken, until *wham!*—that chicken was history. Coyote was no longer drunk. She was off like a shot with dinner in her jaws. Neither of us had time to pick up the gun, and we were both laughing too hard to aim it anyway.

Hosteen Begay told me, "The dumbest coyote with half its brain knocked out has more sense than the smartest fox." If you've ever watched coyotes in action, you know that's a fact. It's their smarts that make coyotes tricksters. If a coyote can't get what he wants by making you laugh, he'll trip you up instead. I remembered that Nelson had admonished me to honor Coyote, and I told Hosteen. "Then you should hear a story Dinehs tell about Coyote," he answered.

Back in the old days of First Man and First Woman, all the fire in the world was up on Fire Mountain, controlled by Fire Man. Coyote, being Coyote, was tired of being cold, and even more tired of eating cold meat. So Coyote, being Coyote, found a couple of birds he thought he might be able to trick into getting the fire for him.

212 • LEWIS MEHL-MADRONA

*"I'll tell you what. You guys are cold, too, right?" The birds hadn't
figured out yet how to fly south for the winter. It was before that time. So
yeah, they replied, they were cold, too. "Tell you what I'm gonna do. All
you have to do is take this little stick to the top of Fire Mountain, catch
some fire, and bring it back. You bring me some fire this one time, and I'll
be glad to give you all you want in the future, any time you want it."*

*The birds were stupid enough to appreciate that deal, so they did what
Coyote said. But Coyote neglected to tell them there were monsters guarding Fire Mountain. Two monsters. With huge eyes that never closed. The
monsters reared up, just as the little birds were about ready to steal some
fire, and singed their tail feathers. Terrified, they flew back home.*

*Coyote said to them, disgusted, "Hell's bells! Do I have to do every-
thing myself?" The birds hung their heads, ashamed, but nothing he could
say could convince them to go back up the mountain and face the monsters. So Coyote went way out to the ocean and collected some beautiful
shells from the seashore. He knew that when you held these shells by your
ears, you could hear the sound of the waves; you could even feel the cool-
ness of the water and the kiss of the breeze. Coyote returned to the foothills
of Fire Mountain and tied some sticks to his tail. Then he ran up to the top
of Fire Mountain. But unlike every other animal who had ever tried this
before, Coyote made a lot of noise as he went, so that the monsters couldn't
help but hear him coming.*

*They shouted, "Hey! Who is making so much noise? What are you,
stupid?"*

*"It's me! Coyote! And yeah, some people say I'm pretty stupid." The
monsters agreed he must be, as they sharpened their claws on some rocks.
"But I like to think I'm just too generous for my own good. Listen, I don't
want nothin' from you. I don't want no fire, if that's what you think. Fact
is, I just talked to a couple of bird friends of mine, who said they saw two
of the loneliest old monsters they'd ever seen up here on this mountain. So
I brought you a present of beautiful shells from the sea. If you hold them to
your ear, you'll be able to hear the waves of the ocean and feel the sea
breeze on your faces. And while you enjoy it, maybe I could stand here
with my back to the fire and warm my buns."*

Hosteen Begay started chuckling as he told his story. There is a long
Dineh tradition of bun jokes, some so corny it's hard to see how anyone
can find them funny. A modern example: "You know how they could
tell Ronald McDonald made it through the sweat lodge? From the
sesame seeds on his buns." I watched a roomful of Dinehs break up at
that one.

The monsters decided there wasn't any harm in Coyote's proposal. Anyway, they'd been up there guarding the fire ever since the world was created. They were tired. All Fire Man ever did was sleep, since he figured the monsters were fierce enough to protect his precious fire. Nobody had ever thought to give the monsters a present before. They thought it might be kind of nice to hear what an ocean sounds like, and to feel a cool sea breeze on their faces. So they accepted Coyote's present. They had a really good time with those shells.

Meanwhile, Coyote had his back to the fire. The fire roared up out of the mountain and licked the sticks that were tied to Coyote's tail. Before the monsters could stop him, Coyote was running down the hill with his tail on fire.

Fire Man woke up and saw what was happening. He took out his fire arrows and started letting them fly. But Coyote was zigging and zagging and dashing and prancing, and doing what a coyote does to get away. And he did! Fire Man gave up trying to kill him when he saw that Coyote was setting the whole mountain on fire. He no longer cared what happened to Coyote. He saw that the people and animals who lived below the mountain were going to have to pay for the fire, and that satisfied Fire Man.

The story's implicit moral is, of course, that every great power comes at a price. But along the way I learned that if I were to dare to follow Coyote's way, maybe I'd be able to steal fire from the gods.

Looking within a chronically ill person's soul and finding the healing resources hidden there can be a little like stealing fire from the gods. Sometimes the coping mechanisms we have learned to deal with an illness end up keeping us sick. People develop habits that nurture and maintain illness. Since, when we are sick, these habits seem helpful, we become extremely reluctant to change them. Often these habits help us manage and contain otherwise unbearable emotion. But if a healer can steal, like Coyote, past a habit's "defenses" (the monsters guarding the fire), he or she might find something that can be used to support the healing process.

It was no coincidence that the years I spent apprenticed, first to Marilyn, then to Hosteen, were the years I was most in need of healing myself. Hosteen Begay knew what it was like to lose a family. His wife had died years before. His children had moved, first to Phoenix, then to Los Angeles. They became modern Navajos. His granddaughter, whom he had never seen, was even in the movies. He was proud of that; others in his clan had seen her on television and told him all about it. To his grandchildren and great-grandchildren, Hosteen Begay was an almost

214 • LEWIS MEHL-MADRONA

mythical character, from another world they had little use for. I worried
that my children were developing similar sentiments about me, but
without the romanticism.

During the months I lived in Santa Fe, I spent five days out of fourteen back in Berkeley to be with my kids. (I also continued to work with
Marilyn while in California.) I kept a small apartment in Berkeley
where we could visit. My kids came out to New Mexico over some of
their school holidays, but they were getting older and more involved in
their social life with their friends, and traveling was not very appealing
to them. My friends were wrong about the desirability of the arrangement I had created, at least from the kids' point of view.

There were other problems. The growing tension with Ellen was
forcing my children to choose sides. And to them I looked like the less
stable parent, running around New Mexico learning Native American
healing and practicing part-time in Albuquerque, while their mother
had a stable practice in Berkeley. The kids were withdrawing from me
to avoid being embroiled in the conflict.

I brought a photograph of my son to Hosteen Begay. It had been
taken several years previously. In it we are sitting on the steps of a coffeehouse. He is young enough to be missing teeth, which his smile
reveals.

Hosteen didn't even look up when I came into the hogan. The
buzzing of a fly abruptly stopped. I set the picture down, and he studied
it carefully. He shook his head as if to say no. I took a seat before him, on
one of the pine stumps.

"You will lose the boy to the mother," he said. "You are not strong
enough to free him. The more you try, the more he suffers. Whatever
you do will only make matters worse. You should let him go. He will
seek you when he is older if you do what's right. That is all you can do."

At the end of the summer of 1985, I returned to Berkeley to be closer
to my children. Though I preferred living in New Mexico, I knew this
would be better for them. I came back to lead some friends in starting a
demonstration clinic for chronic illness. We wanted to be able to practice
either traditional or scientific medicine or both, depending on what was
best for the individual patient. We planned to apply the principles I had
been learning in working with patients who had long-term, disabling
medical problems.

WISCONSIN. The autumnal beauty of rolling, harvested farmland. For
two years I had lived amid these hills and landscapes, a younger man,
searching for purpose and meaning. Then in 1986 I returned to do a ceremony only forty miles from the house where I had lived with a family I

could no longer call mine. I was returning to Wisconsin, having been called to lead my first sweat lodge. My help had been requested. In a way, this lodge represented my graduation.

I was driven to a stone and wood house. Fifteen people, a group of friends who met regularly to create experiences for themselves, had congregated for the lodge. After meeting at Jean Huston's Mystery School, they had continued to meet after completing the program. Friday night I taught them about the gift of the sun. I told the story to honor my teacher; I felt her there in spirit, watching proudly. Silently I spoke to her, thanking her for the training she had given me. I was grateful to her, and ready for what I had been called upon to do.

The wind rose in the night, splattering the windows with a rain so hard it almost sounded like rapid gunfire. The next morning was glorious and cold. Frost covered the ground. I went outside in two sweaters and a coat, and still I was shivering. It took my blood a while to adjust to October in Wisconsin. The early morning sun was too low in the sky for me to feel its warmth. I could see the puffs of my breath in the cold air. My feet were cold, too; my single pair of socks and tennis shoes were not enough for this climate.

I had not yet seen the lodge my friends had built. I had given them instructions for it over the phone. Overall, I emphasized that if they loved the lodge they were building, it would be perfect. I spoke to a giant oak tree beside the house, telling her my intention to lead the lodge. With winter coming, she had lost most of her leaves, her voice. She could only sigh her agreement, acknowledging that I was new but that the spirit of the land would guide me. Any ceremony we did in the name of love would be honored, I heard. The earth had been ignored there for too long. The oak promised to support me, despite my inexperience.

The sun was barely visible on the horizon. Horses stood quietly outside the barn as I walked to the lodge. I passed a swimming pool, went through a backyard gate, and found myself in a magical pine and maple forest. The forest floor was covered with needles and cones. Maple leaves drifted silently to the ground as I passed. I heard the workers building the lodge before I saw its frame, standing in a small clearing, surrounded by the forest. It was magnificent, as beautiful as any I had seen, and as sturdy. I was led to the east-facing door. I could see the sun rising through the pines.

I examined the spot chosen to heat the stones. The opening in the forest canopy was large enough for the sparks to fly through. We trimmed back some branches and arranged stones in a circle around the fire pit. Helpers were enlisted to carry kindling and firewood from the barn. Rocks had been brought from Minnesota, but were dangerous because of their high quartz content (they would have exploded when heated). We searched the forest for some native stones, finding piles beneath trees. Some of the stones were appropriate; they were sufficiently large to hold heat without exploding. We carried them to the fire area.

I gathered everyone together in the house so they could go to work making prayer ties. One man had made prayer ties before; he volunteered to help the others when help was wanted. From the weather of the evening before, I knew that alternating white and black ties were needed to honor the Thunder spirits. The weather forecast had been for cold and rain. The day was cold, but bright and sunny. I chose four other colors, with 101 ties apiece—green for healing, yellow for alertness, red for courage and endurance, and blue to honor the sky and the Star Nation.

I returned to the sweat lodge site with a helper from North Dakota. We made a tipi of kindling, putting pine needles and dried leaves underneath. When the tipi was finished, I invited the woman who had arranged for the lodge to light the fire. Her initial attempts to light the edge of the kindling tipi failed, but when she accidentally dropped a match in its center, the fire ignited and blazed quickly. Everyone laughed. The fire blazed from the southeast, the direction of compassion and alertness. "A mild, wonderful sweat," I told everyone. "The fire has told us." The almost sleeping trees whispered the news of a sweat lodge across the valley to the trees on the ridges beyond. Soon the entire Wisconsin countryside knew of our designs.

After building the fire for the stones, we sat beside it, speaking with it and meditating. It required little direct attention. Two hours after its initial lighting, I gathered the group and their prayer ties and brought them to the lodge. The day was still very cold. I led them sunwise into the lodge. Asparagus ferns covered the ground. I hung the prayer ties and ceremonial robes from the ceiling. My helper brought in a shovel-load of coals. I placed sage on the coals. The shovel was passed around the circle, and everyone blessed themselves with the smoke. I was surrounded by fifteen curious, hopeful, apprehensive faces, about to begin.

With the coals sitting before me, I held the tobacco over the smoke, blessing it and beginning the prayers. A pinch went into the pipe for each of the seven directions. When the pipe was filled, my helper began to bring in the stones, large and white. The first sang to us as it was placed in the center of the pit. As each stone entered, it sang its own song. The robes danced above our heads to the medley of stone songs, and the black and white prayer ties began to sway. After the last stone had entered, I touched the bucket of water to the stones with a prayer that it be transformed into medicine for our healing. My helper entered the lodge, closing the door behind her.

In the darkness, I poured seven dippers of water onto the stone people, to start the purification ceremony. We sang the Four Directions song. The fire had spoken truly: the sweat was relatively mild, and we could remain inside with the door closed for some time. I felt the Christ spirit within the lodge, protecting and healing everyone there. While Marilyn works mostly with feminine spirits, my own primary helper spirit is masculine, although he has told me that in reality he is neither or both. He said I have cast him in a male form for my own comfort.

My usual consciousness had departed. In the darkness a spirit was telling me what to say. Words entered my awareness and were spoken. Action was directed. I responded to what I was told to do. This is the essence of shamanism—the spiritual direction of the moment takes precedence over tradition. I surveyed the hearts and minds around me. Most were open, some were closed. Two of those present would end up leaving the lodge before it was done.

We sat still in the heat and the darkness. Time may have continued outside the lodge; our watches and clocks would have faithfully reported its lapse for any of those who bothered to notice their time of entry. In the timeless stillness inside, yellow, luminous spirit eyes observed our sweat. Materializing in the heat, in the folds of the robes and the prayer ties, in the corners of the directions and from the visages of the stones, they watched and I felt their approval.

The cold eyes of the crow, the watchful gaze of the badger, the piercing stare of the hawk were all to be found in the lodge. Along with those observers was one I hadn't known before—a spry old Indian man, hundreds of years old. He had heard about us on the wind. Our songs drew him. He was the land, the ancestors, the spirits of men and women who lived for thousands of years amid the birch, the maple, and the pine. His countenance was harsh. He was accustomed to desecration. He searched for our faults. Finding them, he smiled. We were amateurs, he could tell. But we were there with heart, mind, and soul, addressing him respectfully, asking his blessing in a sacred manner. We were allowed to continue. He sat among us with his animal brethren. He did not accept us too readily, but he was pleased. How long it had been since the European newcomers, or even the natives of this area, had honored him! Later, the land's owner would pray to purchase the land next door, to protect and preserve it from subdivision. I believe the old Indian heard this heartfelt prayer. One year later she was able to purchase and preserve the land.

The old grandfather's approving nod meant so much to me. I had lived upon this land, filled with a young man's dreams and conflicts. Now I had returned, an older and I hoped wiser person, for another purpose. I had been approved—as were the people around me. While some do sweat lodges to "play Indian," the grandfather of the land saw we were there to worship. We were accepted and blessed, despite our mistakes and inexperience. Whatever is done with love and a prayerful heart is acceptable, imperfect or not, for love is perfect. Without love and worship, a perfect lodge, following all of the traditional ways, would fall flat. Love is the key.

One person left after the first door. As the second began and the prayers moved around the circle, I entered a new state of awareness. I returned to the spot where I had met the spirit of the mountain. There, spirits spoke to me. At the conclusion of the prayers, I delivered messages from those spirits. A raccoon spoke to one man. An eagle with glowing blue eyes directed me to tell another woman to seek the mountaintops but be sure to keep a roof over her head. Another woman was grieving. Three of those she had lost directed me to tell her to seek them in three pine trees. They would be there to comfort her. They were there now on the side of a snow-covered hill.

Other messages came. One young man prayed for the pain in his belly to be released. He was trying to pour all his energy into the earth to stop the pain. The spirit told me that would kill him. His pain would not cease until he stopped trying to give away all his energy. The pain kept a little of his energy inside him, and was all that was preventing his death. The spirit spoke through me, telling him the earth could take care of herself—she didn't need or want the young man's energy. In fact, she had more than enough energy of her own, and he should help himself to it. These instructions were strong and direct. A white luminosity shone over the man's head, reflecting upon his skin. The spirit asked him to pray for life. It did not wish to answer his prayers for death.

As I finished my prayers, a second person asked to leave. His prayer had been short and quiet. As he prayed, I had seen a barren landscape. I could feel his illness. His cells were depleted. I offered him the opportunity to stay with the door open, but he declined. I had hoped he could stay long enough to drink the medicine that would soon be passed around the circle. My heart filled with sadness to sense his depletion and his underlying rage. Its source I could not guess. I prayed that another could reach him.

Later, as I watched him eat several bowls of ice cream, I heard about his insatiable thirst and frequent muscle cramps. I urged him to seek medical attention. Given his symptoms and his size, I suggested he might have diabetes. This made him very angry, but he did see a doctor when he returned home. She confirmed that he was a diabetic, and as a result of her treatments, he is healthier now.

The medicine passed in a dipper around the circle. Everyone took a sip. Then we passed the dipper again, pouring water on our heads to open the crown chakras. We were ready for the third round.

My helper closed the door, and I placed more water on the stone people. This was our purification door, to prepare us to smoke the sacred pipe. Then our prayers would be heard. We sang again. Voices were strong and powerful, reaching toward the heavens. Sweat poured from our bodies and the heat was maintained, steady and even. The third door lasted a long time. The man who had wanted to die finally called out for the door to be opened. It was opened, and the cool air poured inside.

We sat together respectfully, inside the swollen belly of our earth mother. She would send us forth from her womb, like children, purified and blessed. We cleaned our hands and faces to smoke the pipe. My helper drew the first smoke and passed the pipe. When it got to me, I smoked the last of the tobacco, prayed, and let my helper return the pipe to the altar. We were ready for the final door.

In the darkness I felt a great peace descend upon the lodge. I asked everyone to remember that their prayers had already been answered, and that they were well. They had been purified. Now they were free to pray for any they had forgotten, and feel the spirit descending upon us. I recognized the Christ spirit again. Several people cried softly. The drum beat began and we sang the third and final song, sitting quietly for a short time in the darkness before the door opened.

CHAPTER NINE

AIDS and the Spirit of an Illness

IN BERKELEY, in 1987, the new year began under a misty sky, with a steady wind that kept the ocean's white-capped swells moving beneath the Golden Gate Bridge and clear across the bay. I had awoken at dawn to walk along a deserted stretch of piers down by the Berkeley Marina. Between the chill wind and the early hour, I had the piers pretty much to myself.

Not that there weren't other signs of life. Streamlined navy jets were on maneuvers over the choppy waters, accompanied by awkward swarms of helicopters. Thousands of feet higher, vapor trails followed commercial jets westward toward Hawaii and the Orient. A motor-driven yacht was idling a few yards away; I watched its captain leap aboard. His momentum rocked the fiberglass boat against the old automobile tires lashed to the side of the pier. Within half a minute, he had hauled in his lines and cast off from Berkeley's shore. I waved to him and he punched his whistle in reply. Then he turned out of the sheltered harbor, aiming his bow toward the open sea.

The night before, thousands of revelers had lined the San Francisco waterfront across the bay. The holiday had brought work to a standstill. The Embarcadero office buildings were still empty, their lights blackened, the streets beneath them filled with confetti made of shredded calendars, day-planners, and old computer printouts.

I walked slowly along the water, past the fluttering banners of the sailboats at their moorings. I moved on to the part of the marina where only big rocks lined the water. There was a friendly-looking older man sitting on one of the rocks. As I continued past him, I considered speaking but didn't; I had come here to be alone with my thoughts.

I found a large, flat rock, removed enough from the path that I would be left alone. I pulled out my small pipe and a cigar, and arranged them among some crystals and other sacred objects on the piece of bear fur I had carried with me. I badly needed advice from the spirits. Striking a match protected by the palm of my hand, I tried to light a candle.

New Year's morning has always been a time of reflection for me. The year that had just ended, 1986, had been both "the best of times and the worst of times." Our center for holistically oriented treatment of chronic disease, with offices in Berkeley and San Francisco, was working very effectively. We had cancer patients who were improving, with several even in remission. We had seen some dramatic results with rheumatoid arthritis, lupus and other connective tissue diseases, and also with more common problems like depression and asthma. We had AIDS patients who were doing far better than anyone had expected.

But the Center for Recovery from Illness also had serious financial problems. The very success of the practice threatened to close it down. Once we were discovered and championed by the AIDS community, the number of cancellations from patients with other illnesses grew. No matter how many programs existed to teach people that they could not catch AIDS by casual contact, people still shied away from those with AIDS. Even the liberal, educated clientele of the clinic had an aversion to sitting in a waiting room along with AIDS patients, a reaction that had no basis in medical theories of contagion.

The progressive loss of our other patients was draining the life blood of the clinic—for many of our AIDS patients were losing their insurance and were thus unable to pay for services. I could not turn them away. We did not try to collect from those who could not afford to pay, nor did we stop seeing them. The billing clerk gave up fighting with me, while the rest of us tried to carry on business as usual. But the bill collectors had little patience and less sympathy with the altruistic intentions of our impractical practice.

The patients we helped kept me going, along with a wonderful staff. Some were only part-time, but all needed to be paid. On this New Year's morning I felt oddly detached from these money troubles, even numb, as though the mist that was starting to roll in from the bay had anesthetized my anxiety and pain. For now, most of my creditors were asleep, or at least unable to reach me.

After multiple tries at lighting the candle, I gave up; the wind was too strong. I was to be allowed only the quick lightings I could make of sage or tobacco. Using my whole torso to shelter the next match, I managed to light some sage twigs. I waved the smoke over my body. The smell restored some of my sense of well-being but also brought tears to my eyes, for I could hold off the pain and sadness no longer. I sang the Four Directions song. Huddling against the wind again, I struck match after match until I finally succeeded in lighting the cigar. I took a deep drag on the smoke stick to keep the fire from going out, chanting a tribute and a call to Archie.

Here was another of my sorrows. The year before, Archie, still living in Ohio, had been diagnosed with a minor heart condition. Over the phone he told me what drugs his family practitioner had prescribed. The drugs didn't seem to me to be a good match for his condition, and I knew they could have dangerous side effects for a man of Archie's age. I implored him to see a heart specialist I knew in Cincinnati. But Archie declined, not wanting to hurt his GP's feelings by seeking a second opinion. Within a month Archie was dead—probably from a lethal abnormal heart rhythm caused by the drugs.

Though I grieved for him deeply, Archie was in a way still with me. I felt the presence of his spirit returning to me when I performed my ceremonies.

It was a striking irony, and humbling one, that I was powerless to stop Archie from dying of the misapplication of scientific medicine, just when I was taking part in some spectacular successes through alternative healing techniques at my clinic. But I knew Archie would be proud of what I was doing. Too bad, for the clinic, that our successes didn't translate into a more comfortable financial foundation. I imagined Dr. Barbour, my former clinic director in Wisconsin, telling me, "I told you so"—he'd told me that one day I'd regret not paying closer attention to what the management experts had to say about running a healthy practice. He was right. I still did not think the Wisconsin procedure-driven approach was the best one for me, but by studying it more carefully I might have learned something useful to help me through the current financial crisis.

During the work week there were more patients to be seen than time in which to see them. And true to form I often lingered too long with individual patients, leaving myself too tired to worry about business matters at the end of the day. Then, shortly before Christmas, I discovered the newest of my problems. I needed something out of our administrator's closet. She was on vacation, so I opened the closet myself. Reams of unfiled insurance claims fell on top of me, off a high shelf. Many of the claims were past the deadline. I could see where part of our cash-flow problem came from. Forget the patients without insurance— we had not even been billing the insurance companies that could pay.

My so-called friend Dakota, a person to whom I had given full rein over the financial aspects of the business, suddenly disappeared. Our accountant suspected her of embezzling money. The accountant reported her belief that Dakota had a scheme for paying herself on rotating days, so as to receive extra paychecks. She told us about unexplained bonuses, painting a picture that I first rejected but slowly came to believe to be true. I had felt a closeness to Dakota through our discussions of our cultural pasts. Being of Japanese ancestry, Dakota had heard stories of her parents being interred at a camp in California during World War II, which had made her seem expecially sensitive to the plight of Native Americans. Then came the news that Dakota and her three children were living in Marshall Islands, leaving me to wonder if she had planned her departure for months. It appeared that, for the six months prior to her departure date, Dakota had stopped filing any claims, stowing them out of sight on the top shelf in the closet instead.

How do you go on when a friend has betrayed you? I was trapped by my lack of residency training—I did not have the credentials to simply go out and get a job as a doctor. I toyed with the idea of finishing residency, but that was impossible without closing the clinic. I also thought about working as a psychologist, but the salary would have been too low to sustain the personal debt I had incurred to get the clinic going. Unless my creditors showed mercy, only by declaring bankruptcy could I quit the clinic, and I was not yet ready for that.

Sitting by the bay that morning I was feeling defeated, and badly needed to hear what the spirits had to say. I was not happy with the treadmill I was on because of the money I had to generate just to pay the clinic's operating expenses. Some weeks we didn't net enough money to pay me any salary. I usually couldn't imagine changing—surely if I persevered, I thought, things would get better. But this morning I was detached enough in my meditative space to realize that success was not assured. We were equally likely to collapse and close.

Eventually I felt Archie's presence. I could smell him over the smoldering cigar and the salt sea; I was comforted to have him with me. I offered tobacco to the four winds, to the sky spirits, to Mother Earth, to all my relations, and filled the bowl of my pipe. The spray from the waves crashing against the rocks made the pipe even harder to light than the cigar had been; I ran out of matches and had to resort to my "sacred Bic." I offered the smoke in gratitude, praying for a vision from the Spotted Eagle Nation about where next to go with my life. Was it possible to practice spiritual healing within the confines of the medical system and make a living doing so?

I sat on the beach that morning smoking the cigar in prayer, as

Archie and I had done so many times before. I was losing too many battles. I felt that my embittered ex-wife was trying to turn my children against me. It seemed the episode with Dakota would be the final blow that would destroy my practice. Smoking the cigar, I slowly slipped into a feeling of peace. Time would pass; something would change.

Though I relaxed, the spirits were of little help to me that day, or the help they offered wasn't what I expected: there was no encouragement to be had about the clinic. I decided I wasn't getting through very well. Perhaps the drizzling rain like a bad phone connection, was ruining the conversation. Then I noticed that the old man I had seen earlier out on the rocks had come over to stand beside me. "Beautiful day, isn't it," he said when I turned to look at him.

It was hardly turning out to be what most people would call beautiful—more a typical Bay Area day that tourist brochures refer to euphemistically as being "enshrouded in mist." But that particular morning's windswept beauty was a good match to my wistful mood. So I answered, "Right now, it's beautiful to me too."

"Days like this are important, aren't they. To remind us what a blessing sunlight can be. If we never knew sadness, how would we recognize our joys?"

I was a little surprised, out on these slippery rocks, to come across someone as wistful as I was—surprised and intrigued. We spoke a little longer. He was curious about the objects spread before me, and I explained them as I gathered them up. It was one of those conversations you have with strangers, where emotional secrets are shared and explored, though nothing all that specific is said. He talked about how rainy days helped him honor his losses; they helped him let go.

I left his company feeling strangely uplifted. A few steps on, I thought, Why leave it at that? Why not find out where this man is from? I turned on my heel, and the man had disappeared.

There was an ocean behind him, and rocks before and beside him. There was no place a human being could have gone, not in the thirty seconds it took me to turn around. Had I been talking to a spirit? What was his message? Was it to let go? Now I think so, but then I couldn't tell. I felt I had no choice but to keep on with the financially floundering clinic and the whole impossible routine I had established in Berkeley.

I BELIEVE ILLNESSES have spirits. You learn the spirit as you spend time working with it. Minor diseases respond well and quickly to treatments (of many kinds!), but major illnesses are recalcitrant; their successful treatments demand more time, attention, and skill. I spent thousands of hours with AIDS patients and came to know the spirit of the virus intimately.

Perhaps the depression that descended upon me in 1987 made me best able to work with AIDS patients—for the spirit of AIDS is one of despair.

Many will know this or that person with AIDS who is a fighter, and not despairing. I must be clear that I am referring to the spirit of AIDS itself and not the people it possesses. The spirit attaches itself differently to different personalities. The Québecois have a saying about unfamiliar beasts, *Q'est-ce qu'il mange en hiver*—What does it eat in winter? Find out, and the beast won't seem so mysterious. Likewise, to know the spirit of AIDS, we must spend hours with its victims; we must stalk the virus, studying its habits and its ways.

Kelly was one of my AIDS patients. A former actress in her late thirties, from New York, Kelly found her way to our San Francisco office, impressed by our name, the Center for Recovery from Illness. Our symbol was a circle of seven tears, representing the seven types of healers of Cherokee medicine. Among the Cherokee, medicine people work in teams of seven, each member having a different specialty. An easy case would be handled by one healer on his own. If the case was a little bit harder, then a team of three or four would work on it. The most difficult cases were treated by all seven.

We were also a team of seven practitioners. Each of us regarded cases from a Western perspective, but our varied training ensured that our approaches were quite different—different, and complementary. Between us we practiced homeopathy, Chinese medicine, Tibetan Buddhist healing, massage therapy, hypnosis and psychotherapy, and chiropractic, as well as the diagnostic theories and tools of conventional medicine. And, of course, my own skills included the medical views and treatments of the Native American tradition. Given our differences, we had some pretty heated discussions at times over how to proceed with certain patients. One thing we agreed on was not to force our beliefs on patients. We tried to let the patients lead us to what would help them, not vice versa.

Kelly spent the weekend before her first appointment dreadfully sick. It had been perhaps the worst weekend of her illness. But the pain she was experiencing didn't diminish her larger-than-life personality. "I am a martyr," she told me. "AIDS is the Christ. I am the cross, suffering along with the man who is nailed into my limbs." Through the glass windows of the office, I could see that the sky was gray and overcast, making the day seem more colorless than usual. The weather in San Francisco is deceptive. It can be calm and peaceful, but a storm can pick up quickly and sweep across the city—like an AIDS-related infection, exacting the suffering of the individual in full measure.

"How are you suffering, Kelly?"

Kelly looked up. "My whole body is aflame with pain." She stood, began pacing, and said, "I'm searching for something, anything, that will stop this constant pain. Maybe death. Maybe narcotics. Maybe something you can do to heal me." Kelly had obviously once had the outsized body to match her personality. Now she was starting to waste away.

"I'll try to help, but I can't promise I can make a difference. I can promise to do everything I can. How long has it been since you've been sick, how long have you known you had the virus? Start at the beginning. Tell me about your life and everything that's been happening to you."

Kelly sat down again and pulled out a cigarette from her bag. I wanted to tell her not to smoke in my office, but given her anguish, I didn't have the heart to do so. "Doctor," she said, "I got the virus from my lover Thomas. He was an alcoholic, and he must have gotten it from a prostitute."

"You speak of him in the past tense. Has Thomas died?"

"Yeah," she said, pulling a handkerchief out of her bag and dabbing at her eyes. "I still cry over his name. As if his name were Grief. We shared so much of it, him and me." I nodded for her to keep going. "Grief over the life we lost, over what was supposed to be. A whole generation's grief over how we thought we held the world in our hands when we were young, how we told our parents our lives would be different. We would be happy, we would be fulfilled, our dreams would be answered."

The rain began to fall in sheets.

"Then our friends started divorcing," she said. "There were suicides, cancers, so many people dying before their time. Now our generation even has its very own plague. Which of course I had to get, just so I could suffer too."

"You sound very bitter."

"I am. My whole generation is. We've become as broken and as bitter as our parents; the dream has shattered. I've been looking for something to heal me for the past two years. I've gone as far as D.C. for this or that treatment, I've tried all the antiviral drugs, and I haven't found anything that has made any difference at all."

I was listening carefully to Kelly's quest for healing as the wind whipped the rain against the windows. The sky grew darker.

"I have children," she whispered. She found that simple fact almost too painful to voice. "Both in college. They think I'm tainted by this disease, not worthy of respect."

I thought of my own children. I was afraid they also were learning to view me without respect. "Your children must feel grief, too," I said. "They're not too young to experience that. What grief have they known?" I asked. As Kelly answered my question, I considered her response, I also noted that I might have posed the same question to myself.

In my youth, I too thought I would conquer the world. My dreams were shattering, just as Kelly's already had. Once the divorce went through, Ellen and I were no longer civil to each other. Naturally the kids wanted to get out of the middle. The easiest way, they discovered, was to spend less time with me.

I could see how this solved their problem, but it was heartbreaking for me. And I worried what their mother might be teaching them—I didn't imagine Ellen stopped bad-mouthing me simply because I wasn't around. My daughter was older and more able to draw her own reasonable conclusions about us both. My son, though, was younger and more impressionable, and Hosteen Begay's admonishment that I let him go weighed heavily on my mind.

I thought of my last outing with my kids; driving down an old goat path in our '72 Land Cruiser, crossing a rickety bridge that barely held us, and heading south into the Jemez wilderness of New Mexico, where we built a sweat lodge and camped. I missed those moments with them, away from adult conflict. We spent several wonderful days hiking and doing some ceremonies and then we drove out through El Rito, stopping at a family taquerio that could just as well have been in the center of Old Mexico. The top was off the Land Cruiser, and we were all covered in road dust by the time we got back to the civilization of Albuquerque and its airport.

The year before, the last time I visited him, Hosteen Begay had been sitting at the table, sorting rocks. He didn't know how old he was exactly, but his memories stretched back at least eighty-three years, and he could easily have been ninety. He wore a faded plaid shirt and worn-out moccasins, tied only at the top eyelet. Despite his age, his skin was smooth under his white hair. His eyes were smiling, as they always seemed to be.

I asked his advice about a woman I had been dating. I wanted a companion badly. I had lived many lonely, isolated years during my marriage and I thought a new relationship might bring me the kind of intimacy I yearned for. Of course, I would have counseled anyone else against rushing into a relationship for those reasons. Any sudden marriage was bound to exacerbate the conflicts that lay behind the yearning for a relationship. I had to look within and settle those conflicts before I could expect a real, loving relationship. But I didn't see things quite so clearly when it came to myself.

Hosteen Begay put on his glasses and stared me directly in the eyes. Then he smiled and laughed. My ears turned red and my face flushed. "It must be the *bellagana* in you," Hosteen said, still laughing, but not without compassion. *Bellagana* means "white person" in the Dineh language. "Because I doubt you will listen to me. You must stop looking for love. When the spirits want you to have love, they will bring it to you. You must devote your life to work and your children, and though that won't win them back, it will bring you peace within yourself. Shake my hand. Shake my hand so I can feel your resolve."

He stood up and took my hand in his. We did not really shake, but rather he held on to my hand and studied me carefully. "You will not change. For all the other things you have learned, this is the one area where you prefer to remain stupid."

"But, Grandfather," I said, "I need a companion, a half-side."

Finally Hosteen Begay let go of my hand. He took off his glasses. "You have watched too many of those Hollywood movies, the kind my granddaughter acts in." Then he turned to his stove and lit it. He poured coffee into a charred old pot and put it on the burner.

To him the matter was closed. But I needed to hear more. "Is it not right that a man and a woman come together in this way? Is this not what the elders teach us in the ancient stories and songs?"

"Only young men speak so stupidly and without wisdom." He smiled at me gently. His coffee started to boil. "Do not even bother to answer me," he said. "I will be gone soon, before you see the wisdom of my words. You will keep trying to find this thing you call love, like a crazy teenager, until it bites you in the ass. Then maybe you will grow up."

AFTER TWO WEEKS Kelly was starting to feel better. She had begun to explore her inner world and was benefiting from the bitter herbs my Japanese colleague had prescribed. She was taking movement classes and rediscovering the sense of joy that came from using her body. She had given herself permission not to return to a dismal home in Chicago and a job that held few rewards. It was an office job she had taken after her uncertain health made performing impossible.

In consultation with me, Kelly discovered that the ghost of Ted, her first husband, was still haunting her. Ted had been, like Thomas, an alcoholic. Though Ted had been dead twenty years, he remained a terror to Kelly. During the last year of his alcoholic life Ted was already gone, Kelly said. She recalled a malevolent being that inhabited him, an ugly green thing, a violent and sadistic product of the bars and the gutters Ted frequented—a monster from the nightmares of our society's addicted millions. Kelly had essentially lived with a terrorist. He threatened and abused both Kelly and their daughter. Ted had brief moments of sanity, and during these Kelly caught a glimpse of the man she loved, but ordinarily he was trapped behind clouded, monster eyes, and a mouth shut tight over rotting teeth.

Kelly caught Ted once urinating in his shoes. This was quite a statement to the world—"I despise even the ground I walk upon." He was impotent. He wore nothing but boxer shorts almost every day. He had the largest liver ever recorded in his small community hospital's autopsy room.

"Ted has more to do with my AIDS than Thomas, who gave me the virus," Kelly told me. "Ted, or the malevolent spirit that lived within Ted, was everything bad, everything evil, the very essence of AIDS, even though he died before it was discovered. Maybe, compared to him, the viruses are innocent creatures. Maybe they just fill the void that Ted left inside me."

"Can you describe that spirit? How did it get in there?"

"I guess my guardian angels were on vacation."

"Evil spirits can't come in where they're not invited."

Kelly puffed again on her cigarette and nodded. "The spirit of evil that took over Ted just moved right into me when he died. Maybe I wanted the company. Maybe I didn't think I deserved any better." She exhaled her smoke with a profound sigh. "That evil spirit is sure not the Christian devil. He's not that intelligent. He's not that willful. But the gate was open, you know?"

"Who is he?"

"It's hard to say. He has too many faces. One thing's for sure, he doesn't plan so well, he's not that conscious, he's just pure, unconscious evil. Aimless evil. Just this alcoholic, malevolent conglomeration of aimless energy."

Kelly's metaphysics, springing from her lived experience, went far beyond her education. I found what she was saying startling, for the spirit she described was completely in line with the evil spirit Iktomi—a being in the Lakota pantheon somewhat parallel to the Christian devil. Iktomi's primary power stems from misinformation. He tries to get people to believe the wrong things and then live according to them. A success, for Iktomi, would be getting a woman like Kelly to accept the idea that she deserved no better than an alcoholic husband, or getting a man like Ted to believe that misery was all he could expect from life.

"And now this evil spirit has its claws in you," I offered, "wanting to take you down as well. Do you understand what I'm suggesting? Your spirit has turned a little bit mean, too. Just like Ted's spirit. This evil energy is fighting to control you, consume you." This wasn't easy for Kelly to hear. She started to weep, then nodded in agreement.

My secretary knocked on the door and brought me a cup of coffee.

This was her signal to me that the session had gone on too long. As I drank the coffee, and wrapped up with Kelly, I wondered how many people Iktomi had gained power over through disease. How often had he convinced them their illnesses were necessary, deserved, and inescapable?

The alcoholic, I thought to myself, is the symbol of our culture. What does it mean to be an alcoholic? What does it mean to be inhabited by the AIDS virus? To really understand a culture, line up its unhealthy citizens and ask, Who are these people? Where have they come from? Why are they here? Answer those questions, and you will understand the soul of an age.

I LEFT CALIFORNIA for a week in May of 1987. I had been invited to give a workshop on spiritual healing in Zagreb, Croatia. My expenses were paid by the conference organizer, and it was a rare opportunity to meet my counterparts from around the world.

After I finished my opening talk, a young man in the audience stood up, fervently and humbly seeking help for his hospitalized father. The father had a dissecting aneurysm—a weakened and ballooning blood vessel wall of his arm's brachial artery. The condition can result in a sudden and fatal loss of blood. His vascular surgeons were proposing to amputate his arm to prevent his hemorrhaging into the chest cavity. His son believed that as a group we could help his father. I requested that he return after the lunch break with several items his father had handled daily, for use in a ritual.

The son returned with his brother and a handful of their father's personal talismans—a key ring, a billfold, and a photo of their deceased mother. I began the ritual with the Four Directions song, asking the spirits of the west, north, east, and south to notice our circle. Then we prayed. I passed smoldering sage around the room in an abalone shell for all to use to bless themselves.

The son stood near me in the center of the room and related what it was he wanted from the ritual. He then described his love for his father; he spoke of his childhood memories, of wonderful gifts his father had given him, of meaningful experiences they had shared. His brother talked of their relationship in the present, of the father's strong love for the family, and of their own heartfelt hope that he could be well.

When they finished, I asked each person in the room to say some words, either about the sick father or about his or her own father. I asked especially that they keep their speeches simple and direct. When all had finished speaking, I started a prayer for the man. Each person added his or her words to the prayer, which ended with the words of the two brothers.

I filled the sacred pipe with tobacco. Then the two brothers and I smoked for the sake of the father. I called out to the spirits who had come to our circle. If it was possible, I asked, and as long as it was for the greatest good, would they please go over to that hospital and see what could be done. I saw a clear image of the man and of two spirits standing on either side of his narrow hospital bed. The room was white and antiseptic. They reported that his predicament was the tangential result of an earlier life choice, and they weren't sure how much reversal was possible. The father would have to undo a previous decision, and they would try to help, but no guarantees could be made.

I related this to the group, and we sang another prayer song to end the ritual. The next day I learned that the man's doctors had suddenly changed their diagnosis. They said the aneurysm was much smaller than they had previously thought, and so was not as great a problem. By the second day after the ritual the man was discharged and told to return for a followup in a month.

The miracle was expressed physically in a manner the doctors could explain acceptably. This is how many miracles are translated into physical events in this time and culture. The man's doctors could not accept healing, but they could admit misdiagnosis. They reported a probable mistake and let the patient go.

The collective power of everyone in the room, the pure desire of the two brothers, and the power of the two spirits were all components in the miraculous outcome. Everyone had a father about whom he or she cared and could speak. I couldn't take credit for what happened. We as a group couldn't take it either. The spirits did not know themselves if they would succeed. Our group asked respectfully for what we wanted, without demanding, remembering that the greatest good might preclude our desired result. The credit for this miracle belongs to another dimension, which served as a kind of transducer to convert our prayers and desires into a physical event.

Prayer and ceremony hold a magic and power that cannot be denied. It is through ritual that we address the nonphysical energies which surround us, nurture us, protect us, enliven us, and instruct us. It is the simplest way of formally requesting help with our problems.

Soon after I returned to San Francisco, Kelly was ready for a ritual of her own. She had been coming to the clinic twice a week for six weeks. People as dramatic as she was can be easier to lead into ceremony than others—twelve appointments are not many, but Kelly was a quick study. Her life in the theater had prepared her to embrace ritual and ceremony.

She had made a doll of Ted while I was gone, to serve as a robe for the evil energy that had filled him before his death, the same energy that she felt was behind her AIDS. It was a Styrofoam doll, clothed in green felt. Orange yarn hung from the sides of its Styrofoam head. A twisted, dried red pepper made the perfect alcoholic's nose. The arms were twisted, gnarled sticks. The right hand clutched an advertisement's picture of a whiskey bottle and a cocaine vial; the left hand held a sharp knife. Two black boxes served as feet. We carried the doll in a shoebox to China Beach.

We walked down the long, steep stairs leading to the sandy beach while the waves continued their progressive march past us toward the Oakland Bay Bridge. Rocks covered the beach, but not rocks from any native geologic strata; they had been ballast once, jettisoned offshore by nineteenth-century sailing ships. Each time I came to the beach, the tide had washed in new rocks and swept old ones away. Their faces were always changing.

"Who says rocks are not alive?" I remarked, a little self-consciously. I wasn't used to leading ceremonies with people as versed in theater as Kelly. "These rocks dance every night, and the strong waves made them sing." A bare spot beneath some sheer, overhanging cliffs seemed right for our ritual, and I led Kelly over to it. Three large rocks had arranged themselves the night before in a circle for me, Kelly, and the Ted doll. I made a wall of four large and four small rocks to protect from the wind the flames of two small candles. I lit them as Kelly settled down.

The sheer rock wall behind us formed the backdrop for our work. A gull streaked across the sky, its high-pitched cry filling our ears. I thought of photographs I had seen of the area's Indians, who had once lined the harbor and filled the forests hereabouts. "Hau," I heard them say.

Kelly unconsciously nodded.

I soon entered a ritual state of consciousness, a place beneath the surface of usual consciousness, a deeper state of being that isn't rooted in my own personality. It is a state of ecstatic union with nature best communicated through poetry and song, not spoken about. In that state of awareness the rocks truly did speak. The ocean called out to me, and I understood its musical rhythm, the same way I suddenly understood the meaning of the sea gull's cries. I took the sacred crystals from my ritual bag and placed them by the candles. My large quartz healing crystal stood upright in the sand.

In this ecstatic state I knew instinctively where to lay the crystals, and where the candles. I unwrapped my pipe and made an altar for it upon the sand. I put some sage in my abalone shell. Having lit the dried leaves, I passed the shell to Kelly. While she blessed herself with the smoke, a song sang itself to me. It was a crying song, the kind the old ones sang when someone had died. The song was low, very soft, and pitifully sad. I listened to it for a minute or two, then noticed Kelly seemed to be nodding to its cadence, too. I began to hum the tune. Even today the melody has stayed with me. When Kelly returned the shell to me, I purified the pipe's red pipestone bowl and mink-and-bead-covered stem with the sacred smoke. Then I set the pipe down upon the altar with the bowl pointing north.

I sprinkled cornmeal in a circle around us and began to pray. I called upon the Creator and the grandfathers and grandmothers, the earth and the sky, the ocean and the rocks, and the spirit of that place. I named each of the seven directions. I let them know our purpose: "Creator, we have come here to pray for Kelly. We have come to pray about this energy she has carried for twenty years. She does not want to carry it any longer. We pray for it to leave her and come into the robe she has prepared for it. We wish to honor it, we wish for it to be carried into the light, and we pray for protection from this spirit, for it is powerful."

The shoes of the doll began to move. Before I could react, a man was sitting in the circle beside us. He looked as real as Kelly. He wore only a breech cloth and a cloth wrapped around his forehead, and his long, black hair blew with the wind. When he first appeared, the look on his face was one of pure hatred and rage. At first I was so scared, I pretended not to see the figure. I didn't know how to protect us. Then I remembered the song I had been hearing. I knew I had to sing the song to let that spirit go. I began to sing it just as I had heard it. Kelly joined me, and the spirit stood up. My eyes were almost closed, but I was watching him indirectly, through the corner of my eyes; Marilyn had taught me that that's the best way to watch spirits. He stood and walked away from us, toward the ocean. "Thank you for coming, spirit," I said. I felt another wave of fear pass through me.

"Creator!" I called out. "Grandfathers and Grandmothers! Protect us. Mother of Corn, White Buffalo Calf Woman, Sons of the Wind, protect us." I sprinkled cornmeal on the doll and on top of Kelly and me, finally scattering it around us to reshape our circle. "We know that the power of light outweighs the power of darkness. Creator, protect us, and help us transform this energy. Guide it to the light and set it free."

"Wiohpeyata," I prayed, "spirit of the west wind, as you sit in the west in your black blanket, help us with our fears of this spirit, of AIDS, of alcohol and drugs. Help us to honor our fears and to hear the message that our fears bring."

Shaking my bear-claw rattle, I continued. "Waziyata, north wind, as you sit in the north in your red blanket, grant us strength and endurance. Give us the strength to speak to this alcohol spirit and to put aside the gifts he offers. Give us the courage to stand firm on our ground, the strength to walk with sacred footsteps. Help us to walk the good red road behind the sacred pipe. Let us fall neither into jealousy nor into hatred." The spirit, too, was standing still and listening, appearing fearful now himself as he stood at the edge of the sea and sky. A seagull seemed to fly right through him.

"Wiohiyanpata, east wind, as you sit with the rising sun and the Spotted Eagle Nation, help us to see clearly." The man was fading and now I could see the shadows of four figures, hardly separate from the spray of the waves. "We are crying out for a vision," I called out. "A vision of wellness for Kelly. She has come here because she is sick and she wishes to be well. She calls upon you for your help, for your vision. Help us to see how to deal with the spirit of this illness."

"Itokagata, south wind, as you sit wrapped in your white blanket with the White Buffalo Calf Woman, give us love and compassion for each other."

Kelly was listening carefully. "Help me," she said softly, "and all those in my life who were consumed by the alcohol spirit."

"Wakantankan, as you sit above us with the Star Nation, protect us, for we are pitiful in your eyes. Protect us from these evil spirits, from AIDS, from alcoholism, from drug addiction." I wanted to get up and go over to see whether those spirits had really disappeared, but I was too frightened to move. I felt some sense of protection when I sat absolutely still and kept praying. I could feel evil energy all around us, lurking in the shadows, skipping over the waves, flying with the gulls. It still threatened Kelly and me, though not so directly as before.

"Mother Earth, smile up at us as you sit below us. Help us to feel cradled in your arms, for you are our mother. Help us to feel nurtured and loved, help us to feel your healing power, for this is Kelly's prayer. She wishes to be well." I sensed the spirits who stalked Kelly standing in the distance—Ted, her first husband, who had been consumed by evil; Thomas, her last husband, who had died of AIDS and infected her; Suicide, who stood lurking, waiting for Kelly to come to her; and something that I could only call Pure Evil, standing above and behind them all, wavering in the wind. Was this Iktomi? Or the being Christians call Satan? Reflexively I lit more sage to banish the smell of these spirits, which was stronger even than the ordinary stench of dead fish and seaweed on this beach.

"Tunkasila, bless us as you sit in the center of our hearts with all our relations. Help us to know that we are one with all creation."

Kelly seemed to be in pain. I continued praying. "Help us to feel one with the rocks, the water, the creepy-crawlies, the winged ones. Help us to feel one with the four-leggeds. To know we are the brothers of the stone people and the sisters of all creation. Let us give thanks to all the sacred beings."

Finally I stopped and asked Kelly to say her prayer. She asked for knowledge of the spirits, but I knew she didn't need that. Spirits can heal us whether we understand them or not; we just need to acknowledge that they are there, to stop questioning them, because questions are doubts. I barely heard Kelly speaking. I was watching Hosteen Begay. He was smiling and telling me everything would be fine. He was in a position to know, for he had been in the spirit world himself by now for almost a year.

Kelly finished her prayer. Then we sang a song in honor of the spirits who had come to participate in and witness our ritual. I hadn't planned to push for anything as concentrated as a healing today, but I could feel the energy building as we sang. Singing seems to focus the power of the spirit world, the way a magnifying lens can intensify the power of the sun's rays and start a fire. And one thing Kelly knew about was singing. The beauty of her voice was not important to the ritual, though her contralto sound was truly beautiful; I have heard people with ordinary voices sing beautifully too, when they sing with sincerity. Kelly had sincerity and a passionate desire to be well, both lending energy and power to her extraordinary instrument.

When we finished, I addressed the being who now inhabited Kelly's doll. "Spirit of all that has been evil in Kelly's life, evil spirits who filled Ted as he was dying, when his spirit had already left his body, we are here to address you. We are here with Kelly, who asks you now to leave her body and take with you all the illness you have caused. She has housed you for twenty years, and now we pray that you take your leave of her. We ask that the star people guide you along the Milky Road to the Lodge of the Creator, to become one again with the Creator, to be cleansed and purified. Kelly and all her helpers and all the sacred beings demand that you depart. Now get you gone!"

I shouted the last words and then asked Kelly to speak to the spirit, to tell it her intentions in no uncertain terms. Her voice was true and firm, like the younger self she said was hers before she met Ted. She told the spirit to leave.

A gust of wind whipped across our circle. The candles flickered, but the flames held. The ocean's waves rolled in closer toward us. By now it was mid-afternoon, and the sky was still covered by steel-gray clouds that were blowing in from the open ocean. We could hear the rocks shifting beneath the waves. Rain was starting to fall. I asked Kelly to sing a song that expressed her feelings to the spirits. Her operatic voice sounded angelic above the waves while the fog closed in around us, enveloping our ritual circle. A nearby oceangoing vessel blasted its foghorn several times in slow succession, providing an amusingly intempo musical counterpoint to her song. All was still when Kelly finished.

I shook my rattle and began to chant, singing in praise of the spirits. When the song ended, we prayed again—a prayer for each direction, and a pinch of tobacco for each prayer, until the pipestone bowl was full. Then we smoked the pipe. We asked the sacred smoke to carry our prayers skyward, across the Milky Road, to the Creator's lodge.

As the smoke drifted skyward, a palpable relief filled the space between us. I finished our ritual by using a crystal to help clear the blocked energy within Kelly, moving it along her energy lines, channeling energy through it at her points of blockage. Then we offered the doll she had made to the ocean.

We collected all the litter we found while leaving the beach. By the time we made it to the stairway we had quite a collection of aluminum cans and old beer bottles. Kelly labored up the stairs, breathing so hard I worried she might become hypoxic before reaching the top. But she was beaming when we got there, chattering cheerfully as we headed back toward the car.

Ted's spirit had kept Kelly's soul at bay. For years she had not been fully embodied, and that left her open to viral infection. Through the beach ceremony Kelly had rid herself of Ted's influence. That evening her daughter called her to seek a rapproachment, and to ask her mother's forgiveness. For the first time they talked together about the abuse Ted had inflicted on them both, and about Kelly's pain at not having done a better job protecting her daughter. A barrier between them had dissolved.

EARLY NEW AGERS like Louise Hays drew up bestiaries of diseases, arguing that cancer is a body's way of expressing this unhappy idea, mononucleosis that one. Such formulations are simplistic, in that they discount the spirit of the individual. Illness results from a relationship between the disease's spirit and the person's own.

There is also some truth to such formulations. Illnesses *can* be symbolic, though they aren't always. They rarely mean the same thing for two different people. My childhood asthma, as I've mentioned, had to do with my shame at being illegitimate. I sensed my mother's embarrassment and guilt, and knew I was somehow to blame. I felt I did not have the right to breathe—and so my body expressed the idea physically. But too many of my AIDS patient took Ms. Hays's ideas or similar ones to mean they were at fault for their own illnesses. My patients would tell me, essentially, "I read something that says AIDS means x, and x is bad, so that makes me bad, so I deserve AIDS." And so an idea that began as a helpful insight became an obstacle to healing. If AIDS always meant the same thing to every person who had it, it wouldn't be as hard to treat as it is.

But how is anything spiritual expressed by a viral infection in the first place? Looking at how a virus operates provides some clues. A virus sleeps within a cell membrane until the cell can no longer repair and maintain itself. When intracellular conditions deteriorate, the virus awakens—functioning like a tiny catfish, cleaning the cellular debris. During this process, the virus replicates. Infection is the by-product.

Is anything more than physiology involved in a viral infection? A high presence of damaged cells is an open invitation to viral cleanup. It triggers the replication of one of the many viruses related to cancer, AIDS, chronic fatigue syndrome, and other diseases.

Hosteen Begay told me, although not in medical terms, that it is the individual with a compromised spirit who invites illness and infection. Feelings of spiritual emptiness, depression, and doubt generate conditions that encourage internal cellular breakdown. A woman like Kelly, who believes she must take on the evil that has killed her husband, is a woman susceptible to illness. When the psyche doubts, the cell becomes sluggish. Disease can ensue.

Healing requires the soul's participation. Biological healing lags behind the healing of the soul, but surely follows. Hosteen Begay taught me that without feelings of fulfillment, connectedness, and faith, the body cannot maintain health. Humans need their relationships with the land and the spirits if they want to be healthy. Restoring the relationship results in the apparent magic of healing. When God is dead, cells begin to die. When the soul is empty, the cell becomes an empty shell. Hosteen Begay came from the spirit world during the ceremony I held for Kelly to remind me of this wisdom.

When I began her ceremony, I hoped Kelly might end up partially better. Many times ceremonies accomplish only this much—and this is plenty. But because Kelly entered so wholeheartedly into the ceremony, and because the spirits were prepared to help her, a more essential change took place.

I did not make the mistake of many healers, of immediately taking Kelly off her medications. I did taper them off somewhat. A ritual healing engages a person on an emotional level; the exhilaration a person feels afterward may make symptoms completely disappear for several days, but then they can return with a vengeance. Illnesses wax and wane. They have a rhythm, like every other living process.

Kelly had relapses after our ceremony, but she continued in her wholehearted devotion to healing and is still alive at the time of this writing. Is she cured? Not entirely, not yet, but her continued life nine years later is a wonder all by itself.

Conventional medical wisdom says that all AIDS patients die. This is the only reason we permit the use of AZT (azothioprine) or DDI (a newer AIDS drug), for the toxicities of these compounds are extreme—they cannot even gain FDA approval as anticancer drugs. AZT and DDI can help patients, but they also manifest more and more side effects over time, until the effects concatenate and sometimes finish off the project AIDS has begun. Well-behaved AIDS patients take their medicines and slowly but surely die.

What about stubborn AIDS patients? By stubborn, I mean the unconventional patients I came across, like Kelly, like an Australian client who was on the brink of death from *Pneumocystis pneumoniae,* who willed himself to health, which he has maintained for years now. And there are others. Now a genetic mutation has been discovered which permits infected HIV patients to live without developing AIDS. Can the prayers of the many influence the genes of the few?

Then there are those whose anger negates every attempted treatment. Working with AIDS drew several furiously angry patients to my practice. Their fury was understandable, given the political climate surrounding the disease, but it made my work next to impossible. It is not the kind of energy from which healing springs. I know there are activists who urge people to get angry about AIDS, thinking the anger leads to a fighting spirit, but in my experience this kind of anger turns invariably inward; and by blaming themselves for an illness, angry patients can only perpetuate it. Of course, a passive attitude to a disease is no more helpful. Having trust in the possibility of healing is the key, and having trust is neither passive nor aggressive.

One patient, Theodore, taught me much by his example. His opportunistic infections had primarily been intestinal, along with one bout after another with pneumocystis pneumonia. He was suffering terribly and was on the verge of death from chronic diarrhea and malnutrition. He spoke to me about Dr. Imanuel Revici in Manhattan, who treated patients with a controversial phospholipid therapy. I told Theodore that if he believed the therapy would help him, it was worth a try.

Shortly thereafter, Theodore made the precarious pilgrimage to New York to see Dr. Revici. He loaded up on an entire bottle of antidiarrheal medication, and his friends bundled him onto a plane. Upon arrival, the minute he saw Revici, he knew that this kindly, ninety-three-year-old Romanian gentleman would help him. Revici said to him, "Dear, don't worry, you will be well. Don't worry at all."

How this resembles a shaman's comforting words! Theodore's prayers, Revici implied, had already been answered. He would be well. Theodore trusted Revici completely. He stayed in New York for three weeks, seeing the doctor every day. His diarrhea rapidly cleared. His parasites disappeared. He communed with others in the talk-filled waiting room. Sometimes he waited with other patients up to five hours to see the doctor. Newcomers on stretchers and in wheelchairs were welcomed with tales of miraculous recoveries. Theodore recounted that these patients' spirits began to improve even in the waiting room, just from the atmosphere.

The phospholipid injections and oral drops were a liquid sacrament; it was the ceremony of it that drew so many faithful to Dr. Revici's office. A sterile plastic cup became, for a Revici patient, as sacred as the Holy Grail. The American Medical Association and the New York State Medical Board were trying to stop Dr. Revici from dispensing the lipids, but their efforts only made the medicine even more powerful to his devotees. The arduous journey that patients like Theodore had to undertake to get to the lipids also served to overcome any encountered skepticism. I myself doubted there was much, if any, biomedicinal benefit to the lipids, but that didn't diminish their sacred power. When we ingest something sacred, a kind of magic is released within the body. And magic was what Revici was dispensing.

Yes, biomedicine continues to demand a so-called objective evaluation, but how would we design an experiment of Revici's methods? Would a double-blind, controlled trial include the atmosphere of Revici's waiting room and the old gentleman's kindly manner? Would other dispensers of lipids maintain his confidence, accent, and compassion? More likely an objective, white-coated scientist would dispense the sacred drops. But context is crucial to effectiveness, and belief is a vital part of any cure. I suspect that those who believe in a treatment will always produce better results than their neutral counterparts.

The placebo effect is sacred and powerful. Recently I attended a dinner sponsored by the makers of a new antidepressant. The progression of slides bored one woman at the table, a psychiatrist's wife, until a slide appeared comparing the antidepressant with placebo. "My God," she said, "fifty percent of the patients taking placebos improved!" The one person there with no professional interest in the proceedings was properly excited by something the rest of us had seen so often we had forgotten. The

240 • LEWIS MEHL-MADRONA

fact that half the patients improved because of their faith in their treatment was much more exciting than the new antidepressant's results.

The journey, the waiting room, the old, elfin man, the ceremony of the lipid administration were all an inseparable part of Revici's treatment. There is no way to divorce a man from his medicine.

Theodore seemed cured when he returned from New York. Because he had done so well, local Revici advocates convinced him to be a spokesperson for the treatment. Theodore dutifully told his story to an audience peppered with physicians, including me. With full priestly authority, one of the physicians present attacked the foundations of Theodore's recovery. He argued it could only be temporary; he'd seen such brief remissions before. Soon Theodore's T-cells would decline again. The doctor predicted Theodore would relapse by Thanksgiving.

I watched Theodore try to argue, but clearly he had taken the doctor's words like a bullet to the chest. He stumbled over his answers. His color turned ashen. His head dropped. By Thanksgiving he was sick again; by Christmas he was dead.

The prediction proved correct, but not necessarily for the reasons the doctor gave. I know other miracle cures who continue to be well. They shield themselves from the doubting Thomases in the medical professions and the media. They cultivate their trust in their cure in monkish obscurity, guarding the secret of it carefully.

Most people I have known who have been through a miraculous healing experience don't like to talk about it much. There seems to be a sense that talk diminishes the power of the cure. I was once asked to produce a list of people who had experienced miracle cures, who would consent to be interviewed and photographed by *Life* magazine. None of my patients who had been through fairly spectacular cures would consent. And wisely so, I thought. Only those cured of moderately severe illnesses (rheumatoid arthritis, lupus, depression, and the like) were willing to go public. *Life* scrapped the article idea. Moderate miracles don't make good copy, though they are no less important to the lives they touch.

Perhaps reticence, or humility, is a condition of continued health. I've often wondered if comedian Gilda Radner's fatal relapse (she died of ovarian cancer) didn't stem from her advocating alternative cures on the talk-show circuit. Her purpose was admirable, to bring to a wider public a cure that had worked for her, but the spirits do not seem forgiving of too much chatter and speculation. Watching Theodore's health be destroyed by a doubtful—even though not intentionally hostile—audience gave me a glimpse of how difficult it can be to "keep the faith," how easily the faith can be undermined.

My own experience indicates that with serious illness, after whatever treatment, 20 percent of patients will thrive over the long term, trusting steadfastly in their cure and in themselves. I have also observed that fully 75 percent of patients improve at the beginning of a treatment; most then gradually deteriorate. After a year, only the stalwart 20 percent remain. These stalwarts are fringe population. They are difficult to measure, because you will not find them filling out questionnaires in medical clinics. Their convictions have drawn them elsewhere. To a rural, aging, Mississippi Choctaw shamaness, perhaps. To the clinics of northern Mexico. To the lamas of Tibet. These 20 percent keep the supporters of fringe disciplines active, and sometimes proselytizing the majority. And the 80 percent who deteriorate and die as expected give the evidence majority practitioners need to persecute the fringe practitioners, to depict them as charlatans and quacks.

How do the 20 percent thrive? The key, in my experience, is trust. Trust is an implicit, deep faith that leaves no room for doubt or skepticism. "I believe this will work" is not trust's end point; rather, trust's starting point is "I *know* this will work."

Ritual helps human beings to trust. The powerful sensual appeal of ritual prayer, song, and dance allows us to forget our skeptical world view for a moment. We remember that we belong to the earth, as much as any rabbit or deer. Even our movements, our footsteps, honor the earth. Through ritual, the earth honors us back. We are changed by a power that is not our own, an energy that transcends and understands us and engulfs us in its blessing. When we are in harmony with the earth, our cells are in harmony within us. Harmony is the music of healing.

Disharmony produces cellular degeneration, viral infection, and disease—AIDS, cancer, and so on. Never have we been so removed from the harmony of nature as today. Hosteen Begay thought of pavement as the curse of the *bellagana,* because it prevents so many of us from touching the earth during the day. Stress, sadness, or grief can be neutralized or absorbed by the earth, but only if we are in touch with her. If we have lost our connection to the earth, then we are not grounded, and we must endure, without protection, the lightning bolts flung our way.

AIDS PATIENTS CAME to the Center for Recovery from Illness because of our knowledge of traditional, alternative, and allopathic medicines and our willingness to customize medical programs for them, respecting whatever they believed would help them. Given some yet-to-be-regulated insurance practices, most of my new AIDS patients soon ran out of money. I couldn't stomach refusing them treatments when they did. In desperation, I began to charge an up-front new patient evaluation fee of between $400 and $750.

We did fairly elaborate evaluations, so the fee was not out of line with the service provided, but I still cringed at asking for the fee to be paid in cash before the first visit. It seemed at the time a logical way to limit the number of uninsured new patients. But like so many last-ditch efforts to raise money, the plan was doomed. I was too full of fear to see the many alternatives that occurred to me in hindsight. What if, for example, I had given the clinic to the community? I could have offered to let our patients elect a board of directors, who could hire me if they thought what I was doing was worthwhile, and fire me if not. Maybe I let Iktomi blind me to any possible answers—since I was the one responsible for the debt if the clinic went under.

The evaluation fee made one new patient very angry. Russell was a man who wanted to take an alternative treatment popular at the time, which involved frequent injections of a typhoid vaccine. Originally a treatment for syphilis in the era before antibiotics, the typhoid vaccine was thought to help fight AIDS by stimulating the immune system. At the time many patients believed that AIDS was a variant of syphilis, so this treatment had a double appeal.

The problem with it, I explained to Russell, was that not everyone qualified for the vaccine. It might harm anyone whose illness was too far advanced. Obviously I couldn't give anyone a medicine that would cure the disease but kill the patient. I assured him we would offer him other treatments if he didn't qualify for the one he wanted. Russell replied that he was certain I was only using the vaccine, and the evaluation fee, to rip off gay people, since I wasn't gay myself. I found Russell's large size, his dark black skin, and his Brooklyn accent intimidating as he began to talk.

"I do the same new patient evaluation for everyone with any serious illness, not just AIDS," I told him. "I need to know your medical history. I want to do a good physical, review your lab work, do a psychosocial assessment, and review your nutritional plan. This is a holistic center for chronic illness, not an AIDS clinic, not a typhoid-shot clinic."

In the end Russell was denied his sacred typhoid. His psychosocial assessment revealed an early AIDS dementia with an underlying personality disorder. The dementia was probably partly to blame for his paranoid distrust of me. When I told him politely that I could not give him the vaccine, he promptly filed suit in small-claims court, demanding back his $450 evaluation fee, plus $1,000 for "psychic trauma."

Far worse than the sum was the publicity generated in the gay press over this impending court action. A few courageous patients wrote supportive letters to the gay papers about the work the clinic had done, but for the most part I was assumed to be a villain.

It is an unfortunate aspect of the human mind, or of mine anyway, that one unpleasant experience can outweigh ninety-nine rewarding ones. Despite the many people with AIDS I had helped, several of whom are still alive today, the incident with Russell left me drained and unwilling to fight to keep the practice going. Whatever good I had done for the AIDS patients of San Francisco, my work was over. I consulted a lawyer before the court action. He recommended that after settling the case, I face the inevitable, close the clinic, and declare bankruptcy. After all, I had no money even to pay his fees, let alone keep the clinic open. He was representing me gratis, since I had helped his wife heal her lupus.

By Christmas of 1987 I was planning to move to Tucson. I had been offered a position at the University of Arizona. I scraped together what money I had left to rent a U-Haul truck. A heavy rain kept me indoors on New Year's Day, packing boxes and readying the furniture for the move. Early the next day I walked to the U-Haul center on Van Ness and picked up my truck. With the help of friends, it was loaded by nightfall.

I returned to San Francisco in February for the small-claims court action. I started to argue my case to the judge, a gay rights lawyer who worked as a judge one half-day a week. He cut me short. "How much longer does Russell have to live?"

"Probably no more than a year."

"Then give him his money back. Four hundred and fifty dollars is nothing to a doctor. Give it back. No damages." The case ended.

A day later my lawyer filed my bankruptcy. He assured me that this was a perfectly appropriate strategy. I wasn't so sure, but I had run out of alternatives.

March brought my bankruptcy hearing. The case couldn't have been simpler. I had no assets, having spent everything, living on no salary during the clinic's last days. The judge asked me to tell the court how I had come to be penniless. I told him about trying to run a practice whose patients could not pay, whose administrator embezzled, and whose creditors would not create flexible payment plans—because I was a doctor, I was assumed to be wealthy. Finally I told him about the bad publicity resulting from Russell's court action. The judge thanked me and the hearing was over. It had taken less than an hour from start to finish.

Now I had no choice but to let go, as the spirit I had seen by the Berkeley Marina had advised me to do a little over a year before.

CHAPTER TEN

The Vision Quest

I N SOME respects I had bottomed out. I had to start a new life in Arizona on little income. Luckily my friend Alex, from Wisconsin, now lived an hour outside Tucson—he had contributed money to the university in support of my research position. I had the incredible opportunity to further a kind of work that I had been doing on the side since 1980—developing computer models to predict health and disease in the future for individual patients. These models were based on a kind of mathematics called chaos theory then, complexity theory now.

Of course, sometimes I wallowed in my anger at having had to close the clinic's doors. I felt shame at having had to declare bankruptcy, and grief at being at so far a remove—psychological as well as geographical—from my children.

At the same time, after over a year of nonstop stress as I tried to shore up the failing clinic, my new job in Arizona was quite a relief. I embarked upon three of the most productive years of my life. I worked for the Native American Research and Training Center of the University of Arizona, contributing to studies on the incidence of alcoholism and diabetes among Native Americans. I spent mornings at the university, attending courses, searching the library, and writing grant applications. In the afternoon I saw patients. Evenings were mine for writing or studying. I had the time to finish several new studies of my own: using the computer model to predict birth outcome; using hypnosis to turn breech babies; tracing the effects of combining alcohol use with stress and other substance abuse during pregnancy.

I lived near the Tahono O'odham reservation. Slowly but surely I made friends with healers from the rez and a computer science professor from the university named Sanjay, from Delhi. Sanjay soon was much more interested in studying healing with me than he was in his day job, writing database management algorithms for the Human Genome Project. Many weekends my new friends and I attended sweats and ceremonies in and around the reservations of Arizona.

I helped direct a nonprofit organization, Resources for World Health, in Tucson, to support such ceremonies and other types of Native American medicine. Healings can be prohibitively expensive for the average reservation dweller, and some traditional ceremonies were in danger of dying out because few could afford them. Our organization helped provide poor families with the money they needed, so they could participate in traditional healing.

In Arizona I was involved in a novel experiment, building on the multidisciplinary holistic approach that had characterized the clinic in San Francisco. This time my colleagues were native healers from the local reservations. I rented a house out in the desert where clients could stay when they came from Tucson for intensive work. By working alongside these medicine people I continued learning new techniques. I worked with a Yaqui medicine man, a Tahono O'odham one, an Apache practitioner of body manipulation, and a Lakota shaman. One of the great shocks of my life came when I heard that this gentle Lakota man had been imprisoned for killing his wife. From him I learned how sublime and base elements can coexist in a personality. His was a Jekyll-and-Hyde case, the catalyst for the transformation being alcohol.

I was happy with what I was doing in the late 1980s. I was helping people. I led several ceremonies during which the spirits effected some miraculous cures. The price I had to pay for my calmer lifestyle, however, was a low salary. Given my incomplete credentials, the university didn't pay me much. Resources for World Health could afford me only a small living allowance. The money I received from research grants sometimes provided a small stipend for me but most often did not. I was becoming acutely aware of how my failure to finish a residency was limiting my life.

And my children had little patience for my meager income. They were used to better. After the bankruptcy I didn't have much of a material nature left to offer my kids. I remember taking them to a bar for my birthday one year, because the establishment served free food at happy hour, and I could feed us all for the cost of a couple of beers. My son asked angrily, "When are you gonna grow up? When will you ever do something I can be proud of?" To him my work as a healer did not seem worthy of his pride. Soon he was reluctant to come to my desert home at all.

The desert was beginning to claim all my free time. One friend,

Lynch (the Yaqui medicine man), taught me the ways of the desert. From him I learned several Yaqui desert ceremonies, how to pick sacred spots, and how to stalk at night.

This admirable man still ekes out his living in Sun City, Arizona, outside of Casa Grande. Lynch served for twenty years with the U.S. Army. He lives mostly on his retirement, also works part-time at the local post office. Lynch was a tunnel rat in Vietnam. His job was to investigate the warrens of tunnels dug by the Viet Cong, flushing out whatever soldiers or booby traps were lurking down there. This was a terribly lethal occupation, yet Lynch survived—by the grace of God, he told me. He had used all of his Yaqui skills for survival. He came to feel in the pit of his stomach when a tunnel was dangerous and when it was safe. He could smell danger. He could hear a booby trap set to go off. His hands would twitch when there were Viet Cong waiting in the tunnels to kill him.

Lynch is using these same skills now to teach spiritual development. He took those of us lucky enough to know him out into the desert to learn what he knew. We went at night, in the dark. The first thing he did was hide our shoes. "White people always want shoes in the desert," he said, "but I don't let them have them. You can't talk to the desert with shoes on."

Lynch would take urban dwellers far out into the desert of the Tahono O'odham. He would tell them he was about to start a "welcome-to-the-desert" ceremony, insisting that they all take off their shoes for a moment and leave them on the bed of the truck until the short ceremony was finished. While everyone was busy with the ceremony, his wife would drive off in the truck.

Then the panic would begin, and Lynch would play stupid. "You wouldn't believe, Lewis, how worried people get. People care a lot about their shoes. I tell them, 'Oh well, I guess we'd better get going then. There's only one place she knows to meet us; if we start now, we'll be there by morning, and get those shoes back.' They say, 'But I need the shoes now!' 'What for?' I always ask them, and they always reply, 'To protect me from snakes.' And you know what I say?"

"Shoes can't protect you from snakes," I answered, imitating Lynch. "Only God can protect you from snakes."

"You've been spending too much time with a crazy man in the desert, my friend."

I learned to walk barefoot in the desert from the crazy man. I learned to talk to the animals and the insects I found there. I learned to talk—very respectfully, I assure you—to scorpions, gila monsters, and rattlesnakes. Lynch had songs and mantras to sing, to let these beings know we were there, and coming through. Lynch had no fear of these creatures. How could he, after Vietnam? I never could get through the wall of pain that sealed off this part of his experience. He was reluctant to talk about the details of what happened there, but I heard enough to know his terrors had been worse than any the desert could hold for me.

I think this was what drove me further and further with Lynch—because I knew that whatever we could do together was tame compared with what he'd already been through. I don't deny being terrified half the time. Lynch could drive me up to and past the limits of my fear. But I hung in there with him. My feet winced sometimes on hard stones and cactus buds, but I soon learned how to anticipate the next place to step. "Man is his own worst enemy," Lynch was fond of saying. "Snakes are friendly compared to humans."

NATIVE AMERICAN MEDICINE has been practiced on this continent for at least ten thousand years. When the Europeans arrived they found a very healthy people. Foreign plagues and epidemics soon changed that, but didn't change the efficacy of Native American medicine for dealing with illness and chronic disease.

Our traditional medicinal system has always stressed that the soul's processes are seen as being reflected in the outer world. A fire is burning on the mountain. A person is in agony. An awareness comes which dissipates the agony—and rain comes to quench the fire. These events are seen as related. The fire and the rain provide direct messages about the internal workings of the person.

Maybe one reason why this approach is hard for a modern American to appreciate is that there are now so many people living in such close quarters. A fire burns not on a mountainside but in New York City. What message does it bring, and to whom? Nonetheless, I've found Native American medicine to be effective for people from all walks of life, whether administered in urban milieus or the Sonoran Desert of Arizona. I've developed a sense for how the chronic diseases of our modern society can be healed with the treatments of North America's original inhabitants.

Historically, these treatments demand that personal and social transformation precede healing. Wellness is restored when body, mind, spirit, and community are in harmony. For physical, emotional, and spiritual unease—*dis*ease—are not separate phenomena within Native American medicine. All are levels of a central problem that can be shifted, given a sincere desire and a respectful supplication to the spirits.

Tribes are different. Stories vary. My training has been primarily in Lakota and Cherokee approaches to healing, but the key elements of a Native American approach remain consistent from tribe to tribe—the view of the suffering person as being simultaneously matter, spirit, psy-

248 • LEWIS MEHL-MADRONA

che; a member of both a social and an ecological system; a cell in the body of God.

Some ceremonies and therapies have been lost. But many have survived, either through continuous practice or as memories of the oldest community members. You've already read something about the sweat lodges I've performed, of storytelling hypnosis, of the various other ceremonies I've encountered. I have also learned exorcism ceremonies, techniques for body manipulation, and methods for speaking to spirits, choosing herbs, and making diagnoses.

I know much, but the more I know, the more I see how much there is still to be learned. In the coming years I hope to learn to lead the Yuwipi ceremony and to deepen my understanding of the Sun Dance (a ritual performed on a yearly basis to honor the Creator and the sun at the coming of summer). These are some of the things remaining in my personal quest. I will continue seeking visions in the traditional manner and working with people using the tools I have already learned and found useful. My motto is, "If it works, it's good medicine."

Modern medicine has become such a procedure- and prescription-driven enterprise, it is a shame but not a surprise that it ignores ceremony in its treatments. It is incredible, however, that modern psychotherapy also ignores it, given how powerfully our psyches respond to ritual. (Human beings respond so deeply to it that some clients make a ritual even of the weekly talk-therapy session, becoming quite attached to where they sit, how things should start, what it is permissible to say, and so on. But I am referring to rituals consciously and purposefully conducted.)

Ceremonial treatment methods are the most powerful I have encountered. Time and time again I have had the experience of working for weeks with a patient to change a situation, or improve a physical symptom, almost without results. Then we would do a ritual together, and an immutable problem would transform literally overnight. Had this happened only once, I might have thought the ritual was just serendipitously performed right before the symptom changed on its own. But this has happened too often to be dismissed so easily.

In Arizona I started going beyond what I had learned from others; I was developing my own style. I began to take clients outdoors for sessions. Soon I began to incorporate into these sessions some of the formal elements of ceremony that I had learned. Before long, I was using ritual as an integral part of my medical practice. I used it from the first appointment on, no longer waiting to try it until after more conventional treatments had failed.

In working with clients with physical diseases, I learned that a period of intense time together was often necessary to the healing process. Shamans have historically always worked intensively. The work might take an hour, or it might take a week. Typically the sick person came to live with the shaman, or the shaman would journey to live with the patient. Shamans did not set up schedules of meetings with patients. They did not ask them to come by the lodge once a week for an hour's session. Shamans worked with someone until either the person was well or there was nothing left to be done.

AFTER VENTURING a number of times into the desert with Lynch, I became interested in combining such adventures with other work I was doing with clients. Lynch proved a willing accomplice; the two of us eventually led a number of supplicants into the desert on quests such as these. The results were often remarkable.

During my time in Arizona I led a total of 116 patients through intensive healing experiences in conjunction with traditional medicine people. Our patients ranged in age from twenty to seventy-nine years old, with most in their mid-thirties. I was usually the primary or coordinating therapist, creating a treatment plan that met the patients where they stood, then moved them slowly toward a perspective in which traditional medicine could help them.

Patients came for problems they themselves classified as moderately severe. Since insurance rarely covered the cost of the work, or of the native healers consulted in the course of it, no one came who was not very motivated to be healed. All our intensive healing clients had years of outpatient treatments prior to seeing us, most of which had proved ineffective.

We worked with patients with asthma, severe back pain, cancer, chronic fatigue syndrome, diabetes, hypertension, depression and manic depression, neurological problems (including myasthenia gravis), obsessive-compulsive disorders, infertility, nonmalignant gynecological disorders, and pregnancy-related complications. Fifty-six clients reported total cures—which have held true for five years—after doing this work.

At last I had the freedom to work at length with people. Because of the halting course of my fortunes in recent years, I had plenty of time on my hands. Since I developed the program myself, I had no accountants or management experts pressing me to fit more patients into fewer sessions. I was amazed by how much more quickly people got better through intensive work. A sick person seems to need a good push to get going. The rituals we used gave the push, sparking a transformation the patient could be confident his or her healers would be present to support.

The vision quest has always been an important Native American therapy—really more a profound means of self-exploration, whose transformative powers I found, while working with Marilyn, to have value as a therapeutic method. Before a vision quest the seeker purifies himself, through fasts and sweats, in preparation for the journey to the top of a mountain. There he or she sits alone for one to four days without food or shelter, waiting for a vision to be revealed. The vision is always about the self (even though some contain social prescriptions for an entire community). Visions are offered by the spirits as a guide to personal development, and to facilitate healing.

I will use one woman's story as an illustration of what a vision quest can accomplish. Lanny was a woman with whom I had met three times, for one to two hours each appointment, while passing through Denver. (I often flew through the city on my way to the workshops I had been invited to lead in different centers around the country.) We discussed her problem, and she decided to come to the desert to resolve it.

RITUAL SERVES TO create spiritual awareness in order to accomplish a purpose. Lanny had a definite purpose when she came to me in the summer of 1989. She was a thirty-five-year-old woman—the mother of one child, and married to a banker—who had suffered from severe endometriosis for several years. Endometriosis is a pelvic disease in which the lining of the uterus grows outside of the uterus itself into the pelvic cavity. This lining, the endometrium, goes through the same monthly changes as the uterus and "bleeds" into the pelvic cavity during the menstrual period. Pain and other complications result. In Lanny's case, she had recently developed an apparently related ovarian cancer that had spread to six sites in her pelvis.

Lanny had tried several therapies, none effective, at substantial cost. She wanted to work with me for one week to accomplish what she could for her healing. I told her she could stay near my house in the desert outside of Tucson. During that time she would suffer from no other distractions. She would be alone with the desert and with the sounds of the tame and wild animals who lived in the vicinity.

A pair of horses were corralled on the property where we did the healing work. In Arizona, horses are an inexpensive bounty—for one thing, they can live outdoors, which keeps the cost minimal. I was grateful to have the animals there; we rode them on the open land nearby. My roommate was also raising wolves for release in the wild. Two were very tame, almost friendly. It was especially helpful to have the horses and wolves around during healing rituals, as they kept clients in touch with the natural world.

On her first day in Arizona, after Lanny had settled into her room, I listened again to her history and prepared a homeopathic remedy to help her through the week. Lanny had experienced other malignancies besides cancer. She was born to a mother who did not want her. Her father was alcoholic. Her mother would not touch her for the first two weeks of her life, leaving her nurses and her grandparents to take care of her. Luckily, Lanny's grandparents adored her. With them she found some of the comfort that was lacking at home.

Throughout her childhood, her mother scorned and ridiculed her. Hard as she tried, she could not please her mother or gain her approval. At age six Lanny was sexually molested by her older brother Nick. Her mother did not believe what Lanny told her, giving Nick implicit permission to continue abusing his sister. Lanny's grandparents could not protect her from this situation, and her father was too often drunk to comprehend it. Lanny quickly learned to stifle the urge to express her feelings.

Lanny married an abusive husband, had a child and a traumatic divorce, and then was sexually attacked again. Her life experiences supported her distrust of people, particularly men. She had learned to view herself as being unworthy, base, and disgusting. She had no right to have her needs met. She had no right to complain. Her cancer seemed the clear by-product of these many evils. Her life had recently changed, however—through the loving devotion of one man, the banker, she had come to believe that life was worth living. He had inspired her to fight to live.

I began preparing Lanny for the purifying sweat lodge that would precede her vision quest. We went to the medicine circle where journeys begin. The sun was about to set. I laid out the sacred objects in my medicine bag. I sang the Four Directions song. After filling the pipe we prayed to each of the directions. My work was to remove all doubt that she would be well, creating a bridge between her modern expectations and Native tradition. I had to remove my own doubts as well—for when we started I did not have much hope for her condition.

When my prayers ended, I asked Lanny to pray. She was shy and self-conscious about it, as she had not prayed since Catholic girls' school, but the desire in her prayer was unmistakable. I knew the spirits would answer her prayer and said so. The wolves and horses watched us attentively, along with other night creatures hiding beyond the reaches of the firelight.

I began to induce her trance. I instructed her to take slow, deep breaths, and made mention of each of her limbs and muscles in turn, helping her to free them of tension. I began to tell Lanny the Lakota story of the sacred beings. She knew already about the sweat lodge to come, and was afraid of the power and the heat; I began to prepare her for it immediately.

We'll be talking about certain characters in the sweat lodge ceremony. While you're relaxing and resting, I want you to just enjoy yourself, to let yourself go a little, to listen to my words without thinking about them too much. I want to tell you about the beginning, about Inyan, the rock who was present here first, before any other. You will meet Inyan, the rock, when he enters the lodge with the hot stones. Parts of him come in with the heat to doctor us.

Han existed then, also, but Han is more an absence than a presence. Han is the dark, and she surrounded Inyan in the beginning. The dark is the proper milieu for spirits, and it will be dark inside the sweat lodge. We will close the door to honor Han, and give the spirits a place where they can feel comfortable and welcome.

Inyan longed for companionship. He was lonely. He wanted another being with whom to relate. Not Han, who was too shapeless and formless to be satisfying—he wanted another whom he could touch. He consulted with Skan, the Creator, and was given permission to labor and to give birth. You see how change, even at the beginning of the world, begins with dissatisfaction. You are no longer satisfied with your cancer—you deserve better.

Inyan struggled long and hard with that birth. He lost a lot of blood, the blue blood a rock bleeds. Finally, Maka was born, the earth, which covers the rock almost everywhere, except for certain mountains where we can still see Inyan, and except for the oceans, where Inyan's blood flows.

You've given birth, haven't you. You can relate to the pain of the rock as he gave birth to the earth. You will drink the blood of Inyan in the sweat lodge. It will have been transformed. It will have become medicine for you. It will be wakan, or holy, blessed by the three sacred beings in the lodge—Inyan, whom we carry into the lodge to give us warmth, Maka, upon whom we will sit, and from whom we have built our lodge, and Han, who will surround us.

Lanny was beginning to relax. Her breathing was becoming more regular and slow.

There is an old Lakota saying, that men are content with anything. They will sit around the fire and eat or talk or sleep. It is women who are always trying to improve things, to make the world better for their children. It was the same with Maka and Inyan. Right away Maka wanted to improve things. She didn't like the way it was always dark. She wanted to be able to see herself. How could she know if she was ugly or beautiful if there was no way to see herself?

Maka took the matter up with Inyan. He was stumped. He couldn't see a way to resolve her dilemma. How could he, when the world was perpetually dark? So Inyan and Maka called upon Skan, asking for his help with their problem. Thus began the tradition of prayer—of asking for aid from a higher power when our problems exceed our abilities to solve them.

Skan heard their prayers and created light out of darkness. Han parted in two, leaving herself (the dark) beside a companion, Anp (light). Skan asked Han to hide for a while out of Maka's sight, while she adjusted to Anp. With Anp's help, Maka looked at herself. Now she knew what she looked like—and she thought that she was terribly ugly. That's one reason to keep Anp out of the sweat lodge, by the way: so no one can think they are ugly.

Maka asked Skan if she could take the waters, the blue blood of her companion, and adorn herself with them. Skan liked the idea, and blessed it. So Maka took the water and placed it like beautiful jewels upon her skin, forming the lakes, rivers, streams, and ponds. This made Maka happy, and so Inyan and Skan were happy too.

For a while, anyway. Soon Maka had something else to complain about.

"Maybe it's like that at your house," I said. "Maybe you're always improving things, but your husband would be happy to keep things just the way they are."

Lanny laughed almost silently, as she relaxed deeper into a trance.

Maka complained to Skan that everything was always the same. And she was cold. She wanted variety and she wanted warmth. She begged Skan to create something to warm her and soften Anp's blazing light. Skan reflected upon this, finally deciding to make a warming spirit to sit in the sky. Skan made Wi, whom we now call the sun, from parts of rock, earth, water, and himself. Skan put Wi in the sky and there was warmth upon the earth. For a while Maka was satisfied.

But after a time she was unhappy again. The constant heat was uncomfortable. Skan decreed that Wi give all material things a shadow, to provide a pleasurable variety of light; this was a nice thought, but to Maka it was not enough. "Bring back Han," she begged. "Let me have some time away from the heat of the sun. Let me have some time in darkness to recover from the light and heat."

Skan reflected upon this and felt that it was good. The second time was created. Up until now they had been living in the first time, which was perpetual and unchanging. Skan decreed that the second time would con-

sist of regular cycles between Han and Wi. Wanting to get it right the first time, Skan asked Maka what her pleasure was as to the length of each. One complete cycle was to be called a day. After a day was done, Wi was to rest underneath the world and let Han return. Anp was to precede Wi each morning to announce Wi's return. Thus light always precedes sunrise. Maka announced that she was well pleased. All returned to harmony.

Within the lodge, Wi will enter through the heat in the stones. Wi shines upon the trees, who absorb his heat. We cut the trees and transfer the energy of the sun into the stones through fire. Fire comes from Wi. When we light the fire, then Wi walks among us. We will light the fire in the time of Han, or darkness. In this manner we will honor both spirits.

These four are Wakantankan, the great mystery. They are four and they are one. This they cannot even understand themselves, for Wakantankan remains a mystery. We will pray to Wakantankan in the sweat lodge. You might say your cancer is a wakantankan, for it is a great mystery to you. But we will ask what the mystery is, of your cancer. You do not need to know what to do to make it go away. That will be revealed to you. But then you must do it, for a message that comes in a sacred manner must be obeyed. Otherwise you would be an unpleasant sight to the spirits. So you want to be sure you will do what you are told when the instructions come.

Once I was done with the story, I led Lanny on a trance journey, guiding her into her ovaries to learn what had created the cancer. I worked with images to help her discover what her pelvis truly resembled on the inside. We journeyed like the sun across the domain of her pelvis, learning what was in pain and what healing was needed. She was very quiet, responding by moving her finger across her abdomen when she was done exploring one spot and ready to move to another.

Skan creates everything for a purpose. We could not ask the cancer to be removed until we understood what purpose it served, and, with that understanding, could honor Wakantankan without the cancer's help.

I WAS INTRODUCED TO Morita therapy through the writings of David K. Reynolds, and soon became intrigued by the possibility of using it as a bridge between Native American and modern world views. The therapy was developed in Japan around the turn of the century by a Japanese physician named Morita. It is a direct offshoot of ancient Shinto religious practices.

Morita was convinced that patients' disturbances took place in the outer layers of their being, where the personality interacted with the world. He believed that if one probed deeply enough behind the personality, there would be peacefulness and harmony, rather than angst and confusion. After visiting Freud in Vienna, Morita returned home convinced that Freud's theory was inside out. Morita also believed the Viennese doctor was blind to society's role in illness.

Morita therapy required patients to come to a hospital modeled after a retreat. For the first week they remained on complete bedrest, rising only to bathe and receive meals. Patients kept a journal, which the therapist read. The second week involved light, menial labor, permitting an end to the bedrest, and a chance to experience the importance of performing service. A more strenuous form of physical labor began the third week; there were also a number of group educational meetings. These continued in the fourth week, preparing the patient to reenter life.

I was especially attracted to the focus Morita placed on reclusive retreat, giving it central importance in the healing process. The treatment program we devised incorporated aspects of both Morita and Native American philosophies, which I hoped would be helpful to acculturated Americans and Europeans. The work I was doing with Lanny reflects the program I implemented. Now I call it a "healing intensive."

Clients came usually for seven days, and sometimes longer. A few clients came for a shorter time, either to sample the program or because their problems were less severe. For severe problems, a minimum of seven days seemed to be necessary.

The week began with bedrest away from distractions. I asked clients to bring no reading material—no newspapers, magazines, or books. Telephone calls were not permitted, nor was any other communication with the outside world. Likewise, they could not use radios, Walkmans, or televisions. In this way clients were alone with themselves and their journals for hours; insights seemed to bubble up that would otherwise have been kept beneath the threshold of consciousness by the business of living. Adjustment to these rules was amazingly hard for some clients—one indication of how dependent their illnesses were upon distraction.

Each day of their treatment, clients received two to seven hours of therapeutic time. I spent the time reading their journals, asking about what they had written, reviewing art they might have produced on assignment, discussing their experiences and what they were learning. I also used hypnosis and imagery techniques, visualization, biofeedback, body work, and occasionally more conventional psychotherapeutic discussions. I helped clients enter a trance state, and led (and sometimes raced to follow!) their subsequent journeys. I also encouraged clients to make sacred objects and to draw their dreams and trance journey experiences. I introduced them to Native American images, shields, and totems, and the rituals and ceremonies I planned to use. Clients purified themselves in the sweat lodge on the fourth or fifth night. If they were strong enough, they endured a night on top of a nearby mountain on the sixth or seventh night to "cry out for a vision."

When they stayed beyond the first week, I encouraged clients to start taking hikes or walks or to otherwise engage in light physical activity. Morita believed that an active body produced a restful mind. If the first week stressed self-discovery, the second was dedicated to discovery through service.

They also prepared to reenter the world. I taught risk management strategies, along with ways to apply Native American and Moritist philosophy to future problems. There was a continuing emphasis on self-reflection and discovery, and a new encouragement of worship, in whatever manner was most appealing to the client. Clients learned to use worship as support and to rely upon the spirits for help with their problems.

Counseling, psychotherapy, and spiritual practice are similar processes. There is no one correct path for all people. A deep respect is required for the particular path an individual finds is best for him or her. Spirituality can choke growth, as can psychotherapy, when dogmatic adherence is required to one scheme. Most of my clients tended to practice Nature or Asian religions (as these kinds of people were most likely to be drawn to the vision quest), but the Christians and Jews I worked with reported the experience to be of great value to them. And as Lanny was soon to find out for herself, many clients were drawn to their childhood methods of worship.

At the end of the healing intensives I did in Arizona, some people stayed to accompany me and Lynch on a desert survival trek or some other similarly dramatic rite of passage.

ON THE MORNING OF her second day in Arizona, Lanny and I began with body work. Native American body work can involve the very firm massage of blocked areas. Hard tissue contributes to disease. After softening of the tissue, wellness becomes easier to recover. The Apache woman who taught me the technique once called it "Apache torture." We shared a laugh, but her joke name is appropriate: this kind of hard, deep tissue work releases, just as a sweat lodge does, toxins that have been stored in our bodies. The process of release can be momentarily painful.

Lanny lay down. I started with the pelvis. As I massaged pressure points and moved energies, I encouraged Lanny to become aware of images arising from the pelvis. Almost immediately Lanny saw images of her brother molesting her. Those same images had arisen in our meetings earlier that year. Deeper layers existed to her pain. As I worked with her thigh, the kidney meridian in Chinese medicine, images of being beaten by her mother surfaced. The pain lessened as she described those times. She related coming home after being punished in school, only to be beaten by her mother for getting in trouble.

Then I had Lanny lie still and relax. I attached her to a biofeedback machine, so I could monitor her relaxation process. As she released her tensions, slowed her breathing, and entered her trance, I continued the story from the day before.

Skan established domains and dominions for each of the four sacred beings. Throughout each day, they remained in their dominions, having essentially nothing to do. They were bored. They were lonely. So Skan gave each the power to create a companion in whatever manner each desired.

Wi created a disk like himself, only more lovely, called Han-wi, sun of the darkness. He made Han-wi less bright than himself so he could easily gaze upon her, and gave her the night to govern.

Maka created an alluringly and seductively beautiful being, Unk; then Maka gave Unk all her own bad feelings. Maka did her job too well. Unk was so beautiful, Maka was jealous of her. They quarreled violently, so Maka threw Unk into the waters and resolved to live without a companion. But Maka had already set a dangerous precedent, of disowning one's own bad feelings and looking for them in someone else.

Skan created Tate, the wind, for a companion. Tate is formless, like Skan. Tate was created to carry Skan's messages to whoever needs to hear them. Listen to the wind, for there you will hear the voice of the Creator.

Lanny stirred. From far away in her trance she murmured that she was afraid of the wind. She had always feared that the wind would tell her things she didn't want to hear. She didn't known anything about the wind but always worried when she heard it, retreating indoors when it blew too forcefully.

"Try listening to the wind while you're here," I urged her. "Let Tate whisper into your ear for a change. He will tell you what you need to know about your cancer."

Lanny let the sound of the wind outside carry her to the home of her mother, who had died three years before. Lanny saw herself standing, aware of the rage she had never expressed, in her mother's bedroom. She heard the wind whispering, "Forgive yourself."

She saw her mother's pain. She had seen her mother as a vain, mindless alcoholic. Tate told her to look deeper. There beneath the surface was a river of pain. Beneath the surface were the demons Lanny's mother could never confront. These demons eventually killed her, as she gave up all desire to live. The words "be still" came to Lanny. Her mother had often frightened her with the words, demanding that she "be still" while being beaten. "But this 'be still' is different," Lanny said.

"Your mother wanted obedience more than stillness. Maybe what your pelvis wants is a *real* stillness, a brand-new, never-experienced peacefulness."

Lanny cried softly with this realization. Her biofeedback machines indicated that a profound physiological change was taking place. I encouraged Lanny to remain in the hands of Tate. "Let him help you see all that you need to see." Lanny saw herself refusing to admit the death of her mother, guilty at the rage she felt. The wind asked her to breathe out the guilt. Tate would take care of it—he would carry it to the four directions and disperse it across the heavens.

Later that night we did a ceremony around the fire. The night was pitch black. I sang a sacred song. A powerful spirit came from the southwest. Lanny recognized it as the Virgin Mary. She was embarrassed to see a spirit from the Catholic religion she had abandoned, but felt strangely uplifted by Mary's radiance. Lanny had experienced great comfort from Mary as a child. The Virgin Mary said she was still available for Lanny, that Lanny could call upon her at any time, by any name Lanny chose. Whatever Lanny chose to call her, she should remember the peace Mary had brought her; then Mary would come. Lanny sobbingly described hanging on to the legs of Mary's statue in Catholic school and telling Mary of the many cruelties inflicted upon children in her name.

We smoked the pipe. Lanny prayed for the child within herself. The presence of the Virgin Mary lingered, and all the animals in the area were still.

On the third day, I read from Lanny's journal.

> Alex chain-smokes. Every morning I am greeted by the acrid smell of leftover cigarettes. I stand at the corner sink. Behind me sits Alex at the table. The words we say linger in the air as long as the stench of his cigarettes. I know I have to leave him.
>
> I pick up the empty bottles from the night before. I wash the dishes, finding a mundane task to settle myself. I dry them and place them in my handmade cypress kitchen cabinets. It will be

hard to leave them. I finished them lovingly while the myth of our everlasting marriage still held true. There is a gaping hole in the sheetrock beside the cabinets, for a never-to-be-framed spice rack; this is a more accurate reflection of our relationship.

I tell Alex I am leaving. I tell him clearly so there can be no doubts. I hope what I say will infiltrate his clouded thoughts. As I am telling him, his hands close around my neck. He tightens them. I clutch a half-washed plate in terror. What happened to the hands that used to caress my skin so gently?

I'm six. Nick has come into my room. He unzips his pants, pulls something long and floppy out, and tells me to lick it. Do I hear his voice telling me it will taste like ice cream? Do I hear Alex telling me to take it on my hands and knees?

I'm on my knees. Nick's hands are digging into my shoulders. My mouth is full. He smells. He pants, "Harder, harder." Harder what? His hands keep my head and mouth locked onto what has become large and swollen. "Harder. It'll taste like ice cream." But it doesn't taste the way he says, not one bit.

I remember Alex sitting at the kitchen table, wearing green shorts and no underwear. His penis, flaccid and limp, peeks out from the leg of the shorts. I go to my room and lock the door. I will be gone by suppertime. Terror ebbs and flows away. I see how my cancer comes from all my abuse. The endometriosis saved me from having sex with Alex when I could no longer bear him.

I am remembering things I have not thought about in years. Holding on to the Virgin in the school, crying to her about what Nick has done, crying to her about Mommy beating me, crying to her about the nun slapping my hands with the ruler. Telling her that she is my only friend.

Last night I prayed for joy, humor, and a sense of fun. And I pray for my new husband. My real husband. A husband I can trust.

I began the third day's body work with Lanny on her stomach. I worked with her legs first. Images formed of her grandparents, particularly her grandmother. Lanny loved to sleep at their house. Her grandmother died when Lanny was twenty, and that was a real shock. Her grandmother had always been a source of strength and comfort to Lanny. I massaged areas to remove blockage from her legs, pelvis, and back. In visualization, she journeyed to a house inhabited by the spirits of her ancestors, who told her what she needed to know from the past.

She met her great-uncle Ulysses, a kind and jovial Greek immigrant. She met her father's parents, dead before her birth.

I felt the presence of a kindly old man and woman in the room while we worked. Later Lanny announced that Ulysses and his sister had been present, and wondered if I had noticed.

NATIVE AMERICAN CULTURE is rich in experience stories, and lore, but sparse in developed theory. But theory is implied in the teaching tales and the ceremonies. Rituals reinforce the implicit theory without requiring explicit statement. Indian notions of the spirit world, of regression and reincarnation, can be quite different from those developing in the mainstream culture.

It is common to go to a medicine person, be "put to sleep," and find yourself in another time and place. You may appear with relatives or with other beings. It is impossible to say if this kind of trance has always happened; I suspect so, given ancient tales in which journeys take place to the past, or the future, or the spirit world. There is no indication of circular reincarnation within these stories. Native Americans do not believe that after death we are reborn in a new body. We die and enter the spirit world, where we become spirits.

Thus the philosophy of karma, and of the refinement of the soul through successive lives, is foreign to our beliefs. We have one life to refine ourselves as human beings, although spirits continue to refine themselves in their own worlds. Spirits have their own problems, even including domestic squabbles.

When we enter the past or the future, or journey into the spirit world, we meet spirits. We may find ourselves inside another's skull or within the body of an animal, sharing its thoughts, movements, and feelings. But afterward we do not say, "I was a bear in a past life in the seventeenth century," or "I fought with Geronimo in Arizona." This is far too linear for the Native American world view. Rather, we share an experience. "I was with a bear. My spirit mingled with its spirit and, for a time, shared its earthly robe." Where is that place? "Over there." One points vaguely into the distance, meaning the spirit world. Where is the spirit world? "Everywhere and nowhere."

The spirit world is all around us and in the distance. It is where we journey when we look inside ourselves. It confronts us during the vision quest. It receives us when we dream, and sometimes we see it during our waking hours.

Native Americans (those whose cultures are still intact) are in constant communication with spirits. They often see spirits in physical form, and have spirit helpers and guides, power and totem animals, and plants and stones who speak and assist with daily life as well as ceremonies. Their relationship with spirits is perhaps why Native Americans are frequently compared to children. What a shame that modern Americans are forced to deny that relationship as they "grow up," and then must spend so much time, energy, and money learning hypnotic techniques and regression therapies to reconnect to the spirit realm. We all have experience, even if only as small children, of having trees speak, waters murmur, birds sing, and rocks warble to us. These all are relatives of ours, and they bring important messages to us from the Creator.

The Creator and his spirits can also speak through channels. When I was a child in southeastern Kentucky, Cherokee shamans and fundamentalist Christians alike channeled spirits. During religious rituals, spirits spoke through the shaman or the minister. A Christian calls a spirit an angel, but there the differences end. A member of the congregation might speak in tongues, roll on the floor, or otherwise be possessed by "discarnate intelligences" who were often able to give good advice and assist the members of the congregation in their daily lives.

Do we create forms for spirits to occupy which conform to our world views? It seems we must. Native Americans create shapes in accord with what they find surrounding them in nature. Hindus create fantastic shapes, such as the god with ten heads and eleven pairs of arms, or the god with a human body and an elephant head. Christian angels are most often represented as humans with wings. Christ walked in a human form. We create shapes we are comfortable with, and allow a doorway of consciousness to open so that the spirit can enter the shape.

Medicine people are principally concerned with cultivating spiritual well-being. They hold tightly to their faith that the client will heal, and likewise cultivate hope within the client that healing will occur. Like Paul, writing in Corinthians 1:13, they know that faith, hope, and love are the most important gifts of the spirit. Innumerable studies have shown that hope, although not often emphasized in conventional medical practice, is vital for dealing with illness and suffering,[1] and may even be essential for physical and emotional well-being.[2]

The creation of spiritual well-being was always the goal of the medicine people with whom I studied. They believed that physical and emo-

1. V. Carson, K. L. Soeken, and P. M. Grimm, "Hope and Its Relationship to Spiritual Well-Being," *Journal of Theology and Psychology* 16 (1988): 159–67;

2. M. Dufault and R. Vogelpohl, "When Hope Dies—So Might the Patient," *American Journal of Nursing* 80 (1980): 2046–49; and J. F. Miller, "Inspiring Hope," in J. F. Miller (ed.), *Coping with Chronic Illness: Overcoming Powerlessness* (Philadelphia: Davis, 1983), pp. 297–99.

tional well-being would quickly follow. They were constantly engaged in the process of helping sick people envision a future, since you must envision one before you can have one. The ability to imagine a future leads to hope, which requires a certainty that what we seek is attainable. The medicine person turns the attention of the sick person toward the Creator, who is the source of hope; the focus is on reestablishing a person's relationship with the Creator.

THE FOURTH MORNING was cold and bright. A storm front hovered over the Rincon Mountains. Worried that we would have rain, I quickly made prayer ties to the Thunder spirits, asking them to hold back the rain until we could cover the sweat lodge and be sure the fire was roaring. I woke Lanny, and we rushed to cover the lodge—first with sheets, then blankets, then tarps. We placed black and white flags on the altar with cherry sticks to honor the Thunder spirits. I told her I would see her later in the day, and that the lodge was to take place that evening.

Besides requiring clients to do without the distractions of the modern world, I tried to break the hold time had over their lives—more particularly strict schedules and appointments. I told clients to leave their watches at home. I let them know I would not be coming to see them at the same hour every day. Part of the treatment was to help people give themselves over to the experience of retreat and reflection, rather than trying to control it by marking the passing hours. Many people— especially city dwellers like Lanny—found it very difficult to let go of time. When I arrived that afternoon later than she expected, she was furious.

She began shouting at me. "How could you abandon me today, when you know how frightened I am of your stupid sweat lodge?" The room grew darker and colder as she continued. Lanny bared her teeth. Her voice was a low, mean growl. I worried about what might have come over her.

Frightened, I sprinkled cornmeal in a circle around myself to ward off evil, and lit a candle. The earth is the Mother of Corn; cornmeal is a powerful force of good. The candle brought the powers of light and understanding to bear against the powers of confusion and darkness. Lanny kept up a running tirade throughout my preparations. Having made them, I was ready to address the problem directly. I said quietly, "What do you want to do right now?"

"I want to jump up and tear the skin off your face!"

"Let yourself imagine that, Lanny. What would it be like, really, to catch my skin under your nails, to have my blood on your fingers? Give yourself a moment to breathe with that."

Lanny started weeping. The candle guttered. As she exhaled, she released some trapped energy. The room got a little lighter. Lanny's voice was small and frightened when she spoke again. "Sometimes I turn on my own daughter like this. Like my mother turned on me. It's like I'm possessed."

"Maybe you are."

With that, her weeping turned into sobbing; her body shook with the force of her grief. I held her a moment to calm her. Then I started telling Lanny about the Lakota conception of evil, of how it possesses us. Dissatisfaction is what prompts a desire for change, for creation. If creation happens cooperatively, with the participation and approval of all affected beings and spirits, then it is good. Through prayer, we enlist the help of spirits; we must attend carefully to their answers if we expect their cooperation.

As anyone who has sat on a committee knows, cooperation takes time. Evil begins as the desire to shorten the process of creation by bypassing cooperation. If I want you to agree to my project, even though it isn't good for you, I must find your weaknesses and manipulate them. This is what Iktomi does. Iktomi does not have the power to bypass your will entirely—only to trick you into going along with his own plans.

I began telling Lanny about Wakinyan, the Thunder spirits who threatened a storm earlier.

The companion Inyan created for himself was the Thunder spirits. Their form is so terrible that they must conceal themselves within a cloud, or people would go insane merely from glancing at them. But their purpose is noble. They are here to rid the world of filth. They are here to wash away the demons, like the ones who destroyed your mother. Like the ones who want to destroy you.

They come from the west, bringing life, giving rain, sending lightning. The old ones say that lightning will never strike a cedar tree, because the cedar is the symbol of life everlasting. People used to stand beneath cedar trees for safety in a thunderstorm. I don't know if that will work for people who have any doubt—maybe only for the ones who really know it to be true.

In the lodge, we will throw cedar upon the stones. We will fill the lodge with the sweet smell of cedar once it is purified. We will pray to Wakinyan, the Thunder spirits, for cleansing during the lodge. They come from the west, the direction to which we must look for help with our fears.

Iktomi is the son of Inyan and Wakinyan. He is not proud to be the issue of Rock and Thunder, though his brother Ksa, Wisdom, is. Both have queer shapes. Both invoke laughter when they are seen. But Ksa is honored by laughter, where Iktomi has vowed to humiliate all who laugh at him.

Wohpe, the White Buffalo Calf Woman, is always present in the lodge. Her qualities are love, compassion, and forgiveness. She comes from the south. Look to her for beauty and love. I think the spirit you call Mary is the spirit I call the White Buffalo Calf Woman. Try to see yourself through her eyes. If you can, you will see yourself as a beautiful creature to be loved, cherished, and honored.

I wanted to tell you all this so that you will know how sacred the sweat lodge is. All these sacred beings will be with us in the lodge. They will walk among us. If you are afraid, call to Mary. She will be there, if you ask her to come. Mary will hear your prayers, and your prayers will be answered.

That night we planned to enter into the lodge to pray for Lanny's healing. As we prayed before lighting the fire, bats came from the east. I told Lanny about bat medicine, about the bat's ability to see the unseen. An owl came from the west. I told her about owl medicine; owls are messengers from the physical to the spirit world.

The essence of spirit medicine lies in considering the spirit's nature in its pure form. What makes a bat different from any other animal? What is unique about an owl? That gives us a clue to how we would use bat medicine or owl medicine.

There are no concrete definitions in Native American medicine. Within conventional biomedicine, textbooks are written that precisely define conditions and their treatment. When questions arise, textbooks can be consulted for the definitive view. Within Native American medicine, each practitioner develops his or her own way of defining concepts such as "bat medicine" or "owl medicine."

The essence of a bat to me is in its blind vision. The bat uses sonar to "see" past visual appearances. Bats can see through what is superficial to the underlying truth. Owls prowl the night. They can turn their heads completely around and see in all directions. Their acquaintance with night's unseen powers makes owls messengers from the "other side," communicating between the spirits and the living.

I dedicated the north to the Wolf Nation. I call wolf medicine into a ceremony when I think extra energy is needed. I was learning about the ways of wolves from watching my roommate's charges. Wolves are loyal, devoted family animals who run from conflict unless no options exist—then they fight fiercely. Each kind of medicine has its own calling song to attract its attention. I sang the wolf spirit's song, and offered it tobacco and other gifts, asking for its help and blessing.

South was dedicated to the Coyote Nation, whose citizens were already singing for us.

Our makeshift desert lodge was small and gnarly, made from local palo verde branches. Its low dome was covered with the blankets and tarps we'd thrown over the structure that morning, to keep it dry and to retain the heat of the desert lava rocks. A brilliant fire was burning. The sky was dark and cloud-covered, obscuring the moon. We never got the rainstorm—instead, tiny flakes of snow were beginning to fall. The wind was blowing hard. It was cold outside the reach of the fire. When the fire had sufficiently heated the stones, we would pray to the great mystery, asking Wakantankan to answer a question modern medicine could not address.

We smoked the pipe, speaking to the spirits already gathered of our reasons for holding this lodge. Then the snow came in earnest. At first it had been gentle flakes drifting down; before long, it was falling heavily. The spirit of winter had sent us his finest gift. Before the night ended, there were eight inches of snow covering the desert—a rare thing in Arizona.

Two of Lanny's friends from Denver had joined us. Sanjay was my firekeeper. I was passing along to him a tradition that had been passed to me. No one wanted to leave the fire he started. We were transfixed by the pristine beauty of the snow. It covered jackets and coated hair. Occasionally the wolves and the coyotes howled. The horses came closer, curious about what we were doing.

Sanjay brought the coals into the lodge. I burned sage to dispel any evil influence we might have brought inside with us. We blessed ourselves, then the pipe. I prepared the pipe by connecting the bowl and the stem. I prayed to each of the directions, taking a pinch of tobacco and offering it to each in turn. Slowly the pipe filled. When this was done, the stones were brought inside. Sanjay closed the door and joined us. I thanked each person for coming. We thanked the Thunder spirits for the snow and began the songs for the first door.

In the second round, Lanny had a chance to pray. Her prayers were clear and strong. She asked for her cancer to be healed. She prayed to the north for strength in dealing with her disease. She prayed for her mate and her child. She asked the spirits to help expel the evil inside her, and to help her husband adjust to the new woman she would become. Her prayers were thoughtful and sincere.

After the third door, we passed the pipe. We smoked and knew that Lanny's prayers had come true. My spirit grandfather came and cradled Lanny in his arms. After the fourth round we crawled out into the snow, lingering around the fire before we departed for the warmth of the house.

Lanny wrote this about the lodge in her journal:

> The rock people. How do I explain the jolt of recognition?
> Me, in awe, watching the sun from beneath the earth. Me, small

and insignificant, at home in the light of the red-hot stones . . . all the layers of ambiguity of my life. All the gray matter of my brain etched on the walls for me to see.

I let the soft heat of the rock people melt me. Burn through me to my very core. I let the layers of pain and blocked memories begin to dissolve, like liquid salt running down the walls of the lodge. I was the melting salt. I was dissolving, losing consciousness with each moment. Suddenly someone called for the door to open . . .

Dimly understood recognition emerges as to why I was given *Natrum muriaticum* by Lewis.[3] Sea salt. Salt of the earth. Salt of my wounds. Grief of my soul. These were some of the images he mentioned.

To meet the rock people finally. Hard, clear, gray-white granite. Cousins of the salt caves we saw earlier this week. Not for you, to be slowly and relentlessly eaten by the desert rainy season. Rather for you, the intense energy of the fire. Please loan me some of your fire and heat. Mountain granite, do you know how you stirred my yearnings?

A huge rattlesnake appeared at my right side. It sat on the sand, its head close to mine. At first I wanted to back out of the lodge, but its eyes were mesmerizing. It smiled, even while flicking its tongue in and out. It was very strong. Its head rested on my shoulder, and its rattle massaged my foot.

"What message do you bring?" I asked of the snake.

"Don't be afraid to be powerful," he said. "You may use my medicine for your healing. My poison will destroy the bad, leaving only the good."

Spirit of the rattlesnake, I salute you. Fill me, stone people, with fire and heat; fire enough to crack the granite of my heart's hard edges. Then perhaps I can find my health . . .

"She released a lot of pain during that lodge," my spirit grandfather told me. "No wonder it was so hot. What do you expect? When you ask them to share their pain with the earth, and the stone people in the center of the pit—of course it's gonna get hot."

@   @   @

3. *Natrum muriaticum* is a homeopathic remedy often associated with repressed tears and grief. It is simple sea salt, made potent by successive dissolving and evaporation.

THE NEXT DAY Sanjay helped Lanny make a shield containing the most important images from the sweat lodge and her trance journeys. Sanjay asked her to imagine the sacred beings helping her to choose what to depict. He told her that if she called upon them, they would come providing help. On her shield, Lanny painted the rattlesnake and the stone people under the protective canopy of the Virgin Mary's blue robe.

During a healing intensive I encourage clients to represent their fears and internal emotional processes as dolls, shields, objects, or paintings. Fully invested by the client with emotional material, coupled with the power of belief and faith in the ceremonial process, these objects are sacred and useful for the vision quest to come. I frequently remind clients that this art is not for sale and need not be judged. The medium and the result are far less important than the intention to use the art to communicate with the Creator. Personal sacred art is perfect regardless of its appearance, because it expresses a spiritual experience.

When we prepare a sacred object we must try to be sure our minds and hearts are in the right place. When the Dineh make a sacred robe, they raise the sheep whose fleece will be used for the wool apart from the rest of the herd. The sheep are fed special food that has been grown in a separate garden with special attention and prayer. For Lanny, the time she spent making her shield gave her the chance to reflect upon her insights from the sweat lodge the night before.

We talked about these insights before proceeding on to body work. Lanny lay down on her back. I began on the pelvis, particularly above the ischeal wings. This area stimulated memories of her brother molesting her. Lanny recalled him slipping up behind her, grabbing her breasts regularly once they began to develop. Her mother had always turned away, feigning ignorance. Lanny knew her brother did this to tempt a response from her mother, to see how far he could go without challenge. Another region held the memory of her brother and herself in a motel room when she was sixteen. Their parents had gone to dinner with relatives. He got her drunk and tried to force her to have sex with him. She fought him so vehemently that he gave up.

"These are the memories haunting your pelvis," I said. As I massaged the points, I encouraged her to feel on an emotional level what was trapped in her body on the physical plane. Then, to slowly let them go with each breath out. To slowly let the breath of Tate blow through her body and dislodge those memories, to release their harm.

Then I moved to her thighs. Memories of her first husband surfaced. She had wanted to leave long before she did. Frequent bladder infections had followed sex she hadn't wanted. It was easier to just sleep with him than to fight about it. I worked especially along the line of the kidney meridian, which was painful to her on both sides. As memories of that earlier relationship continued to flow into consciousness, the pain lessened. I gave suggestions to help her release these memories, allowing her body to know it did not need to tense up against that husband anymore. He was long gone.

We worked down the legs toward her feet. Again, on the lower legs, the line of the kidney meridian (along the inner side of the lower leg) was the most tender. I rubbed the reflexology points on the feet. We took a short break before I proceeded to work with her back.

Lanny's anger at her brother emerged more fully as I moved up and down her spine. I gave more suggestions to release it, to let it be transformed, as there was no need to hold on to that pain anymore. We traveled all the way down her arms. Vestiges of her mother's hatred clung to her triceps muscles. I finished by having her turn over so I could massage and adjust her neck, finishing with craniosacral techniques.

That night we gathered around the fire. Beginning again with song and prayer, we called upon the Star Nation to help with Lanny's healing. Star crystals had been placed the night before upon the altar of the sweat lodge. Now we took those crystals and called upon that energy to enter her body and complete the cleanup. I chanted and moved the crystal to where it asked to go. I followed its directions, pulling out energy, returning some, absorbing the darkness and spitting it out upon the ground. When we were finished, we smoked the pipe and sang Christmas songs Lanny had learned as a young girl. Then we talked about her brother's self-destructiveness and the preparations he seemed to be making to die. The cancer was holding a part of him alive within her. She acknowledged her need to release him; part of her body still wanted him, part was still refusing him. She clung to him out of fear—including the fear that no one else could ever love her.

We talked about the feeling that her brother was still haunting her pelvis. She saw Nick as the source of her endometriosis, her cancer, and her pain. The endometriosis was something evil that had been put inside her against her will—a violation Nick had anticipated physically. I gave her suggestions to relax and enter an altered state. The fire was burning brightly. I told her I would sing a song to bring in the spirits. I sang the Four Directions song and ended with a special chant to ask the spirits for transformation of pain into health and help. I played the drum as I sang.

We visited the parts of her that wanted to hold on to her brother, and I asked her to look to see how old that part of her was. "Hold the hand of that part of yourself, and tell her you will always be there for her. Whatever she is afraid of losing, tell her she can get from you. You are always there with that younger part of yourself."

Then I asked Lanny to revisualize her childhood, going through each year with different parents—her own parents, had they been healed by the spirits surrounding us, had they been able to grow up whole and pass the best of themselves on to their children. Each year became clearer to her. I asked her to walk forward in time, paying close attention to significant events. When Lanny got stuck at age eight, her helpers guided her through; then she imagined herself all the way to adulthood.

A song ended the visualization. We loaded the pipe with tobacco, giving thanks to the spirits for their contributions and to the Star Nation for sending healing from above.

ON THE SIXTH DAY Lanny was ready for her vision quest. Lynch and I took her out in the desert in my trusty old Land Cruiser. After collecting our ritual supplies, we began the hike into the canyon. The January sun, despite the snow of two nights before, was already hot this morning. The footing was uneven on the dirt and stone. No trail led to our destination, a single tall, dead saguaro on the top of a nearby hill.

That giant saguaro had called out to Lanny in a dream. I had never seen it before, but when Lanny told us of her dream image, Lynch thought of this place and brought us to it. It was within a canyon. The landscape was just what Lanny had dreamed—the cholla-studded hills, the sheer rock faces of the surrounding mountains. Two hawks circled lazily overhead. We threaded our way between prickly pears that taunted us with their spines. Some were gatekeepers—we had to make our way carefully around them to avoid their outstretched limbs.

We were looking for a cave near the saguaro tree, one that Lanny could sit in through the entire night, waiting for her vision to be unveiled. The sky was sapphire blue, cloudless, brilliant. Wi warned us with his heat while Skan, the Creator, looked over us from above. We stepped over an ancient barbed-wire fence. It continued across the hill and into a dry wash where past flood waters had crushed it into a useless heap. Small desert wrens sang in the palo verde trees, following the wash downslope. The desert looked no different that day from how it would have one hundred years before.

Within the desert, time slows. Thirty years pass and a saguaro tree is still a short, stubby pup. Seventy years pass before it grows arms. The sacred beings remain accessible in the desert stillness, listening for our prayers, waiting to answer them. They have been driven from the cities by our cruelty, by our disregard for sacred spirits. We must leave civilization behind if we wish to commune with them.

Pack rat tunnels lined our path. Our feet crunched on the rotting fiber of pieces of the dead saguaro. Its remnants stood like a skeleton on the hillside above us. One of its broken limbs swayed gently in the wind.

"Listen to Tate," I told Lanny. "The wind will tell you how to heal. He is the Creator's companion. He carries messages from the Creator to you." The wind became more powerful. Before long a strong gust was bound to sever the hanging limb of the saguaro, leaving it to fall to the desert floor to decay.

"The earth creates and destroys," I said. "The same creativity that made your tumor will remove it again. Ksa, the spirit of wisdom, will speak to you today. Perhaps he will ride on Tate's wings. Be alert, for he may come when you least expect him."

We reached the ridge and walked along it to the lone saguaro. To the left stretched the narrow defile of the canyon. To the right lay the great valley. Standing beside the saguaro, we saw the stone ruins of an ancient settlement. The tree had called us here to see them—they were invisible from any other place in the canyon. Ksa whispered that this was to be the place for our ceremony. We started down the hillside, sometimes sliding on the loose sand. Once a prickly pear snagged my boot, leaving a gift of its spines. We crossed another washed-out stretch of barbed wire at the bottom of the hill and started upward, trusting intuition to lead us toward the now-invisible ruins at the top.

When we arrived, Wi was midway across the sky path. From the ruins we found a stone mesa outcropping, with a cave inset. Here we would sit and prepare our ritual. A waterfall appeared to the south, from a spring hidden by a large cottonwood and a few smaller trees. From their shade, deer emerged, their white tails reflecting the sun. We counted thirteen before they disappeared into thickets downstream.

I lit a small fire from a twig tipi. I burned sage to purify us. The smoke clung to our clothes and hair like clouds sitting upon the mountain. Lanny was agitated. Small muscles in her cheeks twitched irregularly. I sang the Four Directions song, asking the corners of the earth for help. The words centered Lanny. The earth heard us. The ground beneath us vibrated to match the song. The sun shone a brighter orange, the sky turned a darker blue. When the song ended I prayed aloud to the Creator, asking for help for Lanny, for Lynch, and for me. We all needed healing in our own ways, as humans always do.

Lanny had with her the shield she had made, and prayer ties. The sweat lodge had been the first step in Lanny's purification, and the fast-ing she was doing today was her next. Come nightfall, Lynch and I would leave Lanny alone at this mesa's cave without food or water while she waited for her vision.

That night Lynch and I scaled the volcanic rock that served as the backside of the mountain, carefully placing our bare feet in the right spots. This mountain was clearly a power spot. We discovered another way to the mesa's small cave, following an absolutely perfect sand dune. Wild horses stampeded through the dry wash behind us. They could run all the way from Phoenix to the Mexican border in that old riverbed. During flash floods it probably filled up with ten-foot-high walls of water.

Lynch and I were in search of adventure. When we crossed the top of the mountain we found ourselves face to face with a desert deer. The deer was shocked to see us and promptly froze. I moved to touch it, but Lynch signaled me to let it be. So we sat about six feet from this deer, waiting for it to recover its senses enough to run away. This took about fifteen minutes. It was a slow deer.

We worked our way back down the mountain. What we saw astonished even us. Lanny had left the mouth of the cave and was sitting in front of a large boulder, about five feet from the biggest rattlesnake that I had ever seen. The moon was rising. The rattler shook his tail. Lynch and I froze. He did not want us any closer. We snuck down the hill and worked our way back to within twelve feet of the snake. He began to rattle whenever we moved, so this time we knew to stay put.

I don't think Lanny was even aware of our presence. She had her shield to protect her, with images on it of the rattlesnake, the stone people, and the Virgin Mary. Lynch and I sat through half the night as this drama played out. We were clearly only observers. The snake had come for Lanny. We had no choice but to sit and wait.

At dawn we were still in the same positions. Then, as the sun rose, the snake slowly slithered away to the west. When it was gone, we all stood up and stretched. By the time the sun was high, all the power of the night had dissolved. Night held the power of the spirit world. Day was meant for our conscious, waking hours, where we could sweep under the rug anything that did not conform to our ordinary world view. Night was when truth was spoken.

LANNY RETURNED HOME the next day, with instructions on how to continue her daily meditations, an appointment with the therapist who had referred her, and stones from the desert mesa to remind her of where she had been. Two weeks later, she saw her gynecologist. He kept her in the office for hours, searching for the cancer like a frustrated gold miner, sifting the sands of a streambed others had long since picked clean.

The next day she spent eight hours at the hospital. The gynecologist found only healthy tissue, not even endometriosis. He could easily have destroyed that healthy tissue by his doubt, had Lanny been in a weaker place. But Lanny was strong. Six months after our treatment, she called to let me know her body was free from all traces of the tumor. Eight years later, Lanny remains well. Only the spirits could have pulled off such a miracle.

CHAPTER ELEVEN

Coyote Medicine

THERE IS A DISTINCTION made in Mexico between those individuals descended principally from the Spanish colonials and those who are of native stock. The races are considered as distinct as blacks and whites are in Alabama. I was intrigued to learn, while living in Tucson, that a Mexican half-breed is known as a *coyote*. That fact spoke to me.

Lanny's rattlesnake also spoke to me. Its principal message was for her, but it delivered a short and vital one to me as well. After all, it kept Lynch and me a captive audience all night long. It had plenty of important things to communicate—I wouldn't be surprised to hear Lynch learned something that night too.

At dawn, after the snake had disappeared and we had stretched our aching limbs, I laid out my ceremonial supplies in the proper sacred manner and began a song of prayer for Lanny. The rattlesnake returned. I stopped singing and stood up, to see if the movement would startle the snake enough for it to slither off. I was already in a state of altered consciousness or I would not have had the courage to stand at all.

It was then that I heard the snake's spirit voice in my head. "Stop chasing me," he said. "You've got better things to do. What are you afraid of? The world of medicine? That's the world that's meant for you. You're supposed to take what you've learned *here* back *there*. Why go chasing after some silly rattlesnake in the desert? Go find your shoes and finish up your training." Then the snake was gone.

I sat back down. There, in the mouth of the cave, I could smell the ocean, as well as the unmistakable fragrance of Archie's cigar. Soon I could almost see the waves and hear the cries of seagulls, begging for handouts from the tourists on the San Francisco piers. I was mentally transported to the last urban environment I had lived in, the site of my ill-starred clinic, and what I thought was my final attempt to be a mainstream medical practitioner.

But I had to recognize that my present course could never be completely satisfying. Without being a full-blooded Native American, someone who had grown up on a reservation, I would always encounter some degree of challenge and suspicion from any full-blooded clients. It was a frustrating dilemma. To a shaman like Hosteen Begay, I acted too much like a *bellagana,* and to doctors in a hospital, I was too much like another Hosteen.

The snake's message was clear, though, and true. What the snake pointed out to me was that there *was* a path in modern medicine that I was uniquely prepared to walk. The path that was uniquely mine was that I might share with others in the scientific realm the insights of the shamanic method. I might help return something of art to the science of medicine, maybe even restore the spirit to its central role in healing. Perhaps it would take nothing less than a coyote physician—a bastard half-breed doctor—to bring the two cultures I knew together.

I WONDERED WHAT message Lanny's rattlesnake had borne for her. I knew that they had communed together for hours, and that much of what had passed between them was likely to be indescribable. But I asked to her to try to describe it for me anyway, as long as she didn't mind.

Before her vision quest, Lanny had been prepared to expect that any encounters she had with animals might hold a special meaning for her. When the snake approached the spot where Lanny was sitting, she found herself paralyzed with fear. She resolved her fright by staring into the snake's beautiful eyes. In doing so she noticed that the snake was as intrigued by her as she was by it. She remembered the snake spirit that had come to her in the sweat lodge, and called upon that spirit to send her comfort and strength.

As her fear dissipated, Lanny realized the snake was offering her a means to confront her mother. To Lanny this woman had often seemed a fearsome ogre, one that hurt her unnecessarily. In her mind's eye the rattlesnake mesmerized Lanny's mother with its hypnotic eyes. The snake then engulfed the woman, wrapping its coils around and around and squeezing, like an asp curled around a caduceus. Lanny's mother began to shrink, becoming smaller and less ferocious. Suddenly her mother's spirit stepped out of her skin, radiant and beautiful. The remains of her body had shrunk to nothing. Lanny embraced her mother's radiant spirit, and both of them spoke words of forgiveness and love.

"Now that you have faced your fear," the rattlesnake told Lanny, "you may always call upon me to cleanse you. When you grow fearful of your mother, call my name. I will stand behind you. Your mother will hear my rattle and retreat. You have shown strength and courage in finding me. For this reason I am your ally."

A poisonous snake is a potent image of both danger and healing—the caduceus Lanny saw in her vision is an archetypal symbol of healing. The symbol acknowledges that the process of healing can be dangerous and painful, because both danger and pain accompany power. I told Lanny of a rattlesnake ceremony I learned from the last living shaman of the Mojave tribe, from Southern California. When this old man was a young boy, the Mojave performed the ceremony every spring to appease the deadly snakes in the area for the year to come.

He told me how the men of the village would dig a deep pit, too deep for a snake to escape from. They would set about catching a mess of rattlers, which they cast into the pit. Then the men would don terrifying masks and costumes. Each man carried a shield and a spear. At the shaman's signal, the men rushed at the pit, screaming their war cries at the top of their lungs and shaking their spears. The shaman would stop the men at the last possible moment. "Rattlesnakes!" he would cry. "Evil is no answer for evil. We could kill you all right now if we wanted." At this the men would growl and cry their fiercest cries. Then the shaman would continue.

"We're not going to kill you. But in return, this is what you must promise. That this year, there will be no killing of children. That no women will be killed on their way to get water from the river. That no warriors will be killed on their way into battle. If you agree to this promise, go in peace. If not, we will kill you right now!" Then the men stood respectfully by as the shaman let the snakes go.

This seemed to me such a sensible approach to evil, I told Lanny, I wanted to try it myself. I loved the fact that the ceremony was intended to last for only a year; the villagers didn't expect a simple snake to remember what it wasn't supposed to do any longer than that. The ceremony had an important metaphorical meaning, too, about confronting what we are most afraid of and making friends with it. The ceremony required a personal sacrifice or gift to what we fear, and the willingness to receive back whatever gift our fearsome foe had to offer us. The next time I was scheduled to work with a group of people on a retreat, I resolved to reenact this ceremony with them.

The first time I tried it was during a workshop on spiritual healing.

I found that the participants were too self-conscious to enter into the ceremony enough to make it powerful. Six months later I had the opportunity to try again with a similar group. This time I kept everyone awake all night and performed the ceremony just before dawn. Instead of snakes, we placed dolls and talismans in the pit. We had earlier made these sacred objects to represent our most pressing problems. After singing and dancing all night long, everyone was too exhausted to resist dropping into a trance when dawn rolled around. The ceremony was powerful and had a magical effect on us all.

After working intensively with so many individuals like Lanny, I can make a few general observations. Overcoming the distractions and inertia of daily life seems to be a key to rapid healing. Not only isolation for the client, but an intensive effort on the healer's part, makes a substantial difference as to how swift and profound the outcome will be. The once- or twice-weekly sessions that pass for intensive psychotherapy in conventional circles do not serve all individuals well—I have seen far more accomplished in three eight-hour days than in twenty-four weeks of one-hour sessions.

An intense focus seems to touch off certain healing catalysts. (A catalyst is a substance that enables a reaction to occur at a moderate energy level—within the human body, for example, because of certain catalysts, iron can be melted at 98°F., but outside the body a much higher temperature is required.) Prayer is a healing catalyst. A loving relationship can be a catalyst. A ritual can serve as a catalyst as well.

A ritual must be situated in physical space as carefully as a satellite dish. Its success relies in part upon its relationship to the elementals in the area—earth, sky, wind, rock, water, and fire. A ritual must be properly anchored in respect to the four directions, the four winds, the places of the sun's rising and setting, and the location of any nearby bodies of water.

For a ritual to succeed, its purpose must be clearly stated. I begin any ritual by asking in a straightforward, direct manner for what I seek. I state to the spirits and the elementals present why I have come to that place, what I intend to do, and what I hope to achieve. I endeavor to behave with respect for the spirit of the place where the ritual is held. All senses must be attuned to the environment, to the communication that occurs between the supplicants and the surrounding plants, rocks, and animals.

A prayer must be stated as simply as a hen lays an egg. I remember witnessing a ritual at which one woman, obviously suffering from unbearable private torments, offered prayers for peace on earth, freedom in the Soviet Union, and political accord in Israel. I don't think Hosteen Begay, who was leading the ritual, even knew what the Soviet Union was. He did not understand her prayers. In this, the spirits are the same. They respond to what is said simply and directly, not to abstractions. Help must be requested aloud for a specific, concrete problem, or help may not be forthcoming.

Instead of an end to all war, the woman might more usefully have prayed for an end to the fighting between herself and another. She might have prayed for the land upon which she lived. She might have prayed for the health of the animals living upon that land, or for their abundance. How could any spirit grant the woman peace on earth? That global an experience is formed from the prayers of everyone on the earth, and not just her own. If consensual experience is the result of prayer (and this is what Native Americans believe), then a global experience is the result of global prayers, and we must recognize that one person's prayers may not supersede everyone else's.

When we approach ritual, we must approach it as a transformative process. Through its power the fabric of the cosmos is altered and the horrors of evil are erased. How the alteration is managed is mysterious. Explanations fall short of describing the process—we must take it on faith. We experience without explanation; we *participate*. Experience takes precedence over rational thought.

Ritual rekindles our faith that prayers are answered. We come to ritual with this faith, and we renew this faith by seeing prayers answered. Doug Boyd, author of *Rolling Thunder,* tells how that medicine man would never commence a healing ritual before being satisfied with the patient's purpose for holding the ceremony. The purpose had to hold dignity and meaning for Rolling Thunder. Just wanting to get well was not good enough. The patient had to have a greater good in mind, were he or she to become well. The fulfillment of this higher purpose became the point of the ritual.

In the Lakota sweat lodge ceremony, the leader reminds the participants, after the sacred pipe has been smoked, that their prayers have *already been answered.* He or she does not say that their prayers might now be answered, or to wait and see whether the prayers will be answered. The leader emphatically insists that the prayers *have been answered,* which can be said because of the covenant made between the Creator and the people through the White Buffalo Calf Woman. Through her gift of the sacred pipe and the promise that she made on the Creator's behalf, once the pipe is loaded and smoked in the sacred, traditional manner, the prayers have been answered.

@   @   @

HELP COMES TO those who ask for it. Marilyn taught me that, and it was a lesson I learned again and again while working with my own patients. Their breakthroughs always began with a sincere request for help. Now I needed help. Lanny's rattlesnake had named my own greatest fear—returning to mainstream medicine. I knew that if I were to make a confident return, I first needed to finish my residency.

I did not commit to that inevitable course immediately. First I settled for a less threatening postdoctoral research position at the School of Public Health at UC-Berkeley. There I published scientific papers on my work with AIDS patients and on the computer modeling of health and disease. The freedom to pursue my academic passions was a rare treat. I even took some math classes at UC-Berkeley—just for fun—on stochastic processes and the theory of queues. I also enjoyed being near my children again. But I knew the respite couldn't last—the prospect of residency loomed.

Why was that so daunting? For one thing, eight years had passed since I left Mount Sinai. I wasn't getting any younger. But if I was older, I hoped I was also more mature. One problem I had in the past wasn't so marked now—I was better able to hold my tongue when necessary. I had learned to channel my idealistic fervor into constructive action or resignation—in the words of the prayer AA had made famous, to "change the things I can, and accept what I cannot."

But did I have the stamina to get through a residency? Most of all, could I get through one alone? I had learned the hard way, after several brief and miserable relationships, that Hosteen had been right about its not being a propitious time for me to be in love. I had given up looking for a mate, but I wasn't certain I could carry out my destiny without a partner. So what was I to do?

I prayed for help, and it came from an unexpected quarter. In July of 1990, a year after treating Lanny, I accepted an invitation to give a workshop at the annual conference of the Association for Humanistic Psychology (AHP), which was being held that year at the University of Vermont. My workshop was on integrating spirituality into the practice of psychotherapy. One of the attendees was someone I have since come to believe I was destined to meet.

I arrived in Burlington, Vermont, the day before I was to give my workshop. I had been invited to a gathering of elders at the Sun-Ray Center in nearby Bristol. It was led by a Cherokee woman, Dyanni Yawahoo. Each elder spoke to the assembled crowd. To my chagrin, I was called up to speak—I certainly didn't feel all that old! After a potluck dinner we gathered around seven smaller fires that encircled a central bonfire. Dyanni led a powerful ceremony—her singing and the accompanying drumming were incredibly powerful.

Afterward I sat close to the fire. The surrounding Vermont woods were engulfed in darkness. From behind the fire a woman approached. I did not remember having seen her before, at dinner or during the ceremony. She had an angelic presence. She looked at me with acceptance and total love; I was transfixed. She did not speak but looked into me as if to show me something. I was overcome with sadness and loneliness. Memories of all my past failures in love, all my personal losses, flooded over me. Soon there were tears streaming down my face. Even here among my friends involved in the Native American spiritual world, I was heartbreakingly alone. When I looked up, the woman was gone. I looked for her in the group and could not find her.

I recovered my composure but the sadness stayed with me. I went to find a ride back to my quarters at the university dorm. A woman named Sherry stopped to introduce herself and to invite me to a sweat lodge at her home later that evening. I told her I would come. After returning to my room, I hurried to dress so that I would be ready when some people came to drive me out into the country where the lodge was to take place. But the sadness of the fireside vision came back to me, and when my ride arrived, I thanked them for coming but sent them on without me. I turned out the light and fell asleep in my clothes.

As I was about to begin the workshop the next day, a woman walked boldly into the workshop room, took one look at me, and walked right back out. Several minutes later she came back in, looking a little less certain. I asked her what the matter was. She said she had thought she was in the wrong room. She was a midwife, and knew my name from the many research studies I had published on childbirth and midwifery; she had assumed I would be a much older man. (She had no idea I published the first of these papers at age twenty-one.) She introduced herself as Morgaine.

After the workshop, Morgaine stayed to talk for a moment about my childbirth research. When she mentioned that an old knee injury was bothering her, I volunteered to try some Apache manipulation techniques on it—I wasn't ready for her to leave. I asked her for a ride downtown, and we ended up having dinner together. We talked for hours about our experiences in America's birth industry, and because we enjoyed each other so much, we segued into talking about everything else possible. The next day Morgaine took me to her favorite beach on the shores of Lake Champlain. Champ, the fabled local sea serpent, never made an appearance, but even if he had I'm not sure we would have noticed. As the sun set over the Adirondack Mountains across the lake, I surprised us both by kissing Morgaine. That was the start of our romance.

Morgaine drove me to the airport when it was time for me to leave. She took the risk of telling me how fated our meeting seemed to her. That morning she had spoken to a friend of hers, Sherry, who had invited her to attend a sweat lodge. It would have been her first, but at the last moment Morgaine canceled. We had been invited to the same lodge!

Morgaine had been Sherry's midwife two years before. The two months prior to our meeting Morgaine had spent in solitude, grieving the loss of her only sister, Cathy. Sherry had thought a sweat lodge might do her some good. Sherry was disappointed when neither of us came, but thrilled to hear we met the following day. She announced to Morgaine that we were meant for each other. Morgaine laughed at that, thinking it a bit premature. Her friends were always trying to set her up with men.

Cathy had died shortly after giving birth, of toxic shock syndrome caused by a deadly strain of streptococcus. Toxic strep gained infamy when it killed Jim Henson, creator of the Muppets. The syndrome is also related to the notorious "flesh-eating" bacterial disease. Much later, with the help of a research assistant, Morgaine and I studied the incidence of toxic strep among new mothers. While rare, the condition is almost uniformly deadly. The more virulent strains (M-1 and M-2) are so toxic that no one to date has survived a postpartum infection. It was the M-1 strain that took Cathy's life.

Morgaine had been Cathy's midwife. Morgaine suffered greatly from rumors inside and out of the medical and midwifery communities about her sister's death. Her personal and professional losses were heartbreaking. There is, unfortunately, a shocking lack of knowledge among physicians and other health-care providers about toxic strep.

Tragically, I would attend an almost identical case of toxic strep in a new mother in the emergency room the following year. The woman was talking and laughing with us in the ER when she was brought in, but within ninety minutes she was dead. This brought me closer to understanding how helpless we are in the face of this disease. The immune system of a new mother is already somewhat suppressed from her pregnancy—and even a perfectly healthy young person can die of such a toxic infection within ten hours.[1]

1. A specialist in toxic shock from the University of Minnesota was especially helpful to talk to in the aftermath of these experiences. He has served as an expert witness in cases where there has been doubt raised concerning medical care. Only the

Three weeks before she died, concerned that Morgaine was working too hard, Cathy made her sister promise to do something for herself unrelated to midwifery. Morgaine showed Cathy the brochure that had come for the AHP conference. Morgaine thought it odd that she had been mailed one at all, since it certainly wasn't midwifery literature, but in leafing through the brochure she had recognized my name, then read about the workshop I was leading. Cathy uncharacteristically made Morgaine promise that nothing would keep her from attending.

On the morning of the workshop, Morgaine had no intention of leaving the house to go anywhere. She was awoken by her sister's voice repeatedly reminding her of her promise to "go."

Even before she was fully awake, Morgaine knew this was about going to the workshop at the AHP conference. Morgaine sat up feeling very clearly the presence of her sister. Reluctantly and mechanically she drove to the university, thinking only about keeping her commitment to Cathy.

I WAS TORN AT the airport. I very much wanted to see Morgaine again soon but was terrified at the thought of another failed relationship. Before we parted, I mentioned I would be coming East again, to a medical conference in New York City in October. Perhaps, I ventured shyly, Morgaine might consider coming there to meet me. She said she would think about it.

Once I was back in California, Morgaine and I began talking every night on the telephone like a couple of teenagers. She soon surprised me by asking me if I might want to meet her if she took a week's vacation in San Francisco. Unbeknownst to me, this was a first for her; she had

---

less virulent strains of toxic bacterias can be arrested by timely and massive uses of antibiotics, and even then the illness will create critical, life-threatening conditions, and frequently long-term damage. These bacteria have since gotten a lot of coverage; warnings have gone out to the public to stop asking for antibiotics for minor complaints. Because so many people never finish their prescriptions, a few hardy bacteria never get killed, and the deadlier toxic strains are believed to be descended from them.

The specialist asked Morgaine and me to write about the danger posed to new mothers from these bacteria. Strep bacteria are often carried in the sore throats of a new mother's sex partner. Near the time of the delivery, during the winter/spring sore throat season, care should be taken to avoid oral sex. During that season 20 percent of people test positive for strep throat, and though a virulent strain such as M-1 among those 20 percent of cases will be rare, it may prove to be deadly for the mother.

never taken a vacation away from either her career or her children. I only later recognized and appreciated what an effort she was making, and the personal risk involved.

But even without that awareness, I was falling madly in love. I was a little frightened to be finally expressing the hopeless-romantic side of my character. Once I saw Morgaine again in person the fear quickly faded. I was having the most wonderful time of my life. During our dinners together and our long walks past the gingerbread Victorian houses in San Francisco, Morgaine and I shared our dreams for the future. I was struggling with what to do next. Still reluctant to tackle residency, I was applying for further postdoctoral fellowships and psychology faculty jobs. I really wanted to return to mainstream medicine but wasn't certain I could hack it. Morgaine was convinced I could. To her there was only one answer to my problems, and it seemed simple enough—I must return to my residency and finish what I had started. Just what Lanny's snake had ordered.

But Morgaine was the one who made it seem possible. She told me she was willing to help me, to give me the support I needed to make it through. If either of us had thought carefully about the pressures that residency would put on our new relationship, we would never have made such a leap of faith, but we were certain that love would conquer all. Little did I know how much I underestimated what going back to my residency would require of me, and of us. But with Morgaine's offer to stand by me I started looking through medical and scientific journals for announcements of open positions, and filled out residency applications.

On the day before Morgaine left San Francisco, we took a drive together. I wanted to show her the redwoods of California. We got hopelessly lost but drove on, simply happy to be together. We ended up at Point Reyes National Seashore, where I had spent a peaceful interlude as a medical student so many years before. We stopped at the top of a mountain overlooking the ocean. We both wanted to do a ceremony to bless our relationship. After setting out my supplies and singing the Four Directions song, I could once again smell Archie's cigar. But there was another presence too.

The sun was very bright, and the smoke from our small fire blew into the high brush beside us. From the light and smoke emerged a figure I recognized. The spirit was of the woman who had come to me at the fireside during the elders' gathering in Bristol, Vermont. The spirit spoke to me, and I knew her to be Morgaine's sister, Cathy. She was leaving, she said, now that she knew Morgaine would be taken care of. I was to tell Morgaine that Cathy was happy where she was, and that her purpose and place were far away. She wanted me to assure her sister that

Morgaine would one day find peace about her death. Soon she was gone, but she left behind her a palpable sense of her love for Morgaine.

We sat for a long time looking out over the Pacific Ocean as the sun set and the sky turned red. I described my vision to Morgaine. She was surprised at the accuracy of my description of Cathy's quiet, controlled, and genuinely kind manner. I apologized as I reported Cathy's appearance, for the spirit didn't look at all like Morgaine and I was certain that aspect of Cathy hadn't come through clearly to me. But Morgaine confirmed that Cathy had looked just as I said.

A YEAR AFTER meeting Morgaine, I returned to family practice residency. One month after that, I went to Santa Fe to lead a weekend workshop. Coyotes were in evidence all around the plaza—there were coyote restaurants, statues of coyotes with scarves on their necks, and postcards of them in tuxes doing the tango to the light of the moon. I could tell I wasn't the only one in need of the coyote's energies. Our whole society was looking for something from the scrawny old bastard. I thought of the roles I seemed to have been given to play in the human comedy—and they were the coyote's traditional roles, of survivor, trickster, and clown.

Coyote as clown was apparent in most of the cartoons and images I saw in Santa Fe. Clowns are a valuable archetype for our overly serious society. Coyotes have some qualities we've disowned, because they embarrass us—a frank animal nature and a crude sense of humor. And they're smart, as smart as we are; after all, a stupid beast would never grab our contemporary attention spans, as fractured as they are by the competing demands of a media-saturated culture.

Clown or trickster—in either guise Coyote's wits can get him into trouble. Like most of us in modern America, Coyote has such enthusiasm for his own cleverness that it can override his good judgment—as in the story of Coyote and the burrowing owl. But there are times in our lives when we need the trickster's qualities. There are times when it is best to be sly and clever in the face of something over which we feel we have no control.

When we want to change, for instance. Change sometimes must begin with a surprise, with a sudden break from everyday life. At the beginning of a treatment, a shaman doesn't know (any more than a physician does) exactly what will heal a sick person. She takes it on faith that the person "knows" at some deeper level of consciousness but isn't able to access the knowledge. Sometimes what the shaman will do is throw her client psychically off balance, so that he, while metaphorically "falling," will reach out and grab for something, anything, to stop the

fall. Once he has caught hold of something, the shaman has that something to work with, to base a healing experience upon. It can take a
trickster to create the healing surprise.

Trickster, clown, and, in the end, survivor. Like raccoons and cock-
roaches, coyotes are especially adaptable creatures, willing to live almost
anywhere, able to eat almost anything. Thus they are well suited to living alongside human beings (and all the garbage that comes with us).
The coyote's habitat has spread in this century from the open country
and grasslands of the southwestern United States and Mexico, to Central America, most of Canada, and northern Alaska—in fact, to every
state in the union except Hawaii, and I bet they'll be there before long.
One of them is going to hear how easygoing Hawaiians can be, and
swim over.

Today we need the archetype of a survivor. We need a role model
who can weather the terrific assaults our nihilistic society inflicts upon
the soul, just as Wile E. Coyote, in the world of cartoons, survives every
blow dealt to him by Roadrunner and the latest products of the Acme
Corporation. No matter what happens to him, Wile E. manages to
survive. Somehow he must eat, because he's never shown starving to
death—though he sure isn't eating any roadrunners.

We need a survivor with a sense of humor. We enjoy an animal who
is extravagant in his territorial and propagation habits, at a time when
almost every other animal's horizons are so depressingly shrunken. Coyote is singular. He is a member of the dog family, but he doesn't act like
any dog I've ever seen. Coyote is me—nothing pure, yet something,
maybe even something to be reckoned with.

IN JANUARY OF 1991 I was invited back to Wisconsin by the members of
the mystery school for whom I'd led a sweat lodge five years before. I
was looking forward to seeing these people again, and looking forward
especially to being joined by someone who had never done a lodge in her
life—my teenaged daughter.

The day before the lodge, she and I toured the area. I took her to see
the University of Wisconsin in Madison, where she was considering
going to college. We also saw the church whose basement held the co-op
day care she vaguely remembered, and the farmhouse we had lived in.
Finally we parked the rental car in the lot of the Deerfield Tavern. We
retraced the steps of our old five-mile around-the-block walk. It was
eighteen degrees below zero, so we had a very welcome glass of hot
chocolate at the Deerfield when we were done.

It was healing for me to close the circle with my daughter in this way. Besides literally circling the block again, we reenacted a ritual that had meant a great deal to us both years before. She showed her willingness to try a new ritual, one she knew was of great importance to me, by circling sunwise into the lodge the next day.

While the stones were heating, I told my daughter all about Morgaine. She wanted to know how we met, when we knew for certain we had fallen in love, and where we planned to get married.

Many who spoke that night in the lodge shared their greatest moments of hope and despair. Always, from the greatest tragedies, the greatest opportunities seemed to emerge. Like Morgaine's path from Cathy's death to our life together, like mine from giving up on a life in San Francisco to having a new one in Vermont. Like my daughter's path joining again with mine. I got choked up during the final prayer, because I realized despite all we had been through, I still felt a strong bond between her and me. And now she knew something of what I had been up to all those years. I hope one day to enter a lodge with her brother, to share the experience with him as well.

The sweat lasted an incredible seven hours. Whenever people got too hot, they just leaned back against the lodge's blanket walls. Water vapor from the steam and our own respiration had frozen solid to the blankets. The lodge probably lasted so long because nobody wanted to go back into the freezing night air.

AFTER MARRYING, in the fall of 1991 Morgaine and I moved, with her children, to downtown Houston, where I started a residency. Neither Morgaine nor I really knew what was in store for us. My resident's salary, after taxes, health insurance, and child support, amounted to about $100 a month, a paltry amount that had to be supplemented by working weekends in the ER. Morgaine had left her midwifery practice in Vermont, and it was no simple task to build a new one in Houston. And none of us cared for the only neighborhood we could afford to move into. She and her children couldn't fathom such a mean, ugly city after so many years in the mountains of Vermont.

Residency was at once harder and easier than I had remembered. I did well in my rotations. I was older and very motivated. Given the salary, I looked for a job moonlighting in an area emergency room. But I couldn't get a license to practice in Texas—because on the application, I had answered yes to the question "Have you ever been sued?" I was told I needed to provide the state with records of the suit. But it had been handled in a California small-claims court, which controlled costs by not keeping records. My explanations, and even a letter from the chief judge of the San Francisco Municipal Court, got me nowhere with the Texas Medical Board.

Finally I sought and found ER work in New Mexico, where I was already licensed from my prior stay there. At one point during the year in Houston, I was pulling three weekday shifts of ten hours each, and two shifts of fourteen, then flying to New Mexico to work in the emergency room all weekend long. Catnaps were my salvation. The children saw so little of me they wondered aloud whether Morgaine and I had divorced without telling them.

Just before summer, Morgaine and the kids witnessed a car bombing in front of our apartment building. There was now no question but that we had to get out of our violent and dangerous neighborhood as fast as possible. Morgaine had just learned she was pregnant with Takoda. When she returned to her former home in Vermont for a month's visit, I interviewed at the University of Vermont for a position that had just opened there, and they accepted me. It was there that I finally completed, over the next four years, my long-overdue psychiatry and family practice residencies.

THE DISCOVERY THAT Mexican half-breeds are called *coyotes* added another layer to my already strong identification with the animal. I have called this book *Coyote Medicine* because the medicine I have to offer is a half-breed's offering; it is a product of the two cultures I have shared in. It is a way of practicing health care that is not at present totally at home either on the rez or in the clinic.

What if we consider coyote medicine in terms of Native American spirit medicine, of the healing powers inherent in an animal's nature? If bat medicine holds the power to see past superficialities to the underlying truth; if owl medicine opens lines of communication between our world and the next; if energy and fierceness are the hallmarks of wolf medicine—what are the particulars of the coyote brand?

Coyote as clown reminds us to laugh at ourselves and our problems. Laughter can come only when we gain perspective—a worry that isn't funny to us in the moment may be in a few years, once we are out from under its shadow. When I can get patients to laugh about a disease, or perhaps the foibles that are behind it, I've helped them on the way to the kind of perspective that can result in healing. I'm reminded of the episode with Sylvia Bowers in my psychiatry residency. There a little coyote clowning turned a dangerous patient into a calm but still spirited one.

Coyote as trickster can be useful in generating a healing surprise, a shock that moves a patient from habitual state of illness into another, more precarious one, from whence he or she can "fall" into wellness. It strikes me too how useful stories are to Coyote here—to trick pessimistic clients into unconsciously believing they can be healthy again, despite any convictions they may have to the contrary.

What about Coyote as survivor? The coyote that has extended its domain across the continent is an animal who is adaptable, who will try anything. If we truly want to be healed, we must be similarly willing to try anything that works. If we truly want to be healers, we must be willing to use anything that works, regardless of our theoretical positions. Because if it works, it's good medicine.

For the powers of coyote medicine to win popularity in the mainstream, its practitioners will also need to be survivors, tricksters, and clowns. Clowns, to disarm any establishment foes, and charm them into paying unexpected therapies serious attention. Tricksters, to have their wits about them, to thrive in a hostile environment. And survivors, to persist even when success seems unlikely and the path obscure.

The purpose of finishing my residency has become manifest. After completing my residencies, I was hired as an associate professor of family practice, at the University of Hawaii School of Medicine, on the island of Oahu. The job title is more conventional than my responsibilities: I have the opportunity to set up a clinic that integrates traditional Hawaiian and Asian healing techniques into a conventional medical practice. Because I am now certified in family practice, psychiatry, emergency medicine, geriatrics, and clinical psychology, I am entitled to teach residents and medical students the way I think medicine should be practiced. I have been exposing medical students to the broader view of healing implicit within Native American (and Native Hawaiian) medicine, along with specific techniques such as acupressure, acupuncture, and the laying-on of hands.

My new job is a kind of extension of the intensive healing program I developed in Arizona. In this new setting, I will be conducting rigorous research projects into the results of integrating shamanism and modern medicine. We will explore the limits and preconditions for healing, trying to answer old Grampa Richards's three questions, but with reference to the larger matter of cultural healing. The population on the island includes large numbers of Native Hawaiian and Asian Americans, and both groups have strong healing traditions of their own. I hope I have finally found a place where my own brand of coyote medicine will be welcome.

I look forward to the future and what I expect it will bring, though of course we can never be sure what fate has in store for us—just as I have never been sure, except in retrospect, whether I could help a person who has come to me to be healed. For this reason I pray for the strength to keep my heart open to those who seek out my help. Being a coyote physician—being outrageous at times, even startling—can work only when there is an abundant bedrock of warmth, flexibility, and caring for the client.

One medicine man told me that right now the earth is calling all souls who have ever been Native Americans. Our task is to help in the transformation of people on this continent, ultimately to preserve human life on this planet. He said there simply weren't enough Indian bodies to go around. As a half-breed, I find this position appealing. I believe Native American spirituality is a gift to us from North America herself. It is the natural spiritual path for those who live on this continent. Native American people have been the preservers of this spiritual path for centuries, but they do not own it. No one can own a spiritual path. The proper response to the current interest in Native American spirituality is to correctly transmit this spiritual path to all who wish to learn it. This ensures both its preservation, its accuracy, and its authenticity.

As I finish, I am thinking about what message I would like people to take away from this book. If I had to choose one single idea, it would be: Don't give up. Don't stop trying. Help is always available, whether inside or out of the halls of conventional medicine. Don't give up until you've tried everything there is to try. Help yourself to a little coyote medicine, and thrive.

Index

Sage, burning of, 41, 132, 176, 216, 221, 230, 232, 234, 265, 270
Saguaro tree, 269–70
Sand Hills, 197, 209
San Francisco (California), 147, 167, 220–21, 225, 243, 274, 281–82
Sanjay (computer science professor), 244–45, 265, 267
Santa Cruz (California), 74, 170, 173
Santa Fe (New Mexico), 209, 214, 283
Santa Rosa (California), 123, 149
Scarface (character in story), 197–209
Schizophrenia, 150
Science, spiritual realm and, 35, 56, 118–20, 172–73
Scott (shaman), 126–28
Sea salt, 266
Serotonin, 20–21
Shaking Tent ceremony, 135
Shamans (medicine men and women)
  Buddhist, 140
  dangers to, at sweat-lodge ceremonies, 178, 181
  fees for, 131
  healing surprises by, 283–84, 286–87
  Hispanic, 141–43
  humility of, 122
  incompetent or charlatan, 126–28
  intensive work by, 249
  postmodern view compared to that of, 164–65
  relationships as key to healing by, 145
  spiritual direction of, 217
  training of, 123–26, 131
  where they can be found, 122–23
  See also Healing
Shawnee (Ohio), 64–66
Sherry (woman in Vermont), 279, 280
Shoshone, 35, 57
Shoshoni (Wyoming), 36, 69
Silver Fox, in story, 101–3, 111
Skan (the Creator), 252–54, 257, 269
Sky Badger, 194
Sky Country, in author's vision, 184, 187–90

Smallpox-infested blankets, 89
SMCMC (San Mateo County Medical Center), 21–34, 54, 69–70, 87
Smoke sticks (cigars), 33, 50, 61, 68, 175, 221–24, 273, 282
Snake. *See* Rattlesnake
Snake handlers, 28, 33
Soeken, K. L., 261n
Spider, in author's vision, 184–86, 189
Spirit animals at ceremonies, 133
Spirits
  at ceremonies, 130, 132–35 174–75, 178–79, 217–18, 230–31, 233–36
  channeling of, 261
  helper (swans), 204, 208
  of illnesses, 224, 236–37
  malevolent, 229–30
  methods of speaking to, 248
  Native American communication with, 260–61
  reliance on, for help with problems, 256
  smell of, 234
Spirituality
  in author's healing intensive, 256
  in Native American medicine, 14, 16–17, 29, 90–91, 125–26, 247, 288
  science and, 35, 56, 118–20, 172–73
Spotted Eagle Nation, 172, 195, 223
Stanford University School of Medicine
  author on faculty of, 139
  author's study at, 16, 19–34, 37, 69–70, 71, 73–74
  Native American students at, 35–36
  restricted admissions at, 143–44
Stanway, Andrew, 125
Stepfather of author, 64–66, 182, 191
Stone, Father, 36, 57, 74
Stone giant, in vision, 185, 186, 188, 190, 191
Stories
  of boy and Big Dipper, 37–38, 42
  of buffalo people, 44–48
  of Coyote, 61–63, 101–5, 111, 136–37

Lewis Mehl-Madrona is a research assistant professor of family practice at the University of Arizona School of Medicine, where he is primarily affiliated with the Native American Research and Training Center. He received his M.D. from Stanford University in 1975 and a Ph.D. in clinical psychology from the Psychological Studies Institute in Palo Alto in 1980. Dr. Mehl-Madrona has extensive clinical, teaching, and research experience. He has worked as an emergency room physician at hospitals in California, New Mexico, and Vermont, and as the medical director of the Center for Recovery from Illness in San Francisco. He has served as an associate professor at the University of Hawaii School of Medicine and as a research assistant professor at the University of Vermont College of Medicine at the Universities of Arizona and Vermont. His research interests focus on mathematical computer modeling as a means of aiding clinical decision-making and improving treatment evaluation. He is a recipient of the 1993 Excellence in Research as a Family Practice Resident Award from the American Academy of Family Practice. Dr. Mehl-Madrona is currently helping to create a clinic and training program for the integration of Western and indigenous healing methods.